Recent Results in Cancer Research

Fortschritte der Krebsforschung

Progrès dans les recherches sur le cancer

33

Edited by

Editor in chief

P. Rentchnick, Genève

Springer-Verlag Berlin · Heidelberg · New York 1970

Sponsored by the Swiss League against Cancer

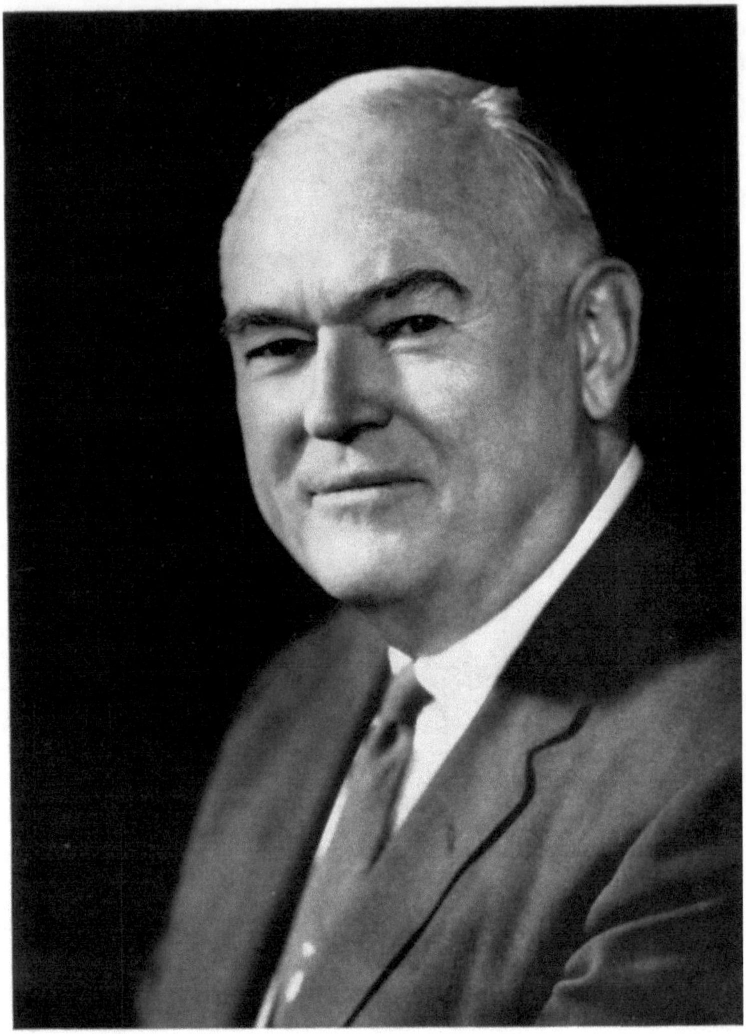

Professor J. G. Kidd, M.D.

Experimental and Clinical Effects of L-Asparaginase

Edited by

E. Grundmann · H. F. Oettgen

With 190 Figures

Springer-Verlag Berlin · Heidelberg · New York 1970

Professor Dr. E. GRUNDMANN
Institute of Experimental Pathology of Farbenfabriken Bayer AG, Wuppertal-Elberfeld, Germany

Professor Dr. H. F. OETTGEN,
Sloan-Kettering Institute for Cancer Research, New York, N. Y./USA

"International Symposium of Experimental and Clinical Effects of L-Asparaginase",
Wuppertal-Elberfeld, 24th—26th Oct. 1969

ISBN-13: 978-3-642-99986-4 e-ISBN-13: 978-3-642-99984-0
DOI: 10.1007/978-3-642-99984-0

Softcover reprint of the hardcover 1st edition 1970

 Title No. 3648

Contents

Part V. Animal Toxicity

Part VI. Resistance Problems

Part VII. Clinical Effects and Side Effects

Opening Remarks

E. Grundmann

Institute of Experimental Pathology, Farbenfabriken Bayer A. G., Wuppertal, Germany

Ladies and Gentlemen,

may I welcome you in Germany, in the capital of the Bergische Land: Wuppertal and in the Pharma Research Centre of the Bayer Comp. I thank you for accepting our invitation. We would like to use the opportunity to renew old friendships and to make new friends.

We all have the duty to look for new possibilities in the treatment of malignant growth and to improve the already existing methods. It is the very nature of malignant disease that all scientific news is taken up immediately and discussed extensively by the public. I also want to emphasize that the public has the legitimate right to be informed of scientific progress even in this subject. But at the same time it must be stressed that the first informations should only come from competent sources, i. e. from experts if a misleading impression is to be prevented. It cannot be denied that particularly about this subject which we are going to discuss here during the next 3 days, more confusion than clarity exists in the general public and even in the medical public. No one in particular can be blamed for this. Nothing appears to be less suited for headlines than the still unanswered questions of the cancer problem, particularly of the treatment of malignancy.

The last question is burdened by the fact that the metabolic difference between malignant cells and normal cells in the organism is minimal and usually only of a quantitative nature. Here the discovery that specific mouse leukemias show a marked sensitivity to asparagin depletion came as a genuine surprise, somewhat of a scientific sensation: for the first time a clear difference between normal and malignant growth became apparent which could be used therapeutically. I am delighted to be able to welcome in this room the discoverers of this difference. In historical sequence these are Dr. J. G. Kidd, who in 1953 made the observation that guinea-pig serum can inhibit the growth of mouse leukemias, then Dr. J. D. Broome, who in 1961 demonstrated in his tissue culture investigations that the inhibitor involved must be the enzyme L-asparaginase. The final piece of information was supplied in 1964 by the Drs. L. T. Mashburn and J. C. Wriston; the inhibiting effect on these mouse leukemias could also be achieved by L-asparaginase obtained from an E. coli source. This at the same time supplied the means by which large quantities of L-asparaginase could be produced. Using this type of L-asparaginase the Sloan-Kettering Institute New York and the Wadley-Laboratory Dallas in particular were able to gather first clinical experiences. I am delighted to be able to welcome outstanding scientists from these 2 laboratories.

Due to the general availibility of the enzyme the number of clinicians gathering experience by this new method increased. Each of the participants made the pleasant discovery that nearly all national boundaries lost their significance and that an international collaboration developed as with no other before. For us in the Bayer Company the collaboration with the colleagues of the Sloan-Kettering Institute New York proved to be particularly valuable, and I would like to use this opportunity to express my gratitude to the Drs. BURCHENAL, PHILIPS, and OETTGEN for this collaboration. I am very glad to welcome all three of you here today. As already mentioned the circle of collaborators extended to very many other countries. So I am in the happy position today to heartily welcome at our symposium in addition to the colleagues from the United States friends from Austria, Belgium, France, Italy, Jugoslavia, Netherlands, Spain, Sweden, Switzerland, the United Kingdom and particularly from East Germany. The purpose of this symposium is to learn of the present state of our knowledge in the sectors of biochemistry, pharmacokinetics, toxicology and experimental pathology and also to exchange clinical experiences gathered so far. We all hope that we shall succeed in this way to set out the possibilities and the limitations of this new therapy. May I thank Dr. GÖTZE of the Springer Publishing Company who is in our midst and will arrange for a speedy publication of this symposium. In addition we hope that L-asparaginase presents only a beginning and that in future other such metabolic differences become comprehensible and will be of practical use.

If we are sitting somewhat close together in this room I would like to take this symbolically for our scientific situation: since particularly in cancer research we all sit in the same boat more than in any other sector of research and we are dependent on each other in success as well as in failure.

I hereby declare the symposium as opened.

Part I
L-Asparaginase and the Asparagine Metabolism

Asparaginase and Cancer—Yesterday and Today

John G. Kidd

The New York Hospital—Cornell Medical Center, New York, U.S.A.

With 14 Figures

Professor Grundmann; Ladies and Gentlemen:

In his letter of invitation Professor Grundmann indicated that he would like me to tell something of how asparaginase was brought into relationship with cancer. I do this with some embarrassment because it entails showing again some slides that a number of you have seen before.

Some years ago I was engaged in a study of an antibody which appears in high titer in the blood of certain rabbits implanted with Brown-Pearce rabbit carcinoma cells. The antibody exerts quite remarkable effects on the living cancer cells, both in vivo and in vitro (1—4). In Figs. 1—4 we can see structural changes brought about by the antibody in vitro in mixture with guinea pig serum, which had been added to the mixture in order to provide hemolytic complement.

In an extension of these immunologic studies I next produced immune sera in rabbits using as antigen suspensions of the cells of Gardner's lymphoma of mice—Lymphoma 6C3HED. Preliminary tests showed that an anti-6C3HED rabbit immune serum, in mixture with guinea pig serum (here too added to provide hemolytic complement), produced a striking regression of established 6C3HED lymphomas in vivo. Controlled experiments soon disclosed that this unparalleled regression could be produced with guinea pig serum alone (Fig. 5). So with successive associates—Jean Elizabeth Todd, Shirley Kauffman, Steven Mohos, Nelson Holmquist, Michel Haddad, Soon Eung Kim, John Broome, and Leslie Sobin—I spent several years studying this interesting phenomenon in some detail [5—12].

We found for example that while serum from normal guinea pigs regularly induced regression of established 6C3HED lymphomas growing in inbred C3H mice, serum from normal animals of other species (horse, rabbit, rat, dog, cat, bovine, etc.) had no such effect; further that while guinea pig serum regularly brought about regression of some lymphomas (6C3HED of C3H mice, Lorenz's Lymphoma II of strain A mice, and the Murphy-Sturm Lymphosarcoma of rats), it did not influence the growth of numerous other lymphomas; and it had no influence whatever on several cancers of other types. Amongst other things, we also found that guinea pig serum had no noteworthy effect on Lymphoma 6C3HED cells when held

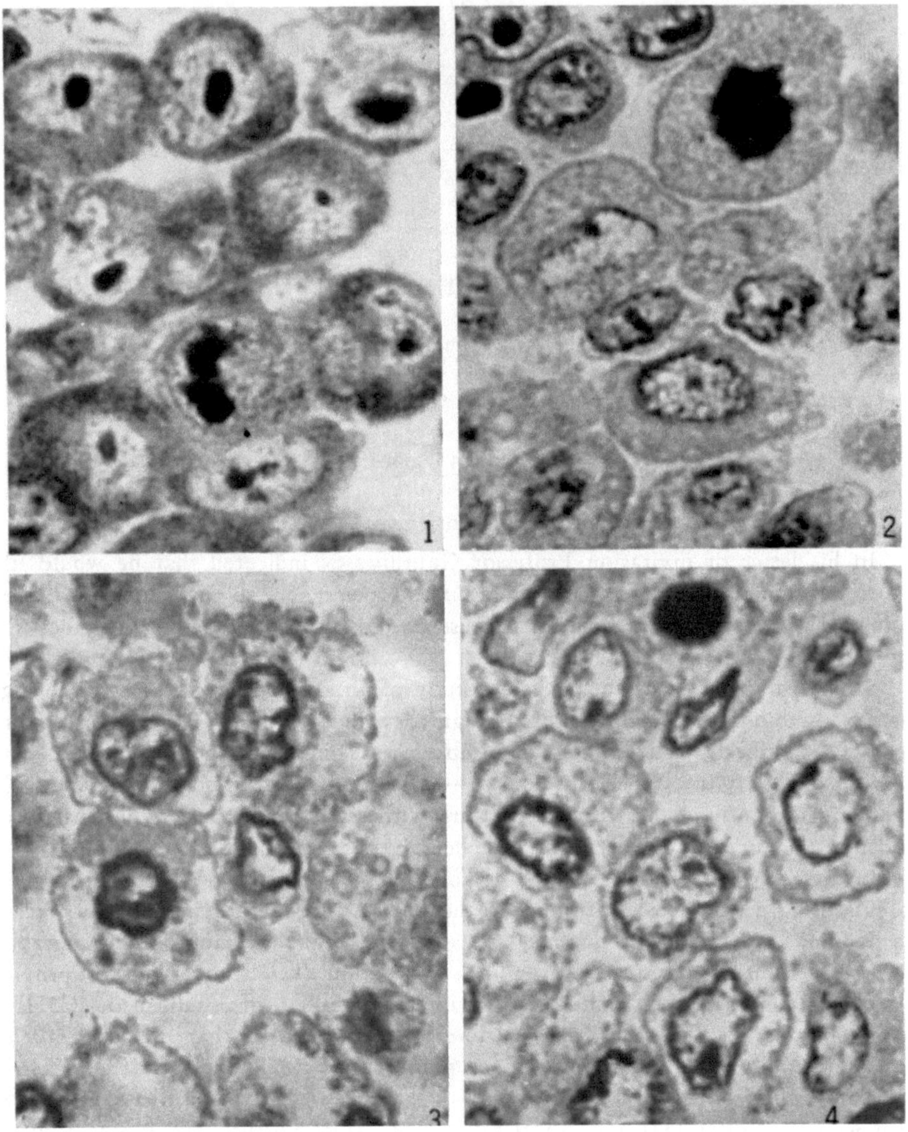

Figs. 1—4. To show structural changes produced in Brown-Pearce carcinoma cells by means of a specific antibody and complement. Fig. 1 shows Brown-Pearce carcinoma cells that had been suspended as individuals in buffered-glucose-Ringer's solution and held in contact with fresh normal rabbit serum containing hemolytic complement during 2 hours at 37° C in vitro Figs. 2, 3, and 4 show carcinoma cells from the same suspension which had been exposed respectively for 5, 15, and 120 minutes during 2 hours at 37° C to the effects of a fresh immune rabbit serum containing the specific Brown-Pearce antibody in high titer. When heated at 56° C for 30 minutes the antibody-containing serum did not produce structural changes in the carcinoma cells under identical conditions

Figs. 1—7 and 11—14 reproduced by permission of the Journal of Experimental Medicine

in contact with them during 6 hours at 37° C in vitro; though when injected into C3H mice in which the lymphoma cells were proliferating in the subcutaneous tissues, the guinea pig serum brought about necrosis of many of the cancer cells within 4—8 hours: thus the guinea pig serum seemed not to act directly but to do something to the host, which in turn effected the regression [6].

Needless to say, I tried hard to identify the active constituent of guinea pig serum. I found early on that the active constituent is a heat-labile protein and that rather more of it is present in a fraction of guinea pig serum containing the beta and gamma globulins than in a fraction containing albumin and the alpha globulins (Fig. 6). But the real identification awaited the observations of BROOME, who worked more or less independently in my laboratory during the period 1958—62. Comparing my finding of 1953—that guinea pig serum contains a substance inducing regression of certain lymphomas in vivo, while the sera of other mammals lack this substance [5, 6]—with CLEMENTI's observation of 1922—that the serum of guinea pigs is a rich source of asparaginase, while the sera of other mammals are virtually devoid of

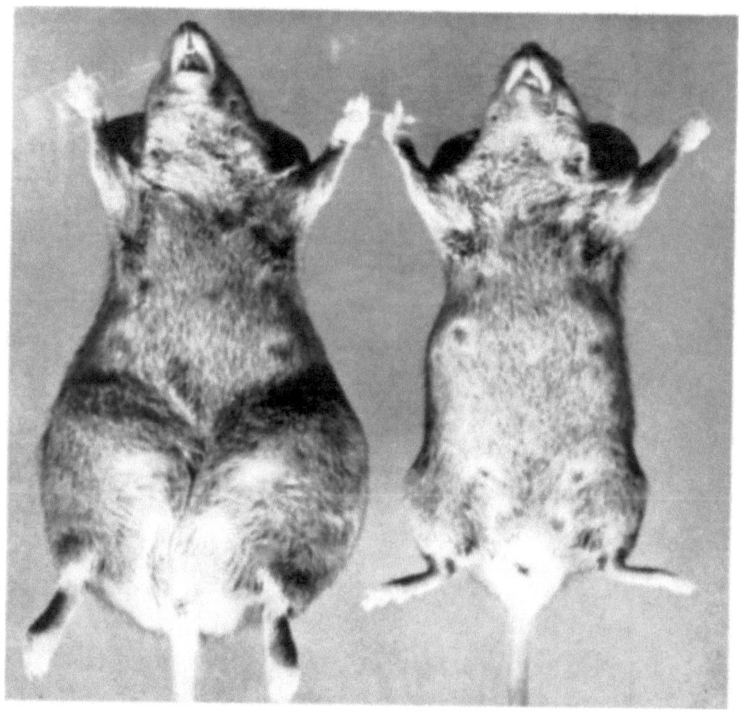

Fig. 5. To show large lymphosarcomas in the groins of a control untreated C3H mouse (left) and their absence from the groins of a mouse given repeated injections of normal guinea pig serum intraperitoneally (right). Both animals were implanted with 6 million Lymphoma 6C3HED-OH cells in each groin on Day 0, and both had bilateral growths measuring 10 to 14 mm across 6 days later. On Days 6, 7, and 8 the mouse on the right was given 1.0 ml of a 3× concentrated guinea pig serum intraperitoneally, with result in prompt regression of its growths. The photograph was made on Day 15. Postmortem examinations disclosed large characteristic lymphomas in the groins of the mouse on the left; no tumors could be found in the mouse on the right

Fractions	Nature of fractions as determined by filter paper electrophoresis: Electrophoretic patterns	Nature of fractions as determined by filter paper electrophoresis: Concentrations of components	Inhibition of lymphosarcoma cells in vivo: 4:1	2:1	1:1	1:2
1. Whole guinea pig serum (experiment A)	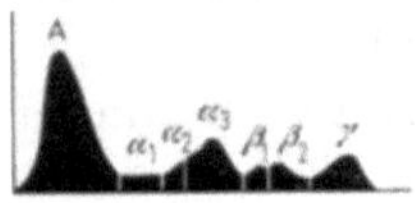	gms-% Albumins A 3.05 Alpha globulins α 1.34 Beta globulins β 0.51 Gamma globulins γ 0.69 Total 5.59		++++	++++	+
2. "E 1.8 M-soluble" (experiment A) 4:1	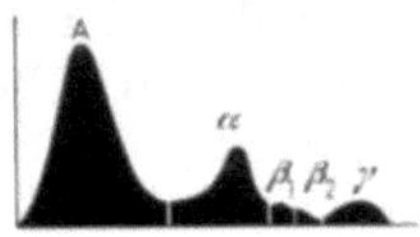	Albumins A 3.41 Alpha globulins α 1.06 Beta globulins β 0.14 Gamma globulins γ 0.28 Total 4.89	++++		±	
3. "E 1.8 M-insoluble" (experiment A) 4:1	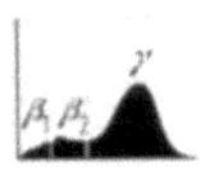	Beta globulins β 0.40 Gamma globulins γ 1.30 Total 1.70	++++		++	
4. "E 2.2 M-soluble" (experiment B) 2:1 Approx.	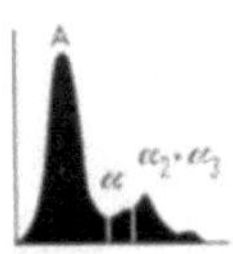	Albumins A 2.62 Alpha globulins α 0.78 Total 3.40		++±	±	
5. "2.2 M-insoluble" (experiment B) 2:1	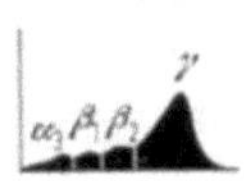	Alpha globulins α 0.18 Beta globulins β 0.47 Gamma globulins γ 1.46 Total 2.11		+++±	+±	±

Fig. 6. An attempt to isolate the active constituent of guinea pig serum fractionation by means of electrophoresis. See text; also [6]

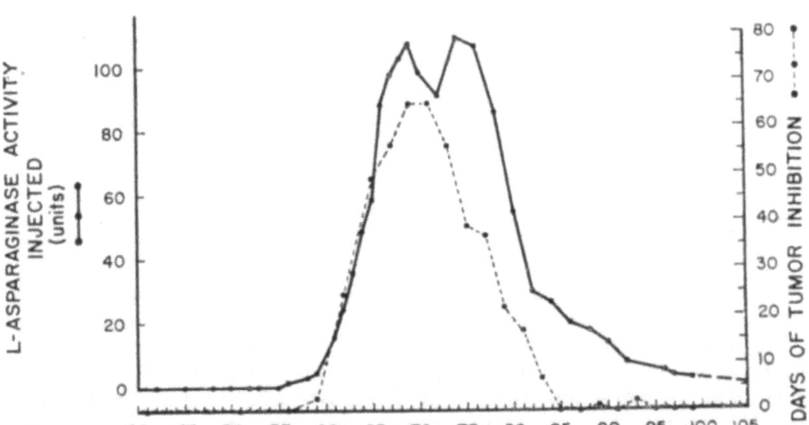

Fig. 7. To illustrate BROOME's successful isolation of the active constituent of guinea pig serum by means of chromatographic fractionation. See [15]

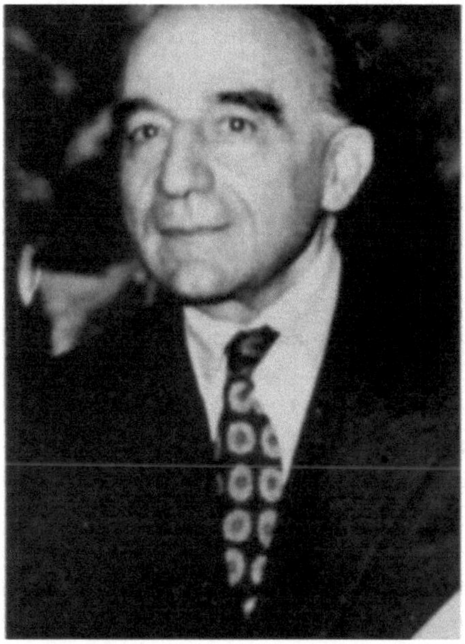

Fig. 8

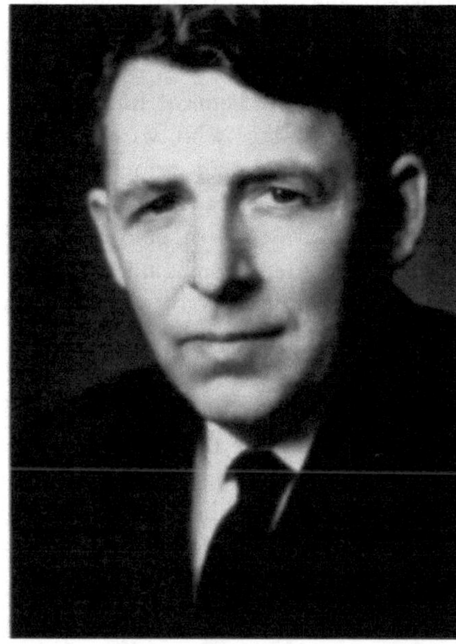

Fig. 9

Fig. 8. Photograph of Professor CLEMENTI of the University of Catania, whose observation of 1922—that guinea pig serum, alone amongst mammalian sera, is a rich source of asparaginase—provided a starting point for BROOME's investigations. Photo generously provided by Professor SEVERI of Perugia

Fig. 9. Photograph of Professor WRISTON of The University of Delaware. With his students LOUISE MASHBURN and TOBIAS YELLIN, Professor WRISTON, who had long been interested in the anti-lymphoma principle of guinea pig serum, promptly confirmed BROOME's biochemical finding. With assistance from JOHN BOYD, MASHBURN and WRISTON then showed that an asparaginase with antitumor properties could be isolated from E. coli B

Fig. 9 a. A recent photograph of Dr. JOHN BROOME who some years ago identified the active principle of guinea pig serum as being asparaginase

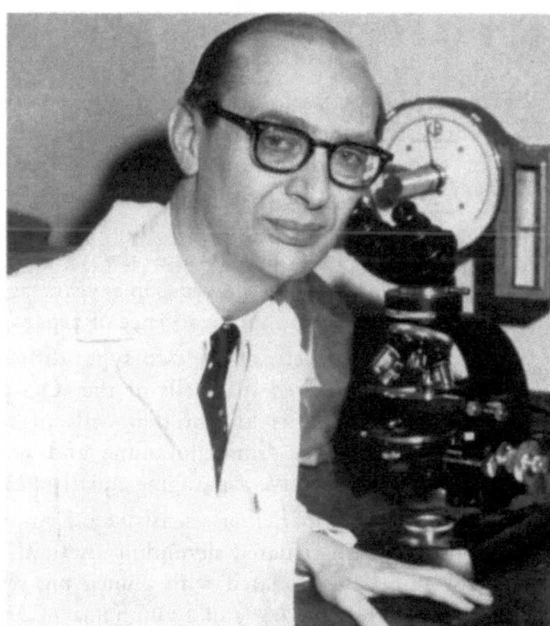

Fig. 9 a

this enzyme [13]—BROOME was led to inquire whether asparaginase might not be the active anti-lymphoma constituent of guinea pig serum. This proved to be so, as his careful studies showed [14, 15, 16].

BROOME's biochemical finding (see Fig. 7) was promptly confirmed and extended by JOHN WRISTON who, with PETER HERBUT, had long been interested in the nature of the antilymphoma principle of guinea pig serum; with two of his students—LOUISE MASHBURN and TOBIAS YELLIN—WRISTON promptly found that the anti-lymphoma principle of guinea pig serum is indeed asparaginase and that the latter can be procured from guinea pig serum in highly purified state [17, 18]. Further MASHBURN and WRISTON, with assistance from JOHN BOYD (another student), soon demonstrated that a highly purifiable asparaginase with anti-lymphoma properties can be extracted from Escherichia coli B (19). I show here photographs of CLEMENTI (Fig. 8), JOHN WRISTON (Fig. 9) and JOHN BROOME (Fig. 9 a).

The findings of BROOME and those of WRISTON and his associates led directly to the production of purified asparaginase in quantity and to the clinical trials of its therapeutic effects, about which we shall hear much during the next couple of days.

The work of THOMAS McCOY and his associates eminently deserves mention at this point. For at a time when EAGLE and other workers had determined that a wide variety of mammalian cells would grow in vitro in the absence of asparagine, McCOY and his associates showed that some cancer cells require exogenous asparagine for growth in vitro while others do not. McCOY's findings were presently extended by others [16, 20]. The concepts they provide are exceedingly useful today in studying the metabolism of asparagine by mammalian cancer cells, as Dr. PATTERSON's findings—to be presented here a few minutes hence—will doubtless make clear.

* * *

Professor GRUNDMANN also suggested that I speak briefly about some of my more recent interests, which have centered largely around the behavior in vivo and in vitro of two types of mouse lymphoma cells: 1) those of Gardner's Lymphoma 6C3HED, which we call Lymphoma 6C3HED-OG, regularly sensitive to the effects of guinea pig serum (asparaginase), and 2) those of Lymphoma 6C3HED-RG1, first transplanted some 15 years ago and always "resistant" to the effects of guinea pig serum [21—23]; BROOME showed some years ago that Lymphoma 6C3HED-RG1 cells grow readily in vitro in the absence of asparagine [16].

It is obvious that cells of the two types differ notably in their asparagine metabolism. It can be inferred that cells of the -OG type are largely devoid of asparagine synthetase and it is known that cells of the -RG1 type can synthesize the asparagine they require from glutamine and other sources. Yet cells of the two types "take up" radioactive asparagine equally [23].

Fig. 10 shows "asparaginase-sensitive" Lymphoma 6C3HED-OG cells heavily labeled in vivo with tritiated thymidine. Actually Dr. SOBIN and I found [22] that in control animals—untreated with guinea pig serum but given tritiated thymidine intraperitoneally—some 60% of Lymphoma 6C3HED-OG cells growing actively as ascites cells became heavily labeled (Fig. 10). By contrast we found that a population of growing -OG cells exposed for 2 hours in vivo to guinea pig serum were labeled in the same proportion with tritiated thymidine but much less heavily (Fig. 11). In addition to the more lightly labeled cells, however, there was a sprinkling (1% or less) of the heavily labeled cells scattered amongst the less heavily labeled ones. We inferred that guinea pig serum (asparaginase) interferes notably and promptly with the synthesis of DNA in populations of growing -OG cells, and that a sprinkling of cells of -RG1 type might account for the 1% or less of the heavily labeled cells to be seen amongst the population. Our findings were confirmed by concurrent liquid

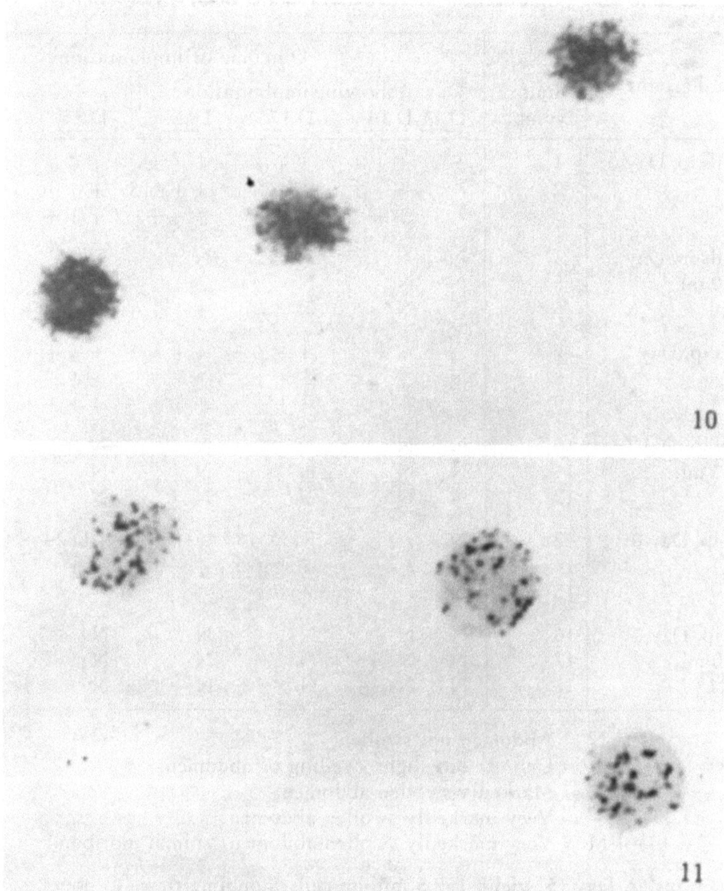

Figs. 10 and 11. Autoradiographs of -OG cells labeled with tritiated thymidine. From SOBIN and KIDD [22]—see text

scintillation measurements, which showed also that the interference with nucleic acid metabolism brought about by guinea pig serum was regularly preceded by diminished protein synthesis, the latter being always conspicuous within 15 minutes following exposure of the -OG cells to guinea pig serum [21—23].

Fig. 12 shows a tabulation of one of our current transfer experiments, in which cells, presumably of "asparaginase-insensitive" (-RG1) type, have grown out following implantation of a population of 1000 of our routine Lymphoma 6C3HED-OG "asparaginase-sensitive" type cells. In numerous experiments of this sort we have now found that we usually get evidence of the presence of a sprinkling of -RG1 type cells whenever we implant 1000 or more of our routine line of -OG cells, and sometimes when we implant as few as 100 cells or less. Through successive transfers

Outgrowth of "asparaginase-insensitive" (?) cells
following implantation of 1000 Lymphoma 6C3HED-OG cells

Experimental groups	Mouse Number	Outcome of implantations Days following implantation: D 11	D 14	D 17	D 22	D 25	D 29
B. 1000 cells ip, Day 0;	1	?	+++	++++	++±	++	N
	2	?	++±	++±	+++±	+++	++
	3	?	++++	+++	++++	+++	++
A. 1000 cells ip, Day 0	4	N	N	N	N	N	N
GPS, 2.0 ml,	5	N	N	N	+++	N	N
Days 0, 1	6	N	N	N	++++	++++	++++M
C. 100 cells ip, Day 0	7	N	++±	++++	++++	++++	†
	8	N	++±	++++	++++	++++	†
	9	?	+++	++++	++++	++++	+++
D. 100 cells ip, Day 0;	10	N	N	N	N	N	N
GPS, 2.0 ml,	11	N	N	N	N	N	N
Days 0, 1	12	N	N	N	N	N	N
E. 10 cells ip, Day 0	13	N	?	K, D, 15 [a]	++++	† D 24	+±
	14	N	?	+++±	++±	++	
	15	N	?	+++			
F. 10 cells ip, Day 0;	16	N	N	N	N	N	N
GPS, 2.0 ml,	17	N	N	N	N	N	N
Days 0, 1	18	N	N	N	N	N	N

N = Abdomen not swollen.
++ = Definite but slight swelling of abdomen.
+++ = Markedly swollen abdomen.
++++ = Very markedly swollen abdomen.
++++M = Very markedly swollen abdomen; animal moribund.

[a] Killed for transfer, Day 15; yield, 157.5 million cells; doubling time, 13 hours.

Fig. 12. Tabulation of a recent transplantation experiment in which cells presumably of -RG1 ("asparaginase-insensitive") type grew out following the intraperitoneal implantation of 1000 of our routine line of Lymphoma 6C3HED-OG ("asparaginase-sensitive") cells see text.

of approximately 10 cells in mice given guinea pig serum we have now procured a "pure lines" of -RG1 type ("asparaginase-insensitive") cells, which seem to grow somewhat better in C3H mice heavily treated with guinea pig serum than in normal C3H mice. We are hopeful but not yet quite certain that we have also established a pure line of asparaginase-sensitive (OG type) cells by similar means.

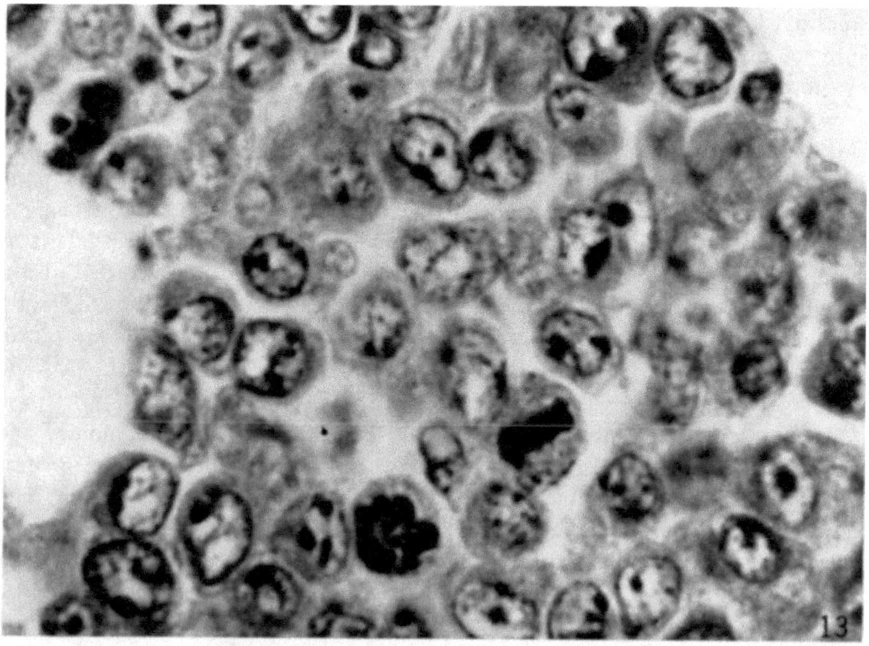

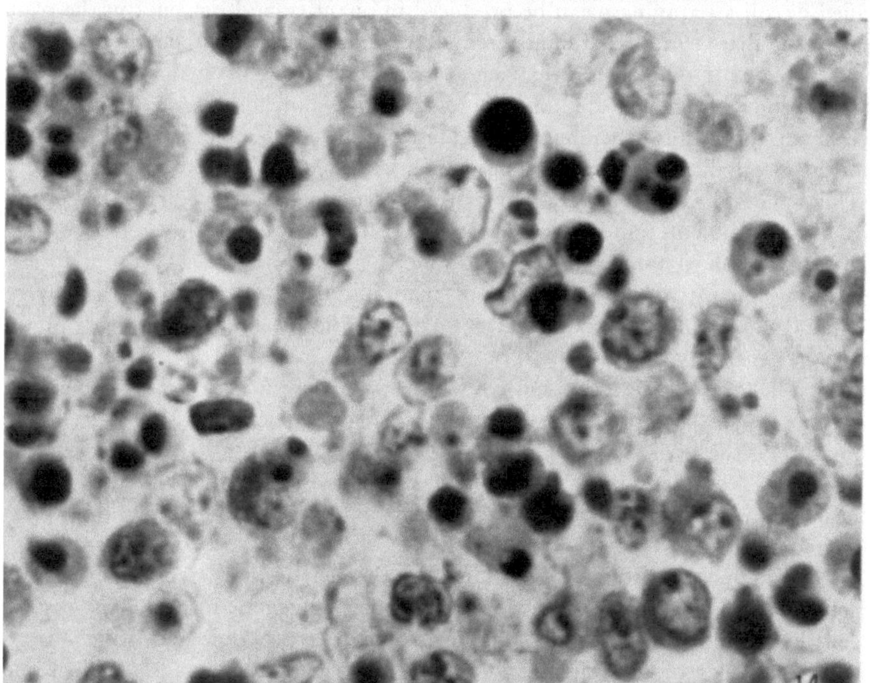

Figs. 13 and 14. Fig. 13 shows Lymphoma 6C3HED-OG cells proliferating actively in the subcutaneous tissues of a normal control inbred C3H mouse 5 days following implantation. Fig. 14 shows necrosis of the cells of the same implantation in another mouse that had been given two injections 4 hours apart of 1 ml of 3 : 1 concentrated guinea pig serum. The animal was killed for histologic study 4 hours after the second injection and 8 hours after the first. See text; also [6]

In this relation I show finally from our older work what happens to "asparaginase-sensitive" cells when you deprive them in vivo of the exogenous asparagine they require for protein synthesis and growth by giving guinea pig serum to their hosts. They promptly starve to death, as Fig. 14 shows.

My theme is that the work of a number of scientists has recently brought asparagine and asparaginase into relationship with cancer, this with some benefit perhaps to man's enlightenment, his spirit, and his well-being. It seems to me significant that these scientists worked as individuals or in small teams, and that their labors were accomplished in widely separated laboratories in the old and new worlds; also that they built their works upon a solid and extensive foundation of knowledge about asparagine, asparaginase, and cancer that had been won previously, bit by bit, over a long period.

Current progress is especially noteworthy. For example, eighteen months ago it was only imagined that E. coli asparaginase might be producible in quantities sufficient for widespread clinical trials against cancers of many types in human beings, and it was questionable whether, once produced, enough asparaginase could be given to a sick human being to starve to death those of his cancer cells that require exogenous asparagine for protein synthesis and growth—this without doing him harm. Today, as this Symposium bears eloquent witness, we know that highly purified E. coli asparaginase can be produced in quantity and not only in the western world; also that, suitably administered, it regularly starves to death those of the host's cancer cells that require exogenous asparagine for survival and growth, this without producing irreparable injury to the host. Furthermore we steadily learn more about the means whereby asparaginase produces its effects in vivo, and more about the metabolism of asparagine in mammalian cells.

This is not to say, however, that a neo-millenium has arrived. For large limitations, large problems, and large questions still abound. In this relation today's scientist may wish to ponder several questions:

Why are many of the leukemias of man initially susceptible to therapy with asparaginase while others are refractory ab initio as, indeed, one may presume, are the generality of cancers?

Can a laboratory test be devised which will show whether a given cancer is composed of "asparaginase-sensitive" or "asparaginase-insensitive" cells, or a mixture of the two?

Why do "complete remissions" induced with asparaginase in cases of acute leukemia regularly prove only transitory? How can this large limitation be overcome?

Is "asparaginase resistance" determined by the genetic character of the "resistant" cells, or is this regulation achieved through some epigenetic means. Can "resistant" cells be altered artificially so that they become "asparaginase-sensitive"?

Will analogues of asparagine, glutamine, or other amino acids, or their metabolites, inhibit the proliferation of cancer cells in vivo?

In light of these and other questions I submit, Mr. Chairman, that the problems posed by asparagine and asparaginase in relation to cancer constitute at once beacons for science and challenges to today's scientists.

References

1. KIDD, JOHN G.: A distinctive substance associated with the Brown-Pearce rabbit carcinoma. J. exp. Med. **71**, 335—371 (1940).
2. — Suppression of growth of the Brown-Pearce tumor by a specific antibody. Science **99**, 348—350 (1944); — J. exp. Med. **83**, 227—250 (1946).
3. MACKENZIE, IAN, KIDD, JOHN G.: Incidence and specificity of the antibody for a distinctive constituent of the Brown-Pearce tumor. J. exp. Med. **82**, 41—63 (945).
4. KALFAYAN, BERNARD, KIDD, JOHN G.: Structural changes produced in Brown-Pearce carcinoma cells by means of a specific antibody and complement. J. exp. Med. **97**, 145—162 (1953).
5. KIDD, JOHN G.: Regression of transplanted lymphomas induced in vivo by means of normal guinea pig serum. I. Course of transplanted cancers of various kinds in mice and rats given guinea pig serum, horse serum or rabbit serum. J. exp. Med. **98**, 565—582 (1953).
6. — Regression of transplanted lymphomas induced in vivo by means of normal guinea pig serum. II. Studies on the nature of the active serum constituent: histological mechanism of the regression: tests for effects of guinea pig serum on lymphoma cells in vitro: Discussion. J. exp. Med. **98**, 583—606 (1953).
7. — TODD, JEAN ELIZABETH: Inhibitory effects of normal guinea pig serum and immune rabbit serum on transplanted AKR lymphomas. Proc. Soc. exp. Biol. (N. Y.) **86**, 781—785 (1954).
8. TODD, JEAN ELIZABETH, KIDD, JOHN G.: Tests for isoantibodies active in conjunction with guinea pig serum against 6C3HED lymphoma cells. Proc. Soc. exp. Biol. (N. Y.) **86**, 865—868 (1954).
9. KAUFFMAN, SHIRLEY L., KIDD, JOHN G.: Effects of guinea pig serum on 6C3HED and AKRLI lymphoma cells implanted in various hosts. Proc. Soc. exp. Biol. (N. Y.) **91**, 164—168 (1956).
10. MOHOS, STEVEN C., KIDD, JOHN G.: Effects of various immune rabbit serums on the cells of several transplanted mouse lymphomas in vitro and in vivo. With special reference to inhibition by an antibody that reacts with neoplastic and non-neoplastic lymphocytic cells of mice. J. exp. Med. **105**, 233—265 (1957).
11. KIDD, JOHN G.: Effects of arsenic-azoproteins on mouse lymphoma cells in vivo. With observations on the effects of other "anti-lymphoma" agents, and on the susceptibility to these effects of lymphoma cells of various types. J. exp. Med. **108**, 665—684 (1958).
12. — Specificity and effects of antibodies that react with antigens of cancer cells. Acta Un. int. Cancr. **15**, 921—923 (1959).
13. CLEMENTI, A.: La desamidation enzymatique de L'asparagine chez les differentes especes animales et la signification physiologique de sa presence dans l'organisme. Arch. int. Physiol. **19**, 369—398 (1922).
14. BROOME, J. D.: Evidence that the L-asparaginase activity of guinea pig serum is responsible for its antilymphoma effects. Nature **191**, 1114—1115 (1961).
15. — Evidence that the L-asparaginase of guinea pig serum is responsible for its antilymphoma effects. I. Properties of the L-asparaginase of guinea pig serum in relation to those of the antilymphoma substance. J. exp. Med. **118**, 99—120 (1963).
16. — Evidence that the L-asparaginase of guinea pig serum is responsible for its antilymphoma effects. II. Lymphoma 6C3HED cells cultured in a medium devoid of L-asparaginase lose their susceptibility to the effects of guinea pig serum in vivo. J. exp. Med. **118**, 121—148 (1963).
17. MASHBURN, L. T., WRISTON, JOHN C., JR.: Tumor inhibitory effect of L-asparaginase. Biochem. biophys. Res. Commun. **12**, 50—55 (1963).
18. YELLIN, T. O., WRISTON, JOHN C., JR.: Purification and properties of guinea pig serum asparaginase. Biochemistry **5**, 1605—1612 (1966).
19. MASHBURN, L., WRISTON, JOHN C., JR.: Tumor inhibitory effect of L-asparaginase from Escherichia coli. Arch. Biochem. **105**, 450—452 (1964).
20. HALEY, E. E., FISCHER, G. A., WELCH, A. D.: The requirements for L-asparagine of mouse leukemia cells L5178 in culture. Cancer Res. **21**, 532—536 (1961).

21. Sobin, L. H., Kidd, John G.: A metabolic difference between two lines of Lymphoma 6C3HED cells in relation to asparagine. Proc. Soc. exp. Biol. (N. Y.) **119**, 325—327 (1965).
22. — — Alterations in protein and nucleic acid metabolism of Lymphoma 6C3HED-OG cells in mice given guinea pig serum. J. exp. Med. **123**, 55—74 (1966).
23. Kidd, John G., Sobin, Leslie H.: The incorporation of L-asparagine-^{14}C by Lymphoma 6C3HED cells: inhibition by guinea pig serum. Cancer Res. **26**, 208—211 (1966).

L-Asparaginase: Early Findings and Current Studies on the Metabolism of L-Asparagine in Lymphoma Cells

J. D. Broome

Department of Pathology, New York University School of Medicine, New York

With 7 Figures

Kidd has described some of his observations on the effect of guinea pig serum in inhibiting the growth of certain mouse tumors, and out of this apparently distant finding we are engaged in the present symposium [1].

I was, of course, very fortunate to have had the idea that L-asparaginase might be the agent in guinea pig serum responsible for tumor inhibition. I have described in an earlier review the sequence of events which led to this [2]. Briefly, after beginning like others in thinking that complement in guinea pig serum might be responsible, my early experiments convinced me that the mechanism of tumor inhibition was not of an immunological nature. I then began to search for other ingredients of guinea pig serum which might be involved. Since a variety of different animal sera were not inhibitory to tumors [1] one could try to find a particular component which distinguished guinea pig serum from these. I began by performing experiments with glycoproteins of guinea pig serum, but these resulted in no success, then I learned that guinea pig serum was an unusual source of L-asparaginase [3]. The first experiment I performed was to try to reverse the tumor inhibitory effect of guinea pig serum by the simultaneous injection into mice of L-asparagine. The results were erratic and inconclusive and success in preventing the tumor inhibitory effect was achieved only considerably later by Ohnuma, Bergel and Bray who added L-asparagine to the drinking water of the mice [4]. Next, I had found that when cells of the guinea pig serum-sensitive lymphoma 6C3HED were placed in tissue culture in Eagle's medium, cells which eventually grew out failed to be inhibited by guinea pig serum when they were subsequently implanted *in vivo*.

In view of our earlier ideas, it was natural to see whether supplementation of the medium with L-asparagine would prevent this process. Indeed it did. The cultured cells now retained full sensitivity to guinea pig serum. These experiments provided a specific clue linking the tumor inhibitory effect of guinea pig serum with asparagine metabolism in the tumor cells. I was unfortunately unaware at the time of two important earlier studies. Neuman and McCoy had shown that for the Walker carcinosarcoma, glutamine and asparagine were necessary for growth *in vitro* [5]. McCoy et al. had also shown that asparagine-independent variants could eventually grow out of cultures of the Jensen sarcoma deprived of the amino acid [6]. Clearly, my results with lymphoma cells were closely similar to theirs. Later I spent some time purifying guinea pig serum asparaginase and I found that enzyme assays could be correlated with tumor inhibitory activity. The final proof of identity of asparaginase with the tumor inhibitory agent of guinea pig serum was the work of WRISTON and his colleagues, who obtained the enzyme as a pure protein and demonstrated that it was powerfully inhibitory to tumor growth [7, 8]. Later, the same group showed that asparaginase from an entirely different source, namely from *Escherichia coli* was a strong tumor inhibitor. The availability of such a source has made much further progress possible.

One of my aims more recently has been to try to understand how asparaginase inhibits tumors and the nature of asparaginase-resistance. I intend now to consider some current and incomplete studies to this end.

L-Asparagine Synthesis in Cells of Lymphoma 6C3HED

We have shown that cells of Lymphoma 6C3HED sensitive to asparaginase have a much lower capacity to synthesize asparagine than have resistant variants [9, 10].

When cells are incubated in tissue culture medium containing a labeled amino acid the amount of this amino acid incorporated into protein can be measured. In this

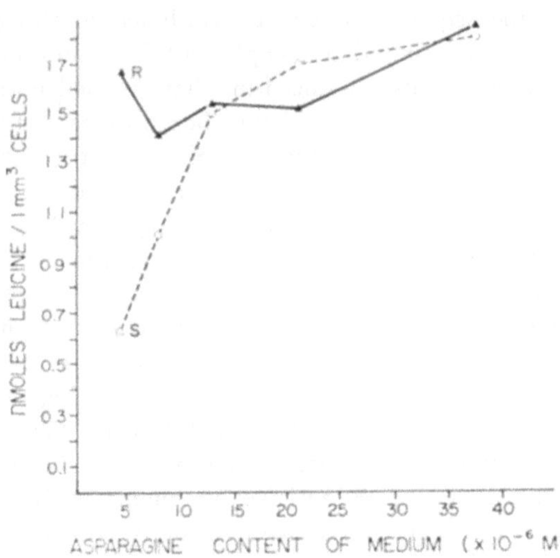

Fig. 1. Incorporation of exogenous leucine into proteins of Lymphoma 6C3HED

Figs. 1—4 are reproduced, by permission, from Journal of Experimental Medicine

way leucine incorporation has been measured in the presence of varying concentrations of asparagine. It can be seen from Fig. 1, that with asparaginase-resistant cells a constant rate of leucine incorporation occurs even though the asparagine concentration of the medium is reduced to 4.5×10^{-6} M. With asparaginase-sensitive cells, on the other hand, leucine incorporation falls when the asparagine content of the medium is less than 13×10^{-6} M. Since we have found that leucine is metabolized in detectable amount by these cells only for protein synthesis, the decreased incorporation at low asparagine concentrations indicates, with certain provisos, a decreased rate of protein synthesis.

Similar experiments can be performed using labeled asparagine, as shown in Fig. 2. It will be seen that through a wide concentration range, the asparaginase-sensitive cells take up more asparagine from the medium than do the resistant cells. If experiments are performed using simultaneously asparagine labelled with C14 and

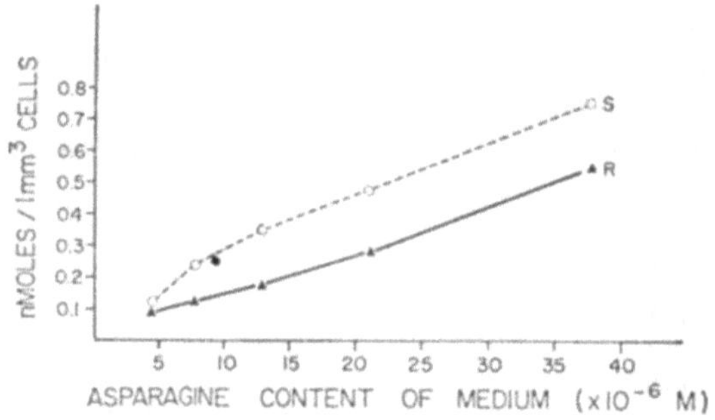

Fig. 2. Incorporation of exogenous asparagine into proteins of Lymphoma 6C3HED

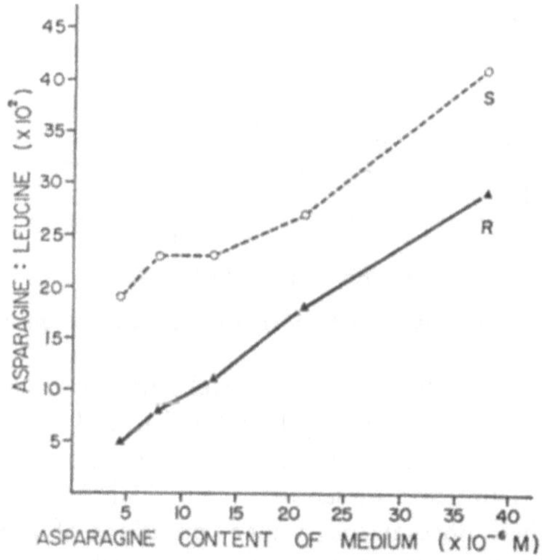

Fig. 3. Ratio of exogenous asparagine to leucine in proteins of Lymphoma 6C3HED

leucine with H3 it becomes possible to measure the ratio between amounts of these two amino acids which are incorporated from an exogenous source into cell proteins. It will be seen (Fig. 3) that the ratio can be varied in the resistant cells in a virtually linear fashion. But with sensitive cells, although some variation is possible, it is clearly limited.

As we saw earlier, below an asparagine concentration of 13×10^{-6} M leucine incorporation is decreased. With certain provisos, these observations imply that asparaginase-resistant, but not sensitive cells can freely compensate for a decreased availability of exogenous asparagine by making an increasing amount of endogenous asparagine available for protein synthesis. This will be true, of course, in resistant cells only if proteins containing the same (or higher) asparagine : leucine ratio are synthesized under the various conditions. Evidence that this condition is met has been discussed elsewhere [10].

The experiments now described shows a further point. The fall which occurrs in the ratio of exogenous asparagine : leucine incorporated into protein indicates that the endogenous asparagine used in protein synthesis cannot be in free equilibrium with that entering from the medium.

The ability of asparaginase-resistant cells to utilize endogenous asparagine with high efficiency in protein synthesis is further demonstrated in experiments in which the level of free asparagine in the lymphomas has been measured during asparaginase treatment *in vivo*.

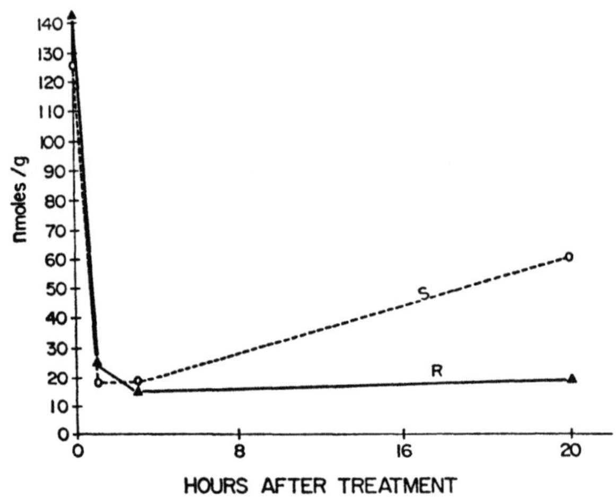

Fig. 4. Free asparagine content of 6C3HED tumors treated with L-asparaginase

In both kinds of tumor the asparagine level falls to virtually the same extent (Fig. 4). A late rise in sensitive cells may be related to cell necrosis. Thus in resistant cells protein synthesis continues with intracellular levels of free asparagine which are inadequate for this function in sensitive cells. This is explicable if in resistant cells the protein synthetic mechanisms, under conditions of asparagine deprivation, do not depend on asparagine drawn from the whole cell pool. It suggests that there is a close linkage between asparagine synthesizing and utilizing systems.

Patterson and Orr have demonstrated an asparagine—synthesizing system in cell-free extracts of the Jensen sarcoma and other tumor cell lines [11]. We have found that although this system cannot be detected in asparaginase-sensitive lymphoma cells, it is readily found in extracts of resistant cells [9, 10]. In these cells the enzyme appears to be cytoplasmic. How, then, is it possible to account for the particular efficiency of utilization of endogenous asparagine in protein synthesis?

To attempt to answer this question we are currently examining the transport RNA of tumor cells, first to see whether a particular linkage can be demonstrated between t-RNA and the asparagine synthetase already found in the lymphoma cells, and secondly to examine whether the t-RNA may be involved in another route of asparagine biosynthesis. We have been particularly attracted to the second course by the finding of WILLCOX and NIRENBERG that in a microbial system glutamyl t-RNA may be enzymatically converted to glutaminyl t-RNA [12].

Studies on t-RNA Species of Cells of Lymphoma 6C3HED

We have prepared t-RNA from cells of Lymphoma 6C3HED following with few modifications the method of YANG and NOVELLI [13]. 15 ml of packed cells, obtained from ascites tumors, yield 150—250 A_{260} units of t-RNA.

The preparation of amino acyl t-RNA synthetase has involved more difficulty. Cells of Lymphoma 6C3HED are not readily disrupted in homogenizers of the Potter or related kinds; freezing and thawing is highly effective for this purpose, but nucleases are normally liberated into the solution.

However, after examining a number of sublines of the lymphoma cells which have been passed through tissue culture we have succeeded in obtaining sublines which yield extracts lacking in nuclease activity. Using such cells we have prepared amino acyl to t-RNA synthetases by the method of NISHIMURA and WEINSTEIN [14], t-RNA has been charged with labelled amino acids by the method of YANG and NOVELLI [13].

It will be seen from Fig. 5 that the charging reaction occurrs rapidly, reaching completion at 5 minutes and afterwards the amino acyl t-RNA appears stable. The

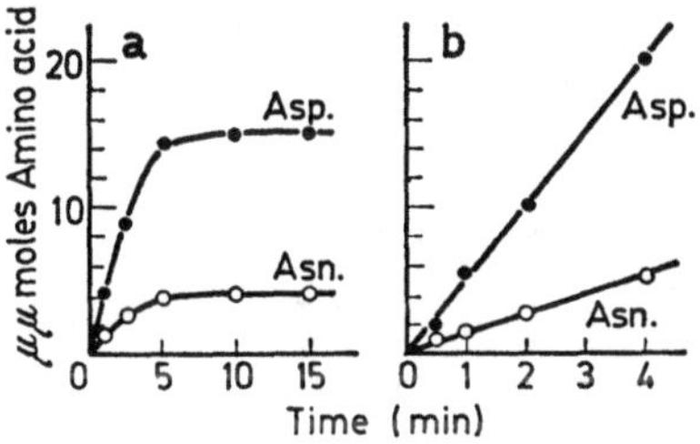

Fig. 5. a) Rate of formation of aspartyl (ASP) and asparaginyl (ASN) t-RNA. Each point represents acylation of approximately 0.3 A_{260} units of whole t-RNA, conditions of reaction were otherwise as described in table. — b) Dependence of amino acyl t-RNA formation on the amount of t-RNA in reaction mixtures

total amount of amino acid reacting with t-RNA bears a linear relationship to the amount of t-RNA in the reaction mixture. t-RNA preparations from asparaginase-sensitive and resistant lymphoma cells accept a variety of amino acids (Table). Here the preparation from asparaginase-resistant cells had a rather higher acceptor capacity than had that from sensitive cells, and particularly for aspartic acid.

Amino acyl t-RNA's prepared as described above have been fractionated chromatographically. After charging the t-RNA, reaction mixtures have been extracted with phenol and the aqueous layer applied to DEAE cellulose. Proteins, particularly any residual nuclease are removed it 0.25 M sodium chloride. t-RNA is eluted in

0.65 M sodium chloride and precipated with ethanol. It is finally applied to a column for reverse phase chromatography [13].

It will be seen from Fig. 6 that label from asparagine appears in 3 peaks, and that the t-RNA species appear the same in preparations both from asparaginase-sensitive and resistant cells. The first 2 species appear to be specific for asparagine,

Table. *Amino acid acceptor activity of t-RNA derived from cells of lymphoma 6C3HED*

L-amino acid	Acceptor activity of t-RNA (μμ moles/A_{260} unit)	
	From asparaginase sensitive cells	From asparaginase resistant cells
Aspartic acid	58.0	78.0
Asparagine	42.6	53.4
Arginine	124.4	138.6
Leucine	109.4	133.8
Threonine	60.6	77.2
Valine	60.6	61.2

t-RNA (1.0 A_{260} unit) and amino acyl t-RNA synthetase preparation from asparaginase-resistant cells (0.5 mg protein) were incubated at 37° C in 1×10^{-2} M ATP, 5×10^{-3} M Mg^{++} and 5×10^{-2} M Tris (pH 7.5) with approximately 1×10^{-5} M C14-labeled amino acid, in a total volume of 0.5 ml. Samples removed at 5, 10 and 20 minutes were precipitated in cold 5% trichloracetic acid and the precipitate collected on Millipore filters.

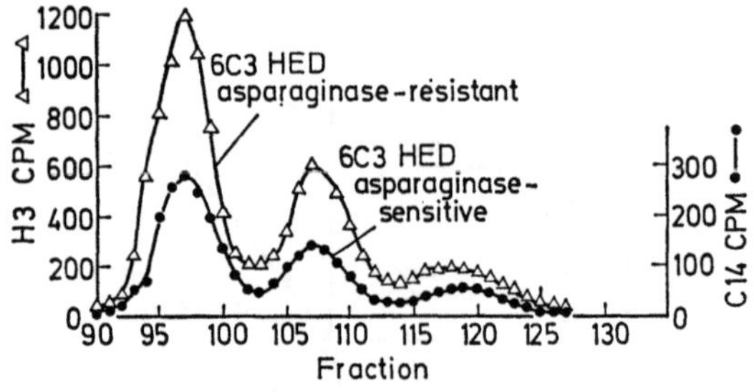

Fig. 6. Elution profile of asparaginyl t-RNA's of lymphoma 6C3HED by reverse phase chromatography

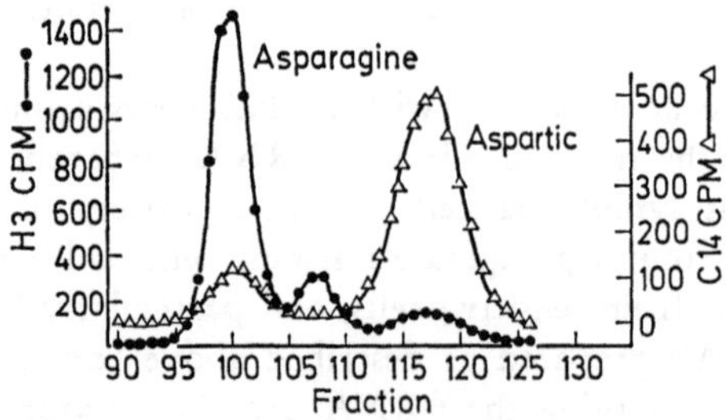

Fig. 7. Elution profile of asparginyl and aspartyl t-RNA's from asparaginase-resistant cells of Lymphoma 6C3HED

but in the case of the third species there is some doubt. Aspartic acid produces 2 peaks of charged t-RNA (Fig. 7) and the larger occurrs at the same position in the elution profile as does the third peak from asparagine. We have found that a small amount of aspartic acid is formed from asparagine under the conditions used for charging t-RNA, and this final peak may be aspartyl t-RNA.

Thus far then, we have demonstrated only similarities between the t-RNA species of asparaginase-sensitive and resistant cells. Our experiments have not yet shown the means by which asparagine biosynthesis may be linked with utilization in protein synthesis. It is hoped that with the methods now developed this objective may be accomplished.

References

1. Kidd, J. G.: This symposium (1969).
2. Broome, J. D.: Trans. N. Y. Acad. Sci. **30**, 690 (1968).
3. Clementi, A.: Arch. int. Physiol. **19**, 369 (1922).
4. Ohnuma, K., Bergel, F., Bray, R. C.: Biochem. J. **97**, 321 (1967).
5. Neuman, R. E., McCoy, T. A.: Science **124**, 124 (1956).
6. McCoy, T. A.: Maxwell, M., Irvine, E., Sartorelli, A. C.: Proc. Soc. exp. Biol. (N. Y.) **100**, 862 (1959).
7. Mashburn, L. T., Wriston, J. C.: Arch. Biochem. **105**, 450 (1964).
8. Yellin, T. O., Wriston, J. C.: Biochemistry **5**, 1605 (1966).
9. Broome, J. D., Schwartz, J. H.: Biochim. biophys. Acta. (Amst.) **138**, 637 (1967).
10. — J. exp. Med. **127**, 1055 (1968).
11. Patterson, M. K., Orr, G.: Biochem. biophys. Res. Commun. **26**, 228 (1967).
12. Wilcox, M., Nirenberg, M.: Proc. nat. Acad. Sci. (Wash.) **61**, 229 (1968).
13. Yang, W. K., Novelli, D. G.: Proc. at. Acad. Sci. (Wash.) **59**, 208 (1968).
14. Nishimura, S., Weinstein, I. B., Biochemistry **8**, 832 (1969).

Studies on the Control of Asparagine Biosynthesis in Mammalian Tissues

M. K. Patterson, Jr.

Biomedical Division, The Samuel Roberts Noble Foundation, Inc.,
Ardmore, Oklahoma 73401, U.S.A.

With 6 Figures

Among certain malignant tissues, sensitivity to L-asparaginase (ASNase) [1] appears to be related to the nutritional requirement and biosynthesis of L-asparagine (ASN) [7, 9, 14]. With other malignant or normal tissues the relationship is not clear. From the early studies of the *in vivo* effects of ASNase by Kidd [10] and the *in vitro* nutritional requirements for ASN by McCoy et al. [11] and others [3, 15], it became apparent that under certain injection regimes or culturing conditions nutritional variants could be derived from the parent population. These variants no longer required ASN for growth and were resistant to ASNase. A similar phenomenon now appears to prevail following the clinical use of ASNase on human malignancies. A second anomoly existed in normal tissues. Those normal tissues tested showed no requirement for ASN and a resistance to ASNase, but only limited L-asparagine synthetase (ASN SYN) [4, 8, 17, 20].

Addressing ourselves to the problem of variant development, two mechanisms were proposed. Variants developed either as a result of cell selection or through a cellular enzyme adaptation capable of enhancing ASN synthesis. To pursue the problem of the former, cloning techniques were employed; for the latter an assay system for ASN SYN was developed [17, 18]. Jensen sarcoma and the Walker 256 carcinoma were selected as model systems because both have an *in vitro* requirement for ASN [12, 13], are sensitive to ASNase [6, 15], and give rise to variant cells.

On the basis of our studies with cloned populations, it was concluded that the Jensen sarcoma variants were derived by a cell selection process and that the selected cell population arose through mutational events not necessarily related to ASN deprivation [16].

Experimental

Concomitant with the cloning experiments, changes in ASN SYN activity during ASN deprivation were studied. Fig. 1 shows the increase in enzyme activity and

[1] Abbreviations: ASN, L-asparagine; ASNase, L-asparaginase, amidohydrolase E.C. 3.5.11; ASN SYN, L-asparagine synthetase, E.C. 6.3.1.1.

labeling index (pulsed thymidine-^{3}H) during the growth curve of the Jensen sarcoma cultured in McCoy's 5 a medium devoid of ASN. The increases in these two parameters would be compatible with the proliferation of a selected cell population. Similar curves were obtained when cells were cultured in the presence of ASNase. The level of enzyme has remained a stable characteristic of the variant throughout several hundred transplant and subculture generations [17]. If cells derived from exposure to ASNase were subcultured into media devoid of ASN or continued in the presence of ASNase medium, ASN SYN activity of these cells was greater than the activity

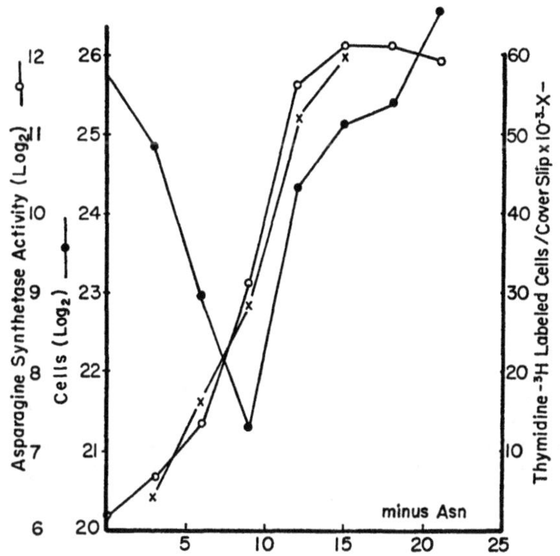

Fig. 1. Relationship of asparagine synthetase (— o —) and labeling index (— x —) and cell populations (— ● —) to time of exposure of cultured Jensen sarcoma cells to asparagine deprivation

of the cells grown in the presence of ASN (Fig. 2). At the end of 7 subcultures each population was subcultured into the different experimental media (Fig. 3). Cells derived from the ASN medium exhibited over a 2-fold increase in ASN SYN within 3 to 5 doublings when subcultured back into the ASNase medium. Cells continually cultured in ASNase medium showed a 2-fold decrease in ASN SYN when subcultured into ASN medium. Subsequent subculturing of the cell populations revealed that ASN SYN was adapted but only within the limits defined in Fig. 3. For instance, continuous subculturing for 32 passages of the variant cell line in the presence of ASN failed to repress activity to the levels observed in the parent cell population.

In light of these observations it was of interest that several investigators reported studies suggestive of *in vivo* adaptation of asparagine synthetase in normal and malignant tissues. Arfin [1] reported that in liver of embryonic chick, ASN biosynthesis decreased as maturation occurred. Becker and Broome [2] reported that injections of ASNase into hepatectomized rats inhibited the first but not the second mitotic wave. They suggested an increase in ASN biosynthesis in the regenerating liver. Broome [4, 5] and Prager [20] found increased ASN SYN in tumors treated with ASNase. Our studies, summarized in Table 1, showed that during experimental

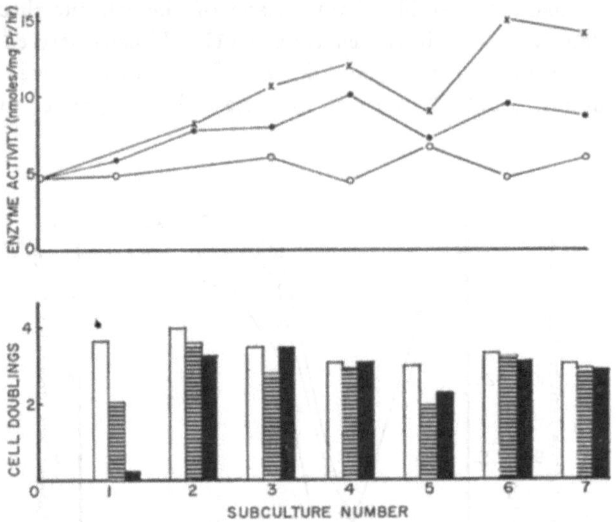

Fig. 2. Cell doublings (bar graph) and asparagine synthetase activity (symbols) of cell populations derived from Jensen sarcoma cultures previously exposed to L-asparaginase for 21 days and then subcultured into medium containing L-asparagine (open bars; — o —), devoid of L-asparagine (cross bars; — ● —), or medium containing L-asparaginase (solid bars; — x —)

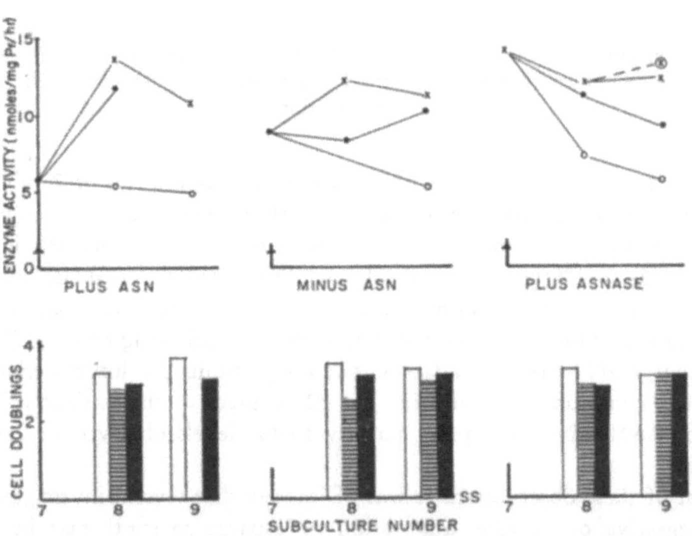

Fig. 3. Cell doublings and asparagine synthetase of cell populations derived from cultures described in Fig. 2 and after 7 subcultures. Each population was then subcultured into experimental medium. Symbols are the same as those for Fig. 2

procedures designed to create a demand for ASN, biosynthesis of the amino acid increased in the liver [19]. In the assay system used, no correlation between ASN SYN and endogenous liver ASNase was observed.

Table 1. *Rat liver L-asparagine synthetase*

Conditions	Relative enzyme specific activity [a]				
Normal	Age (days)				
	—3	2		7	60
	51.0	15.6		6.00	1.0
Tumor bearing	Tumor growth (days)				
	7		10		15
Jensen sarcoma	2.16		3.50		6.63
JA sarcoma	1.61		2.26		4.28
Walker 256	5.20		6.27		12.1
WA carcinoma	2.32		4.34		10.4
L-Asparaginase injected (50 I.U./Kg B.W.)	Hours after injection				
	12	24		36	48
	2.26	3.39		2.90	1.09
Hepatectomized	Regeneration (days)				
	0.5	1.0	2.0	5.0	7.0
	2.44	4.04	3.19	2.39	1.63
Dietary minus ASN	Days on diet				
	5		10		15
	7.13		7.36		5.50

[a] Normal adult value = 1.0.

For study of the mechanism involved in the control of ASN SYN, the increase in the enzyme activity following injections of ASNase was selected. Normal animals and animals bearing intramuscular transplants of the Walker 256 carcinoma (7 days) were given a single intraperitoneal injection of 50 I.U. of *E. coli* ASNase or saline and sacrificed at various time intervals. Table 2 shows the average body, organ, and cellular parameters over a 48-hour period after injection of ASNase. With the exception of spleen weights, injections of ASNase had no effect on the parameters listed within the 48-hour experimental period. Spleen weights and ASN SYN of tumor hosts decreased to normal values within 6 hours after injections. ASN SYN expressed as nmoles/mg protein/hour was 1.03 for normal spleen, 2.61 for tumor bearer, and 1.09 for tumor bearer injected with ASNase.

The relationship between clearance of injected ASNase from the serum and the activity of ASN SYN in the liver of normal and tumor-bearing animals is shown in Fig. 4. The decrease in rate of clearance in the tumor-bearing animals depicted in the graph was also noted in animals bearing the Jensen sarcoma. The peak activity of ASN SYN, shown in Fig. 4, and serum ASNase could be maintained for at least 7 days in normal animals by twice daily injections of ASNase. This suggests a direct role of serum levels of ASN in altering the ASN SYN levels of the liver.

The relationship of thymidine-^{3}H incorporation into DNA and valine-^{14}C incorporation into protein and the ASN SYN activity of the livers of normal and tumor-bearing animals given a single injection of ASNase is shown in Fig. 5. The values

Table 2. *Effects of L-asparaginase on body, organ, and cellular parameters*

	Normal		Walker 256	
Measurement	Saline (10)[a]	ASNase (11)	Saline (10)	ASNase (11)
Body Wt. (gms)	227 ±13[b]	230 ±10	249 ±17	241 ±13
Liver Wt. (gms)	7.0 ±1.5	8.1 ±0.8	10.6 ±1.5	9.7 ±1.5
Tumor Wt. (gms)	—	—	26.1 ±4.1	18.1 ±2.5
Spleen Wt. (gms)	0.62 ±0.10	0.58 ±0.11	1.14 ±0.11	0.64 ±0.10
RNA (mg/gm)[c]	18.0 ±5.8	12.1 ±1.3	17.7 ±3.1	14.6 ±1.8
DNA (mg/gm)[c]	4.87 ±0.56	4.32 ±0.46	3.73 ±0.57	3.78 ±0.44
Protein (mg/gm)[c]	157 ±16	150 ±11	146 ±8	140 ±7
Nuclei (10^{-6}/gm)[c]	228 ±9	226 ±29	170 ±28	200 ±22

[a] Number of animals in each experiment.
[b] Standard deviation.
[c] Liver.

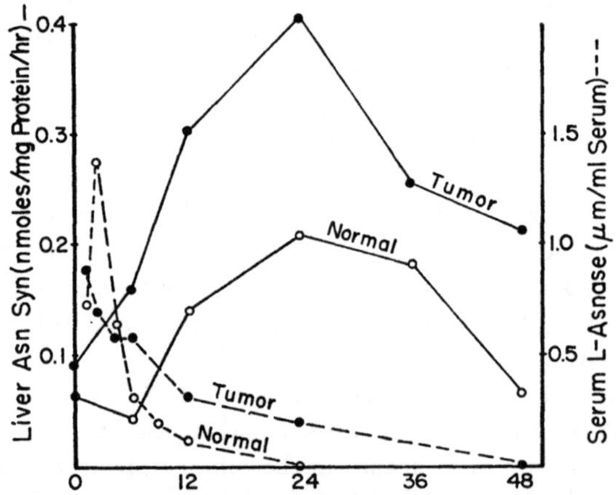

Fig. 4. Liver asparagine synthetase and serum L-asparaginase levels of normal and Walker 256-bearing rats at different time intervals following a single injection of 50 I.U. of *E. coli* L-asparaginase

plotted are the ratio of experimental to control (saline injected) values. The relative activity of the TdR³H incorporation into DNA decreased within 12 hours after injection and approached normal values by 48 hours. Valine-^{14}C incorporation decreased 50% in both the normal and tumor-bearing animals within 6 hours after injection. By 18 hours the tumor-host values were similar to those obtained from the control group. The values for the normal animals injected with ASNase, however, remained low but were approaching the control values 48 hours after injection.

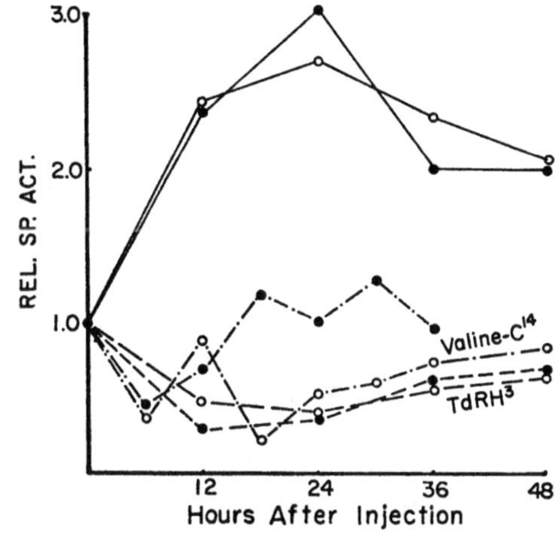

Fig. 5. Relative specific activity of liver asparagine synthetase (—), protein (—·—·—), and DNA (— — —) following a single injection of L-asparaginase. Valine-^{14}C was injected at 10 μc/100 gm B.W. and tritiated thymidine at 100 μc/100 gm B.W. 30 minutes before sacrifice. Solid symbols represent tumor-bearing values and open symbols normal animals. Relative specific activities = ASNase injected/saline injected; specific avticity expressed as cpm/mg protein for valine-^{14}C, cpm/mg DNA for TdR³H and nmoles asparagine/mg protein/hour

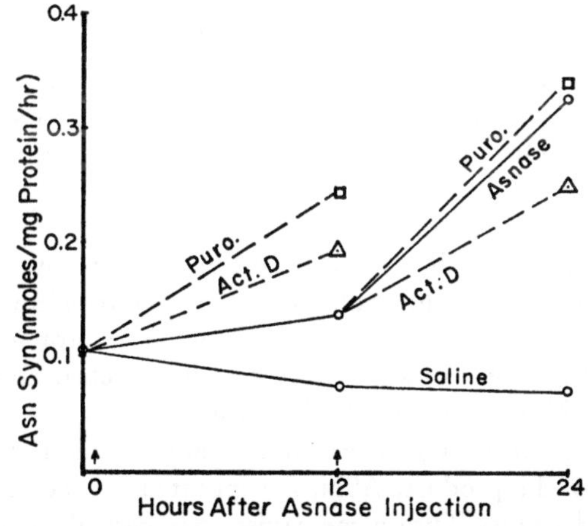

Fig. 6. Liver asparagine synthetase activity of animals injected with 10 mg puromycin/gm B.W. or 200 μg actinomycin D/100 gm B.W. 30 minutes before or 12 hours after a single injection of 50 I.U. of *E. coli* L-asparaginase. Arrows indicate time of injection of inhibitors of protein synthesis

In both the tumor-bearing host and normal liver a 2- to 3-fold increase in the ASN SYN occurred following the ASNase injection. A similar 2- to 3-fold increase was seen in animals fed an ASN-free diet for 5 days and then given an ASNase injection. Although the significance of the effect of ASNase injection on protein and DNA synthesis is not clear, their inhibition does not influence the increase in ASN SYN.

To study the effect of protein inhibitors, puromycin (10 mg/100 gm B.W.) and actinomycin D (200 μg/100 gm B.W.) were injected 1 hour before or 12 hours after a single injection of 50 I.U. of ASNase (Fig. 6). An unexpected, but not without precedence [22], increase in the ASN SYN activity occurred in the animals injected with the protein inhibitors 1 hour before the ASNase injection. Puromycin injected 12 hours after the ASNase did not affect the subsequent increase, whereas actinomycin D inhibited the increase by 20%. Although these are preliminary results using only one level of protein inhibitor, the level used is considered sufficient to block known inducible enzyme systems [21]. It appears, therefore, that protein synthesis is not a requirement for increased ASN SYN activity of liver that follows ASNase treatment.

Discussion

The irreversible changes of ASN SYN during ASN deprivation of the Jensen sarcoma support the conclusion that a nutritional variant, which no longer requires ASN, results from changes in cell population [16] and not by an adaptation of the enzyme. That ASN SYN of the variant population is a reversibly adaptable enzyme, however, was demonstrated by its response to depletion and repletion of ASN in the culture media. The change in enzyme activity, limited to a 2- to 3-fold increase or decrease, was dependent upon the experimental culture conditions. Similarly, ASN SYN of liver showed adaptive changes under experimental conditions designed to create a demand by the host for ASN. Increases in enzyme activity of the liver of up to 12-fold for tumor-bearing animals, 7-fold for animals fed diets devoid of ASN, 3-fold in regenerating liver, and 3-fold following injections of ASNase were observed. The additional 2- to 3-fold increase in enzyme activity observed in the liver of tumor host or animals fed diets devoid of ASN suggests two mechanisms of control of ASN SYN. One mechanism reflects the proliferation of a host tumor, changes in dietary ASN or the demands of regenerating liver, and a second reflecting the indirect effect of ASNase on the tissue.

Gross changes in the animals, organ, or cellular parameters were not observed following injections of ASNase into normal or tumor-bearing animals. The relationship of the decreased valine-^{14}C and thymidine-^{3}H into protein and DNA to the increase in ASN SYN in liver following ASNase is not clear. Inhibition of protein synthesis, however, did not inhibit the increase in ASN SYN and suggests that induction by new enzyme synthesis was not required. An alternative mechanism, feedback inhibition by the product, ASN, is supported by the current data, as well as by other published studies. Such a mechanism has been demonstrated in cell-free systems of tumors [4, 18] and liver [8].

The increased ASN SYN in livers of animals hosting tumors, fed an ASN-free diet, or undergoing regeneration is currently under investigation.

Addendum

Recent results using more frequent injections of actinomycin D (100 µg/100 B.W. at 0 and 6 hours) and puromycin (10 mg/100 g B.W. at 0, 4, and 8 hours) inhibited the increase normally seen in rat liver 12 hours after a single injection of 50 I.U. of L-asparaginase. In light of these observations, induction of new enzyme synthesis by the drug would appear to be a possible explanation for the increase in liver asparagine synthetase activity. The increases noted in Fig. 6 of the text appear to be a "rebound" of synthesis 12 hours after injection of the inhibitors of protein synthesis.

Acknowledgment

The author wishes to acknowledge the excellent technical assistance in these studies of Mr. G. R. Orr, Mr. M. D. Maxwell, Mr. E. Conway, Mrs. H. Johnson, and Mrs. E. Brown, all members of the Nutrition Section of The Noble Foundation. My thanks to Dr. Morris Zimmerman of Merck Sharp & Dohme, Rahway, New Jersey, and Dr. Joseph Hill, Wadley Institutes of Molecular Medicine, Dallas, Texas, for the generous gifts of *E. coli* L-asparaginase.

References

1. Arfin, S. M.: Asparagine synthesis in the chick embryo liver. Biochim. biophys. Acta (Amst.) **136**, 233—244 (1967).
2. Becker, F. F., Broome, J. D.: L-Asparaginase: Inhibition of early mitosis in regenerating rat liver. Science **156**, 1602—1603 (1967).
3. Broome, J. D.: Evidence that the L-asparaginase of guinea pig serum is responsible for its antilymphoma effects. II. Lymphoma 6C3HED cells cultured in a medium devoid of L-asparagine lose their susceptibility to the effects of guinea pig serum *in vivo*. J. exp. Med. **118**, 121—148, (1963).
4. — Studies on the mechanism of tumor inhibition by L-asparaginase. J. exp. Med. **127**, 1055—1072 (1968).
5. — Schwartz, J. H.: Differences in the production of L-asparagine in asparaginase-sensitive and -resistant lymphoma cells. Biochim. biophys. Acta (Amst.) **138**, 637—639 (1967).
6. Dolowy, W. C., Schrek, R., Henson, D., Cornet, J., Brown, E.: Effects of guinea-pig serum on the Walker 256. Nature **218**, 1028—1031 (1968).
7. Hill, J. M., Roberts, J., Loeb, E., Khan, A., MacLellan, A., Hill, R. W.: L-asparaginase therapy for leukemia and other malignant neoplasms. J. Amer. med. Ass. **202**, 882—888 (1967).
8. Holcenberg, J. S.: Guinea pig asparagine synthetase. Biochim. biophys. Acta (Amst.) **185**, 228—238 (1969).
9. Horowitz, B., Madras, B. K., Meister, A., Old, L. J., Boyse, E. A., Stockert, E.: Asparagine synthetase activity of mouse leukemias. Science **160**, 533—535 (1968).
10. Kidd, J. G.: Effects of arsenic azoproteins on mouse lymphoma cells *in vivo* with observations on the effects of other antilymphoma agents, and on the susceptibility of these effects of lymphoma cells of various types. J. exp. Med. **108**, 665—684 (1958).
11. McCoy, T. A., Maxwell, M., Irvine, E., Sartorelli, A. C.: Two nutritional variants of cultured Jensen sarcoma cells. Proc. Soc. exp. Biol. (N. Y.) **100**, 862—865 (1959).
12. — — Kruse, P. F., Jr.: The amino acid requirements of the Jensen sarcoma *in vitro*. Cancer Res. **19**, 591—595 (1959).
13. Neuman, R. E., McCoy, T. A.: The dual requirement of the Walker carcinosarcoma 256 *in vitro* for asparagine and glutamine. Science **124**, 124—125 (1956).

14. Oettgen, H. F., Old, L. J., Boyse, E. A., Campbell, H. A., Philips, F. S., Clarkson, B. D., Tallal, L., Leeper, R. D., Schwartz, M. K., Kim, J. H.: Inhibition of leukemias in man by L-asparaginase. Cancer Res. 27, 2619—2631 (1967).
15. Patterson, M. K., Jr., Conway, E., Whittle, W., McCoy, T. A.: *In vitro* effects of guinea pig serum on the Jensen, JA-1 and JA-2 sarcomas. Proc. Soc. exp. Biol. (N. Y.) 119, 5—9 (1965).
16. — Maxwell, M. D., Conway, E.: Studies on the asparagine requirement of the Jensen sarcoma and the derivation of its nutritional variant. Cancer Res. 29, 296—300 (1969).
17. — Orr, G. R.: L-asparagine biosynthesis by nutritional variants of the Jensen sarcoma. Biochem. biophys. Res. Commun. 26, 228—233 (1967).
18. — — Asparagine biosynthesis by the Novikoff hepatoma. Isolation, purification, property, and mechanism studies of the enzyme system. J. biol. Chem. 243, 376—380 (1968).
19. — — Regeneration, tumor, dietary, and L-asparaginase effects on asparagine biosynthesis in rat liver. Cancer Res. 29, 1179—1183 (1969).
20. Prager, M. D., Bachynsky, N.: Asparagine synthetase in normal and malignant tissues: correlation with tumor sensitivity to asparaginase. Arch. Biochem. 127, 645—654 (1968).
21. Russell, D. H., Snyder, S. H.: Amine synthesis in regenerating rat liver: extremely rapid turnover of ornithine decarboxylase. Mol. Pharmacol. 5, 253—262 (1969).
22. Taylor, E. W.: Control of DNA synthesis in mammalian cells in culture. Exp. Cell Res. 40, 316—332 (1965).

Part II
Preparative Aspects

Isolation and Crystallisation of L-Asparaginase from E. coli

E. Rauenbusch, K. Bauer, W. Kaufmann, and O. Wagner

Biochemical Laboratory, Farbenfabriken Bayer A.G., Wuppertal, Germany

With 5 Figures

In summer of 1967 the first reports of remissions of acute leukemia in patients treated with L-asparaginase extracted from E. coli were published in the USA [9]. But these were only rare cases owing to the scarcity of the pure enzyme. It was therefore necessary to develop a technical process for the production of the enzyme.

According to Mashburn et al. [7] and Roberts et al. [10] the most suitable starting material for the enzyme is the bacterium Escherichia coli. Roberts et al. [10], Campbell et al. [4] and Schwartz et al. [11] showed that there are two types of asparaginase from E. coli which are different in their pH optima of enzyme activity. Only type 2 with optimal activity at neutral pH values is useful in chemotherapy. I should like to mention that we did not notice asparaginase of type 1 in our preparations.

Our test is based on the determination of ammonia which is released from asparagine by the enzyme. In the manual test the ammonia is measured colorimetrically after addition of Nessler's reagent according to the method of Meister [8]. One unit corresponds to one μ mole of NH_3 liberated per minute at 37° C at the pH optimum of 7.2. In the automatic determination with the Technicon Autoanalyzer the old Berthelot-reaction of hypochlorite and phenol with ammonia to indophenol-blue is used [6, 2]. In this case the enzymatic reaction is carried out at pH 5.0 in order to be sure that we are measuring only the type 2 enzyme. The type 1 enzyme has a very low activity at pH 5 [3].

As soon as we had obtained our own enzyme, we realized that it had some unusual properties which we had to consider and which could be partially utilized for the purification procedure.

1. L-asparaginase is very stable in aqueous solution in the pH range from 5 to 9. At room temperature under sterile conditions the enzyme activity is preserved for weeks. At higher temperatures in the range of 60° C the enzyme loses its activity within 1 hour, but can be stabilized by addition of glycine and polyethyleneglycol (Fig. 1).

2. Despite this stability there was some trouble with highly dilute solutions which are necessary for assay purposes. The values were not reproducible and in most cases too low. The reason lies in the adsorption and inactivation of the enzyme on surfaces.

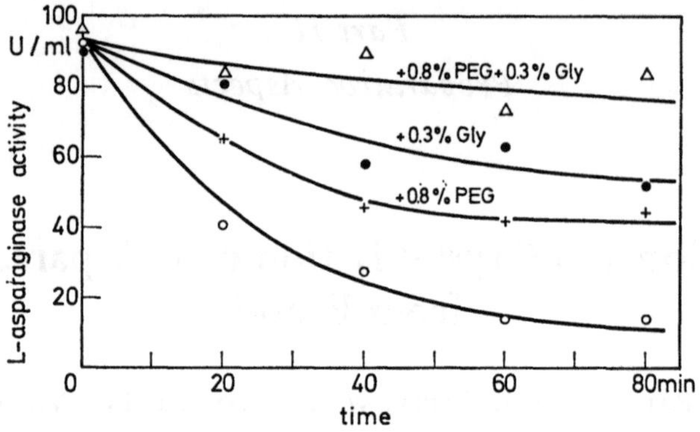

Fig. 1. Stability of L-asparaginase in 0.1 M-Tris-buffer pH 8.0 at 60° C with and without addition of Polyethyleneglycol (PEG) and Glycin (Gly)

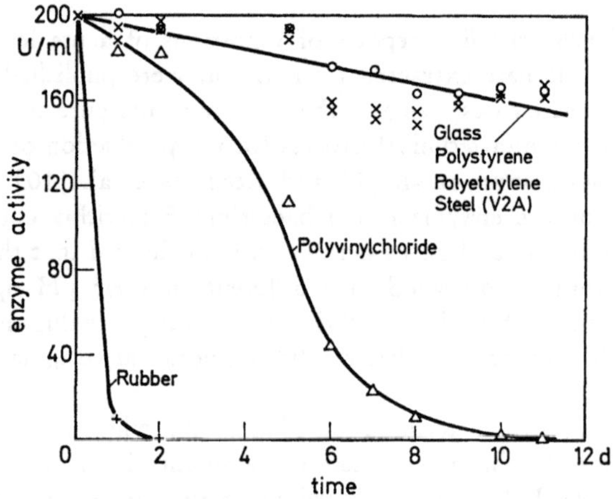

Fig. 2. Stability of L-asparaginase in M/15 Phosphate-buffer pH 7.2, in tubes of different material at 30° C

Table 1. *Inactivation of L-asparaginase in M/15-phosphate-buffer pH 7.2 at room-temperature*

Conditions	Glass beads (g/20 ml solution)	Enzyme activity In buffer (U/ml)	In buffer +0.01% Brij 35 (U/ml)
Solution at start		0.86	1.04
A 1. 1/2 h stirred	10	0.68	0.99
2. 1/2 h shaken	10	< 0.1	0.98
3. + Brij 35 (0,01%)	10	< 0.1	—
B 1. 1/2 h stirred	20	0.45	0.97
2. 1/2 h shaken	20	< 0.1	0.97
3. + Brij 35 (0.01%)	20	< 0.1	—

Fig. 2 shows that rubber is the most destructive surface material whereas glass is one of the least harmful materials. But even glass is not completely free of inactivating properties. If a diluted solution of asparaginase is shaken with glass beads, the activity is lost (Table 1). The addition of a non-ionic surface active agent such as Tween 80 or Brij 35 in concentrations of 0.01% preserves the activity of the enzyme. Therefore we use Brij 35 routinely for our enzyme determinations. Other authors had similar experiences and recommend the addition of gelatine or albumin [5, 13].

Table 2. *Stability of L-asparaginase in the presence of organic solvents*

Solvent	Buffer (0.05 M)	pH	Enzyme activity in % after 20 h at 30° C	68 h at 30° C
20% methanol	tris	8.0	103	97
20% methanol	acetat	5.0	88	98
20% ethanol	tris	8.0	94	93
20% ethanol	acetat	5.0	94	81
50% ethanol	tris	8.0	30	30
50% dioxane-1.4	tris	8.0	81	75
50% tetrahydrofuran	tris	8.0	30	15

L-asparaginase activity at start 35 U/ml

Table 3. *Fractionation of L-asparaginase with acetone*

Fraction	Acetone (%)	Total activity (U)	Specific activity (U/mg protein)		Yield (%)	
1	0—30	430	1.2		1.1	
2	30—35	15,800	63.9	45.5	39.5	71.3
3	35—40	12,700	33.6		31.8	
4	40—45	1,120	1.0		2.8	
5	45—50	170	0.2		0.4	
Original material	—	40,000	10		=100	

Table 4. *Fractionation of L-asparaginase with polyethyleneglycol (PEG) at pH 5.1*

Fraction	PEG (%)	Total activity (MU)	Specific activity (U/mg protein)	Yield (%)
1	0— 6	1.4	69	0.9
2	6— 8	1.1	98	0.7
3	8—12	114.0	232	71.3
4	12—17	6.7	43	4.2
Original material	—	160.0	96	=100.0

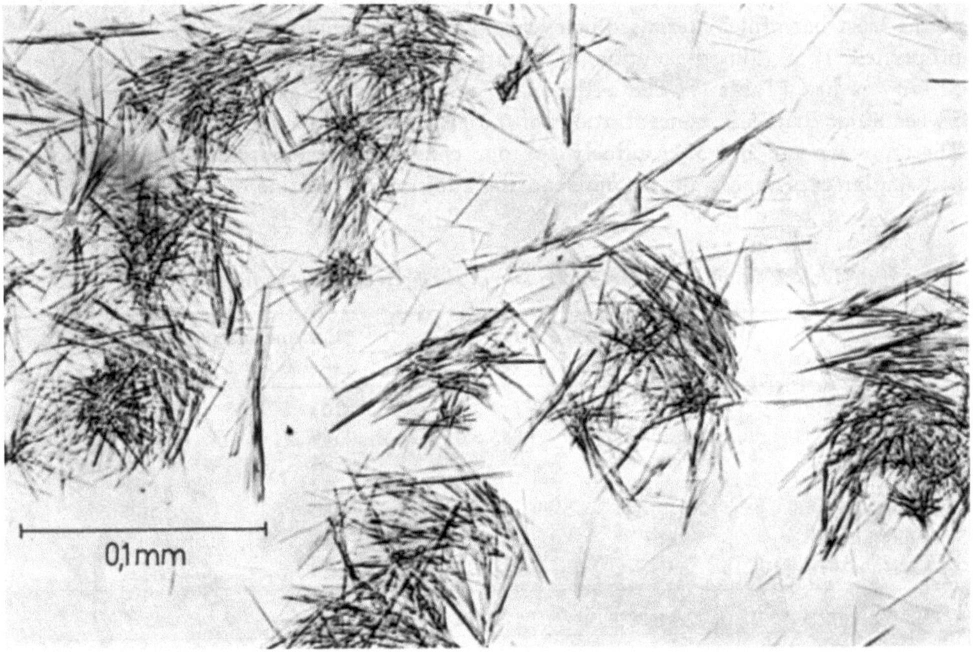

a

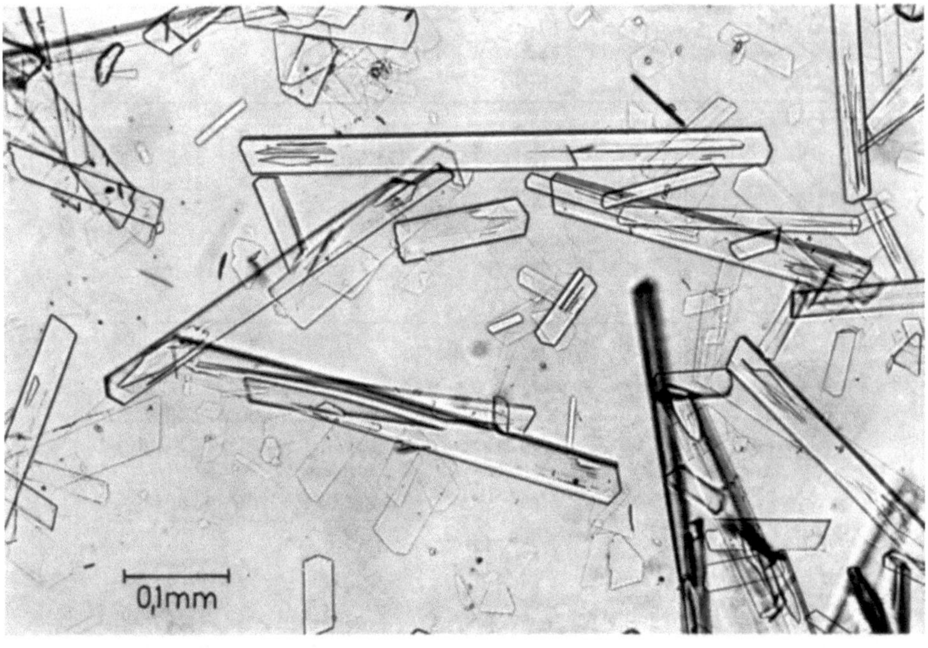

b

Fig. 3 a and b. Crystalls of L-asparaginase A from aequous solutions with polyethyleneglycol

3. The enzyme is relative stable in the presence of organic solvents such as acetone, alcohol and others. For example in a solution with 20% methanol at 30° C the enzyme activity is preserved for at least 3 days (Table 2). This stability is essential for a successful fractionation of asparaginase with organic solvents. Table 3 shows an example for a fractionation with acetone. The rise in specific activity from 8.3 to 44.6 U/mg is 5-fold.

Similar results are obtained by fractionation with 1.4-dioxane, 2-methylpentane-diol-1.4 or polyethyleneglycol. The latter method, which had been used for serum fractionation [1], is especially favourable for the fractionation of rather pure materials at the isoelectric point near pH 5 (Table 4). If a starting material of about 100 U/mg of protein is carefully fractionated with polyethyleneglycol the main fraction reaches a specific activity of about 200 to 230 U/mg of protein with yields of 70 to 80%. When this material is refractionated in the same manner the specific activity rises to 240—260 U/mg of protein [12]. These high specific activities cannot be attained by fractionation with acetone.

The success of the simple fractionation-method was rather surprising. About one year ago when the fractionation was carried out more slowly, a quickly sedimenting precipitate was noticed which, under the microscope, was crystalline. Fig. 3 a shows a relatively quickly fractionated precipitate. By careful processing crystals of about 0.5 mm length can be obtained (Fig. 3 b).

Crystallisation was also achieved in other solvent systems, for example in 1.4-dioxane, 2-methylpentanediol-1.4 or ethanol [3]. The latter process has also been published by scientists of the Eli Lilly company [5].

Production Process

The production of L-asparaginase begins with the fermentation process of the E. coli ATCC 9637 in 30,000 l vessels (Table 5). After about 12 hrs, when growth has finished, the cells which contain the enzyme are harvested by centrifugation and

Table 5. *L-asparaginase-production scheme I*

Process	Total activity (MU)	Specific activity (U/mg protein)	Yield (%)
Fermenter (30,000 l)	200	2	100
↓			
cells			
↓ acetone treatment			
Damaged cells			
↓ extraction with water			
Solution	70	10	35
↓ precipitation with acetone			
Crude asparaginase	50	18	25

suspended in acetone. By this process the cell membrane is damaged and during the following extraction with water L-asparaginase goes into solution. The cell debris are removed by centrifugation and the enzyme is precipitated by the addition of acetone.

The suspension is centrifuged, the precipitate collected, washed with acetone and dried in vacuum. This crude asparaginase preparation has a specific activity of about 20 U/mg protein.

Further purification (Table 6) is achieved by repeated fractionation with polyethyleneglycol. In the last 3 steps the enzyme crystallises spontaneously. The number of the last steps varies from batch to batch because sometimes the desired purity is reached earlier than in other cases. The pure enzyme is again dissolved, glycine is added, the pH adjusted to 7.2 and the preparation is sterilized by filtration. Under aseptic conditions the solution is then filled in flasks and lyophilized. The commercial name of this product is "Crasnitin".

Table 6. *L-asparaginase-production-scheme II*

Fractionation with polyethyleneglycol	Total activity (MU)	Specific activity (U/mg protein)	Yield (%)
Crude asparaginase	250	18	100
1. fract.	200	96	80
↓			
2. fract.	138	180	55
↓			
3. fract. (1. crystallisation)	100	250	40
↓			
4. fract. (2. crystallisation)	75	270	30
↓			
5. fract. (3. crystallisation)	58	275	23
↓			
sterile filtration, lyophilisation			

L-asparaginase was also prepared from other strains of E. coli. The enzyme from the B-strain (ATCC 11303) has a different electrophoretic behaviour from that of the strain ATCC 9637. This will be discussed in the following paper.

Criteria of Purity

1. The main criterion of purity is the specific activity. The purest preparations have a maximal specific activity of about 280 U/mg of protein. The commercial product with 250 to 275 U/mg of protein has 89 to 98% of the maximal specific activity. This does not mean that there are 2 to 11% of contaminating proteins but rather aggregated molecules of asparaginase with a lower specific activity. These aggregated forms are found in all lyophilized or even crystallized preparations.

2. The preparations are further monitored by electrophoresis on acetyl cellulose (Cellogel). Fig. 4 shows an example of the commercial product.

3. In addition, the batches are characterized by immunoelectrophoresis in agarose-gel. Fig. 5 shows that there have been large improvements in the purification procedure but there are still faint lines representing other proteins. Our goal is, of course, to remove even the last traces of impurities.

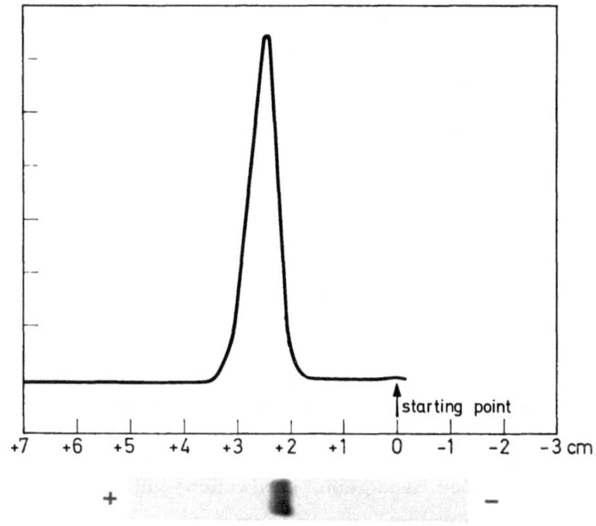

Fig. 4. Electrophoresis of a batch of L-asparaginase A on acetyl cellulose in 0.1 M-veronal-buffer pH 7.82

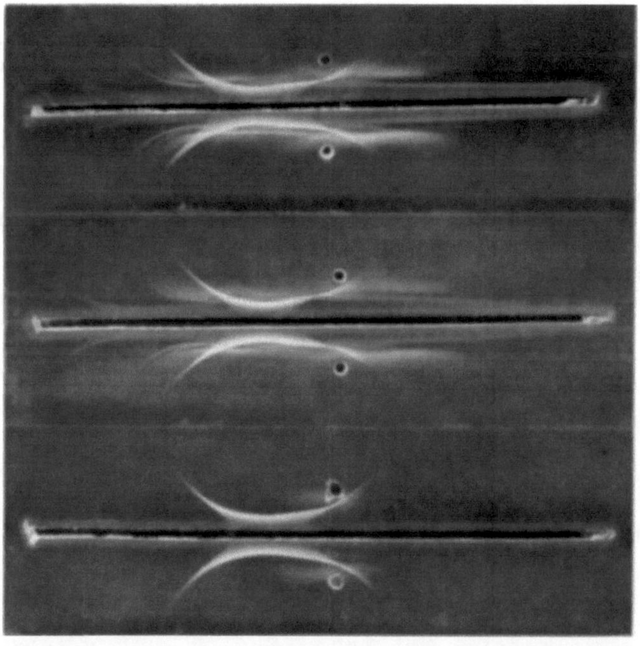

Fig. 5. Immunoelectrophoresis of L-asparaginase. From top to bottom: The electrophoresis of the product after the 1st, 2nd and 3rd crystallisation is shown. 1 µl of a 10% solution of L-asparaginase was used in the upper part and a 20% solution in the lower part of each electrophoresis

4. The pyrogenicity of every batch is tested in rabbits in doses up to 1000 U/kg. According to 'Deutsches Arzneibuch 7' the sum of the squares of the rises in temperature of 8 animals has to be lower than 1.6.

In closing, all members of the team wish to express their thanks to Prof. AUHAGEN for his interest and valuable contributions, and to our technical personnel for their skilful work.

References

1. ALBERTSSON, P.-A.: Partition of cell particles and macromolecules. New York: Wiley and Sons 1960, p. 154—155.
2. ARENS, A.: Private communication 1968.
3. — RAUENBUSCH, E., IRION, E., WAGNER, O., BAUER, K., KAUFMANN, W.: Isolation and properties of L-asparaginases from Escherichia coli. Z. physiol. Chem. **351**, 197—212 (1970).
4. CAMPBELL, H. A., MASHBURN, L. T., BOYSE, E. A., OLD, L. J.: Two L-asparaginases from Escherichia coli. B. Their separation, purification and antitumor activity. Biochemistry **6**, 721—730 (1967).
5. HO, P. P. K., FRANK, B. H., BURCK, PH., JR.: Crystalline L-asparaginase from Escherichia coli. Science **165**, 510—512 (1969).
6. LASH, E. D., SCHWARTZ, M. K.: Automated determination of L-asparaginase. Clin. Chem. **14**, 798 (1968).
7. MASHBURN, L. T., WRISTON, J. C., JR.: Tumor inhibitory effect of L-asparaginase from Escherichia coli. Arch. Biochem. Biophys. **105**, 451—452 (1964).
8. MEISTER, A.: Methods in Enzymology. Eds.: S. P. COLOWICK and N. O. KAPLAN. New York: Academic Press 1955, p. 380—383.
9. OETTGEN, H. F., OLD, L. J., BOYSE, E. A., CAMPBELL, H. A., PHILIPS, F. S., CLARKSON, B. D., TALLAL, L., LEEPER, R. D., SCHWARTZ, M. K., KIM, J. H.: Inhibition of leukemias in man by L-asparaginase. Cancer Res. **27**, 2619—2631 (1967 a).
10. ROBERTS, J., PRAGER, M. D., BACHYNSKY, N.: The antitumor activity of Escherichia coli L-asparaginase. Cancer Res. **26**, 2213—2217 (1966).
11. SCHWARTZ, J. H., REEVES, J. W., BROOME, J. D.: Two L-asparaginases from E. coli and their action against tumors. Proc. nat. Acad. Sci. (Wash.) **56**, 1516—1519 (1966).
12. WAGNER, O., BAUER, K., IRION, E., RAUENBUSCH, E., KAUFMANN, W., ARENS, A.: Polyäthylenglykol zur Anreicherung und Kristallisation von L-asparaginase. Angew. Chem. **81**, 904—905 (1969).
13. YELLIN, T. O., WRISTON, J. C., JR.: Antagonism of purified asparaginase from guinea pig serum toward lymphoma. Science **151**, 998—999 (1966).

Biochemical Characterization of L-Asparaginases from E. coli

E. Irion and A. Arens

Biochemical Laboratory, Farbenfabriken Bayer A.G., Wuppertal, Germany

With 10 Figures

To obtain further information on the properties and structure of L-asparaginase, highly purified, crystalline enzyme preparations were used for the following investigations.

First we noticed a significant difference in the electrophoretic behaviour of the two apparently homogeneous asparaginase preparations A and B (Fig. 1). On cellulose acetate strips (5 hours at pH 7.8), asparaginase B migrated further towards the anode than asparaginase A. The determination of the isoelectric points at an ionic strength of 0.1 gave values of 4.8 for asparaginase B and of 5.0 for asparaginase A [1].

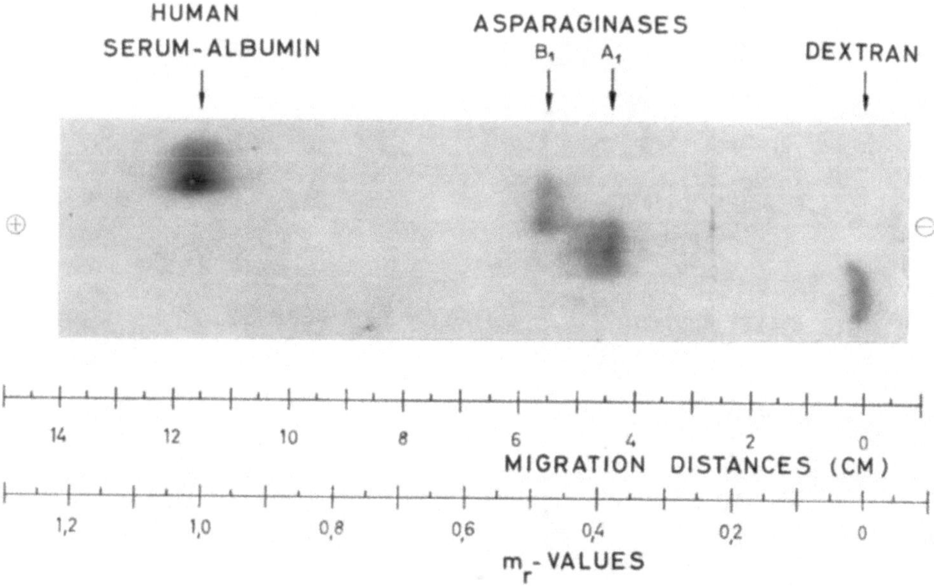

Fig. 1. Relative electrophoretic mobilities of asparaginases A and B

Asparaginase A

A_0	A_1	A_2	A_3	A_4	B_1
3,7	45,1	22,3	20,4	7,5	1,0

Asparaginase B

A_1	A_2	A_3	A_4	B_1	B_2	B_3	B_4
4,1	1,9	4,7	5,3	51,2	26,2	6,0	0,6

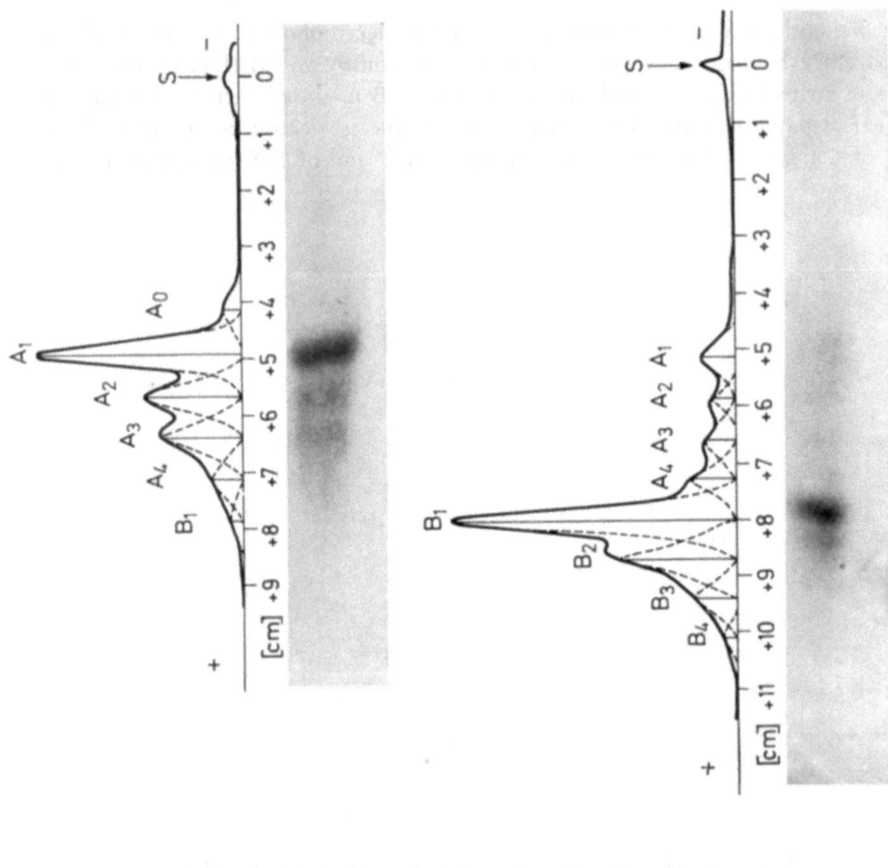

Fig. 2. Prolonged cellulose acetate electrophoresis of asparaginases A and B

Prolonged electrophoresis for 15 hours at pH 7.8, however, resulted in a completely different pattern (Fig. 2). The seemingly single zones separated into several equi-spaced bands, their isoelectric points differed by just 0.05 pH units. Since all these bands had the same specific enzymatic activity we can exclude the presence of inactive, contaminating proteins. The direct comparison shows that both enzyme preparations are composed of several components with the same net charge. Their percentage composition is given beside each electropherogram. If these electrically similar bands consist of chemically identical compounds—and as we will see later we have good reasons to assume this—then we can conclude that asparaginase A contains B components while asparaginase B contains A components (A_1—A_4). Since the isolation and purification procedure was essentially the same for both preparations and these differences were already noticeable in crude preparations, we think that these components are in fact isoenzymes and not artefacts of the isolation procedure. Obviously both E. coli strains produce the same isoenzymes, the only difference is their different distribution. It is evident that asparaginase B in comparison with A is composed of more of the acidic isoenzymes.

The different net charges of the single isoenzymes can be easily explained by a different acid amide content. So far all our analytical data point to this assumption [1], though a final proof has to await individual isoenzyme separation.

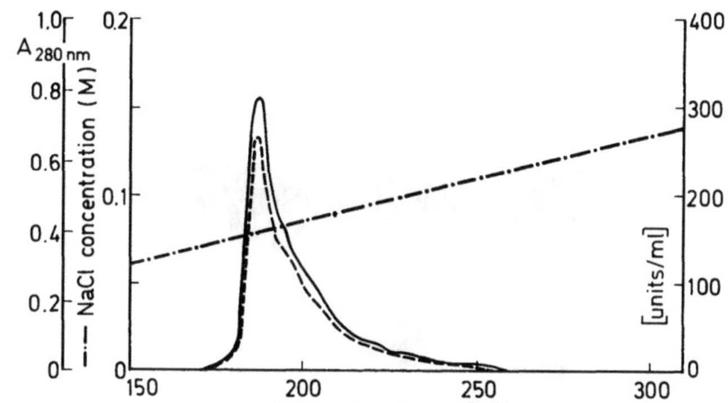

Fig. 3. DEAE-cellulose column chromatography of L-asparaginase A (0.01 M Tris, pH 8.0; NaCl-gradient; column 1.5×90 cm). —— Absorbance at 280 nm; — — — Enzyme activity (units/ml)

Fig. 3 shows the elution pattern of an asparaginase A preparation chromatographed on a DEAE-cellulose column. A beginning separation into the different isoenzymes is indicated by the asymmetric profiles of the protein as well as of the activity curve. However neither variations of the buffer nor of the gradient lead to a complete separation of all these isoenzymes. The most promising results in this respect were obtained by the isoelectric focussing technique. Attempts at preparative isolation using Ampholine carriers with small pH ranges are currently underway.

To determine the molecular weight, the enzyme preparations were chromatographed on Sephadex G 200 columns and thinlayers in comparison with several reference compounds [1]. Fig. 4 shows a typical elution pattern resulting from such a column chromatography. Usually 2 smaller peaks A and B and a main peak C are obtained. Fraction C with more than 80% of the total protein has the highest specific activity and corresponds to a molecular weight of about 120,000. Fractions A and B have considerably lower specific activities and correspond to molecular weights of 240,000 and higher. Dialysis and lyophilization, however, seem to influence this distribution. Rechromatography of the individual peaks shows that the conversion from one fraction to the other is at least partially reversible.

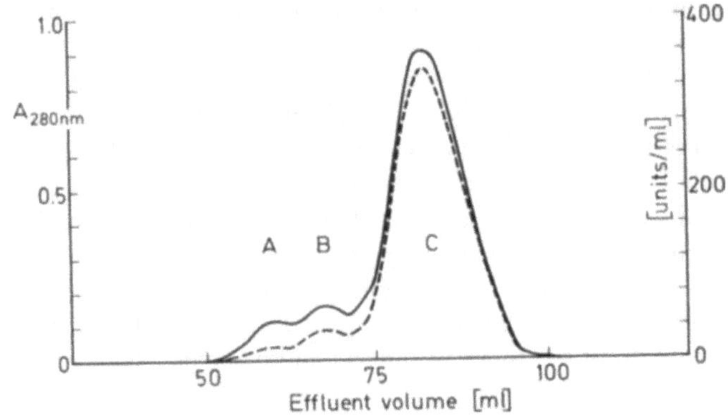

Fig. 4. Sephadex G 200 column chromatography of L-asparaginase A (0.05 M Tris, pH 8.0+0.1 M NaCl+0.01 M glycine; column 1.5×90 cm). —— Absorbance at 280 nm; — — — Enzyme activity (units/ml)

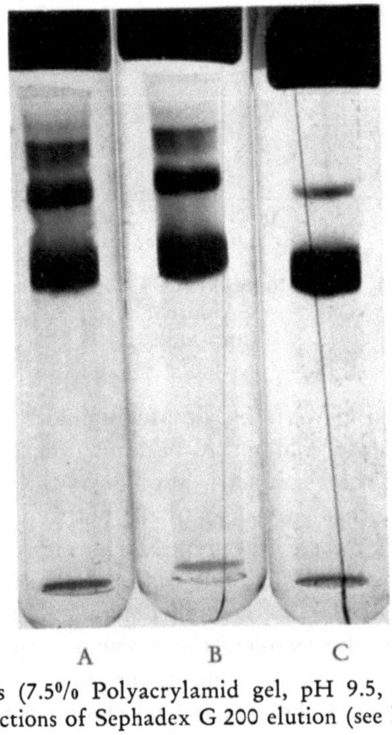

A B C

Fig. 5. Disc-electrophoresis (7.5% Polyacrylamid gel, pH 9.5, coomassie blue). Lyophilized fractions of Sephadex G 200 elution (see Fig. 4)

This fact is also evident from disc-electrophoresis (Fig. 5). The lyophilized fractions of the Sephadex G 200 column show again higher and lower molecular weight components. One therefore can assume aggregation and dissociation equilibria.

Asparaginase in 0.1—1% solution shows, in the ultracentrifuge, a uniform molecular weight of about 127,000 ($S^0_{20\,w} = 7.5$ S) (Fig. 6). At higher and lower protein concentrations more than one peak is observed, whereas in the presence of 8 M urea a single, symmetrical peak with a $S^0_{20\,w}$ value of 1.5 S, corresponding to a molecular weight of about 21,000 is found even at various protein concentrations. No differences were found between asparaginases A and B [2].

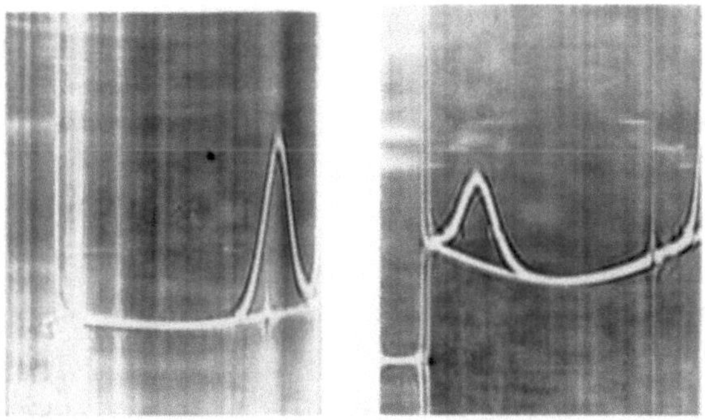

a b

Fig. 6 a and b. Ultracentrifugation of L-asparaginase A. a 1% protein; 0.1 M phosphate buffer, pH 7.4; 20° C; 60,000 rmp; 87 min. b Same conditions as a+8 M urea; 119 min

The amino acid composition of the asparaginases A and B, based on the minimum molecular weight of 21,000, is essentially the same and in good agreement with the values published by WHELAN and WRISTON [3]. Neither carbohydrates nor metals could be detected. The only difference between asparaginases A and B is most likely a different acid amide content, but exact ammonia determinations are unfortunately rather complicated.

H-Leu-Pro-Asn-Ile-Thr-Ile-Leu-Ala-Thr-Gly-(Gly?-Val-Ile-Ala-)---
1 2 3 4 5 6 7 8 8 10 11 12 13 14

Fig. 7. N-terminal amino acid sequence analysis of L-asparaginase A and B (Phenylisothiocyanat-method)

The N-terminal amino acid sequence, shown in Fig. 7, reveals no difference between the primary structures of asparaginase A and B for the first 14 residues. The only N-terminal amino acid is leucine, which suggests that the asparaginase molecule has a single chain structure. At present, however, we cannot exclude the possibility of there beeing other chains having their N-terminal ends blocked. From quantitative end group determinations a molecular weight of about 35,000 is calculated. This result, however, conflicts with the values found by other methods; at present, there is no definite explanation.

Table 1. *Amino acid compositions of L-asparaginases A and B from E. coli*

Amino acid	Asparaginase A	Asparaginase B	Asparaginases A and B		Values in literature [3] in moles amino acid per 22170 g of protein
	Moles amino acid per 21000 g of protein (average or extrapolated)		Nearest integral number of amino acid residues per minimal molecular weight [f]	g Amino acid residues per 100 g of protein [g]	
Lysine	13.02	13.18	13	7.91	14
Histidine	2.02	1.85	2	1.30	2
Ammonia	18.07 [a]	—			—
Arginine	4.79	5.02	5	3.71	6
Aspartic acid	31.00	30.76	31	16.94	30
Threonine	19.68 [a]	19.71 [a]	20	9.60	20
Serine	9.71 [a]	10.04 [a]	10	4.14	10
Glutamic acid	13.01	12.58	13	7.97	14
Proline	8.03	7.88	8	3.69	8
Glycine	17.04	16.96	17	4.61	18
Alanine	19.87	20.13	20	6.75	20
Half cystine	1.00 [c]	1.07 [c]	1	0.48	1
Valine	20.28 [b]	20.47 [b]	20	9.41	20
Methionine	3.27	3.29	3	1.87	4
Isoleucine	7.92 [b]	7.83 [b]	8	4.30	8
Leucine	13.83	13.62	14	7.52	14
Tyrosine	7.06	6.58	7	5.42	8
Phenylalanine	5.10	5.01	5	3.49	6
Tryptophane	1.26 [d] 0.87 [e]	1.20 [d]	1	0.88	2

– means: NH_3-values not determined.

[a] This value is calculated by extrapolation of the semilogarithmic plots of the recoveries of 22, 40 and 70 hours hydrolysates against time to zero time of hydrolysis by the "method of least squares."

[b] Maximal recoveries.

[c] Determined as cysteic acid. Correction was made for 5% loss during the oxidation procedure.

[d] Estimated from the UV-spectrum of an asparaginase solution in 0.1 N NaOH.

[e] Determined in an alkaline hydrolysate.

[f] The minimal molecular weight of asparaginase A is 21062. For calculation one NH_2-, COOH-terminal group and one cysteine residue was assumed. The molecular weight was corrected by subtracting the difference of 0.985 between —OH and —NH_2 for each amide residue.

[g] The amino acid content in % was calculated from the integral numbers of amino acid residues per minimal molecular weight.

The C-terminal amino acid of asparaginase seems to be tyrosine (Fig. 8). Tyrosine is released by carboxypeptidase A in a very rapid reaction. Under these conditions no other amino acids are liberated. Some other variations are currently being studied.

WHELAN and WRISTON [3] found one cysteine residue per molecular weight of 22,000 after reducing the enzyme with dithiothreitol. This value is in good agreement with our value for cysteic acid. With the native enzyme, however, we were not able to detect any free sulfhydryl groups. Furthermore specific sulfhydryl group inhibitors like iodoacetamide, N-ethyl maleimid and p-chloromercuribenzoate did not influence the enzymatic activity.

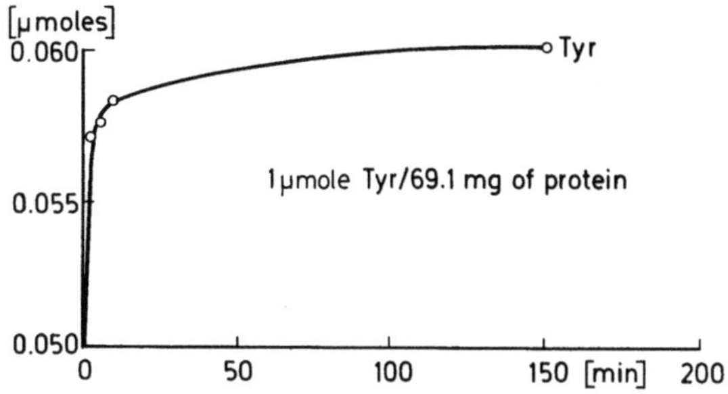

Fig. 8. C-terminal amino acid analysis of L-asparaginase A (carboxypeptidase A, pH 8.5, 30° C, substrate : enzyme = 2800 : 1 w/w)

Of great importance might be the lack of complete substrate specificity of the E. coli asparaginase. As seen in Table 2, various asparaginase preparations exhibit a measurable activity towards L-glutamine. This L-glutaminase activity cannot be separated from L-asparaginase activity. A rather constant percentage between 3 and 4 is obtained for the preparations at all stages of the purification procedure, of the heat inactivation experiments and even for the modified products to be mentioned. These data strongly suggest that the hydrolysis occurs at the same active site of the protein. This conclusion was also drawn by CAMPBELL and MASHBURN [4] from their extensive studies with several asparaginase preparations. Whether this L-glutaminase activity is favorable during the treatment of tumors or disadvantageous because of a reduction of the glutamine level in the body remains an open question.

Table 2. *Substrate specificity of L-asparaginases*

Type of preparation	L-asparaginase Act. (U/mg)	L-glutaminase Act. (U/mg)	L-glutaminase Act. × 100 / L-asparaginase Act.
L-asparaginase A; semipure	160	5.2	3.25
L-asparaginase A; pure	232	7.5	3.23
L-asparaginase A; pH 7.2; 60° C;1 h	223	7.4	3.32
L-asparaginase A; pH 7.2; 60° C; 3 h	144	5.3	3.69
L-asparaginase A; pH 7.2; 60° C; 11 h	92	3.0	3.26
L-asparaginase B	234	8.9	3.81
L-asparaginase X	205	7.2	3.52
L-asparaginase Y_1	242	8.2	3.39
L-asparaginase Y_1	209	8.1	3.88
L-asparaginase Y_1	168	5.6	3.34

Several reasons, for instance the longer in vivo half-life of the more acidic asparaginase B made it interesting to modify the asparaginases by selective and limited chemical reactions. Two examples shall be mentioned briefly. Fig. 9 shows the electrophoretic behaviour of a partially deaminated asparaginase A, the socalled asparaginase X. Analytical investigations [5] showed, that the α-NH_2 group of the N-terminal leucine and one equivalent of the ε-NH_2 groups of the lysine residues are removed. This naturally leads to the more acidic properties of the asparaginase X. No enzymatic activity is lost.

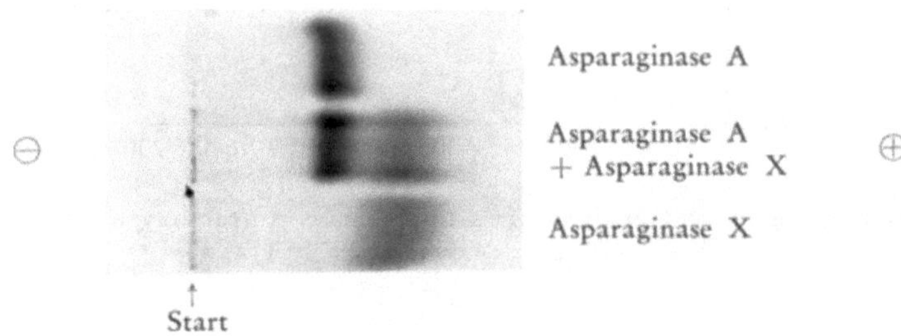

Fig. 9. Cellulose acetate electrophoresis (2 µl of 2% solutions, veronal-Na, pH 8.7, J = 0.05, 3 h 140 V)

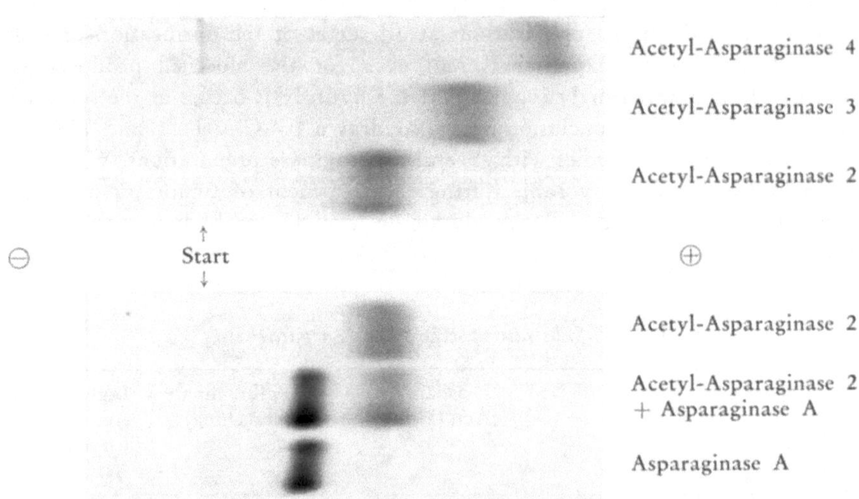

Fig. 10. Cellulose acetate electrophoresis (conditions as in Fig. 9)

Another possibility is given in the acylation reactions. Fig. 10 shows the electrophoretic behaviour of 3 acetylated preparations (asparaginases Y_1) with a different acetylation degree in comparison with asparaginase A as starting material. It is evident, that the acidity increases with an increasing acetylation degree. On the other hand the specific enzymatic activity decreases gradually with the increasing acetylation degree.

With these and other reactions we were able to prepare a large variety of asparaginase derivatives all having still enzymatic activity but different physico-chemical properties.

References

1. Arens, A., Rauenbusch, E., Irion, E., Wagner, O., Bauer, K., Kaufmann, W.: Isolation and properties of L-asparaginases from E. coli. Z. Physiol. Chem. **351**, 197 (1970).
2. Scholtan, W.: Personal communication.
3. Whelan, H. A., Wriston, J. C., Jr.: Purification and properties of asparaginase from E. coli B. Biochemistry **8**, 2386 (1969).
4. Campbell, H. A., Mashburn, L. T.: L-asparaginase EC-2 from E. coli. Some substrate specificity characteristics. Biochemistry **8**, 3768 (1969).
5. Wagner, O., Irion, E., Arens, A., Bauer, K.: Partially deaminated L-asparaginase. Biochem. biophys. Res. Commun. **37**, 383 (1969).

Some Physicochemical Aspects of L-Asparaginase Therapy *

L. T. Mashburn and L. M. Landin

Research Institute of the Hospital for Joint Diseases,
Mount Sinai School of Medicine, New York City 10035, U.S.A.

With 10 Figures

Clinical trials of E. coli asparaginase have been carried out with enzymes supplied by several companies [1—4]. The length of time the enzyme remains in the circulation of the host, is apparently a function of the source of the preparation [5]. In early attempts to detect the difference between two such samples (one from Bayer and one from Squibb), each was subjected to gel filtration on a G-200 Sephadex column. Identical activity patterns were obtained with each sample being divided into two peaks of activity. On disc electrophoresis the activity was separated into three bands which seem to represent a major band of monomer, an intermediate band of dimer, and a small band of trimer at the top of the gel. Each enzyme preparation was also subjected to isoelectric focusing, a procedure which separates compounds through a pH gradient according to their isoelectric point regardless of molecular size. Suprisingly, very different patterns of activity were obtained (Fig. 1).

The Squibb material was focused as a single peak having an isoelectric point at pH 4.97. However, the Bayer sample showed substantial heterogenity of enzyme activity with a shoulder at pH 5.05—5.1, a peak (Peak I) at pH 5.31, another peak (Peak II) at pH 5.47 and a small but very reproducible shoulder/peak at pH 5.6—5.65. The dashed line in this figure and in Fig. 2 represents the glutaminase activity multiplied by 10. Notice that in all cases the pattern of glutaminase activity parallels that of the asparaginase.

Since the Squibb material had a longer half life in patients as well as in the mice which were studied, these results raised several questions. (1) Is one of the several peaks of the Bayer material more stable in the body than the others? (2) Is there an interaction of the patients' serum with the enzyme? and (3) Do samples from other suppliers have the same pattern of activity as either of these preparations or is each preparation distinct as a result of the particular purification process or the substrain of E. coli used.

---

* Supported by National Cancer Institute, Grant Number CA 08765.

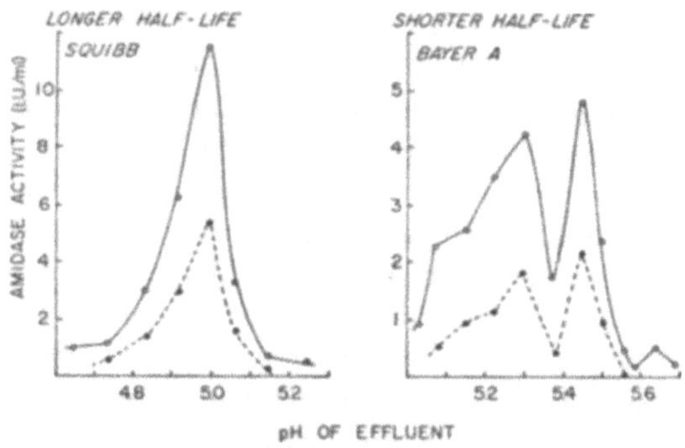

Fig. 1. Isoelectric focusing of L-asparaginase, E-2 from E. R. Squibb and from Farbenfabriken Bayer AG. The electrofocusing procedure was carried out on an Ampholine column (110 ml) according to the instructions provided by LKB Instruments using Carrier Ampholyte of narrow range (pH 3—6 or pH 4—6). One hundred units of enzyme was applied to the column midway in the gradient and focused for 66 hours at 700 volts. Two ml fractions were collected and pH as well as enzyme activities were determined on a suitable aliquot of each fraction. Enzyme assays were carried out in a total volume of 2.0 ml containing 1.0 ml of Tris-HCl buffer (0.05 M, pH 8.6), 0.5 ml substrate solution and 0.5 ml enzyme (aliquot diluted with the same Tris buffer). The pH of the incubation was adjusted to pH 8.6 whenever necessary. The substrate (L-asparagine, L-glutamine, D-asparagine) solutions were each 0.04 M in Tris buffer (0.05 M, pH 8.58). After incubation at 37° for 30 min., the reaction was stopped by addition of 0.2 ml trichloroacetic acid (1.5 M). The liberated ammonia was collected by aeration and evaluated by Nesserlation

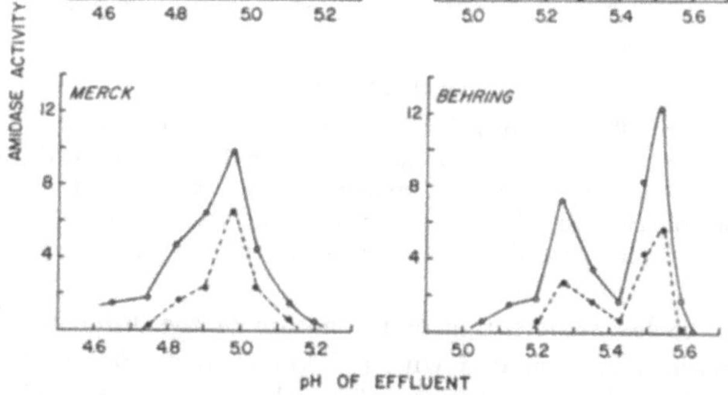

Fig. 2. Isoelectric focusing of L-asparaginase, EC-2 from Tokyo Kyowa Hakko Kogyo, Co. Ltd., Eli Lilly Research Laboratories, Merck, Sharp & Dohme Research Laboratories, and Behring. The procedures used are described in legend to Fig. 1

Starting with the last question first, a number of different samples[1] of asparaginase were surveyed to ascertain the variation of isoelectric focusing patterns. The samples seemed to fall into two groups. One similar to the Squibb preparation and the other more like the Bayer material (Fig. 2). All samples have been normalized for 100 units of activity put on the electrofocusing column so that the degree of stability to the procedure can be evaluated. In all cases, focusing was carried out for 66 hours at 4°. The material from Kyowa Hakko gave a pattern almost identical to that of the Squibb enzyme with the optimum at a slightly higher pH. Whereas the material from Merck seemed to have a shoulder of activity between pH 4.8—4.9 in addition to the peak at pH 4.97. Notice that the patterns obtained with the material from Lilly and that from Behring are similar to that of the Bayer sample in that two peaks of activity with isoelectric points between pH 5.0—5.5 are present. However the isoelectric points of the Lilly asparaginase are slightly more basic than those of the Bayer enzyme. Neither of these (Lilly or Behring) seem to have the first shoulder of activity seen in the pattern from the Bayer sample. The magnitude of that shoulder varied considerably among batches of the Bayer product, however (see Figs. 1 and 3). This variability is apparently a matter of the stability of that peak to the electrofocusing procedure. The recovery of activity of all of these enzymes was from 45—65% with the materials of the shorter half life (Bayer type) always being the lower.

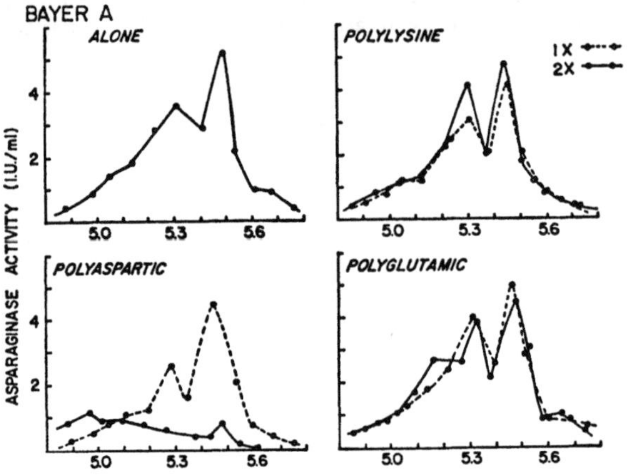

Fig. 3. The effect of Polyamino acids on isoelectrofocusing pattern of L-asparaginase-Bayer A. Samples of Bayer A were preincubated for 1 hr. at 4° with an equal quantity (w/w) o — — — o or two times the amount (w/w) ●———● of polylysine, polyglutamic acid, or polyaspartic acid. Control sample had nothing added (ALONE). Isoelectrofocusing procedures used are described in legend to Fig. 1

In an effort to learn something of the nature of the different peaks of activity, the Bayer material was incubated with polyamino acids for one hour at 4° before subjecting it to electrofocusing (Fig. 3). When the enzyme was preincubated with an

[1] We are indebted to Dr. Chester Stock and Dr. Herbert Oettgen of Sloan Kettering Institute and to Dr. Edward Ginnan of Eli Lilly Co. for the samples used in this study.

equivalent amount (on a weight basis; dashed line) of polylysine, no difference in the pattern of activity was seen. However, when twice that amount (solid line) of polylysine was used, Peak I appears to be more stable to the focusing procedure, although no change in the isoelectric point was observed. Likewise, polyglutamic acid in equal quantity had no effect. However, at the two fold level the shoulder at pH 5.1 is much more evident and therefore, apparently stabilized to the electrofocusing. Polyasparatic acid on the other hand, seemed to render Peak I less stable even at equal weight basis, and when double that amount was incubated with Bayer A before electrofocusing, very little activity was recovered. That which was detected, however, did have a different pattern: Peak I is now at pH 4.95, which is the area of activity of the single peak obtained when L-asparaginase prepared by Squibb, Merck or Kyowa Hakko was subjected to electrofocusing; while the position of Peak II remains the same as before. The loss in activity seen here is apparently the result of polyaspartic acid rendering the enzyme less stable to the electrofocusing procedure since the enzyme, when incubated an equal time (66 hours) at 4° with that amount of polyaspartic acid, retains 95% of its activity. Therefore, apparently, polyaspartic acid can complex with the enzyme in such a way that it is denatured or destroyed when subjected to an electric field while polyglutamic acid could form no such complex.

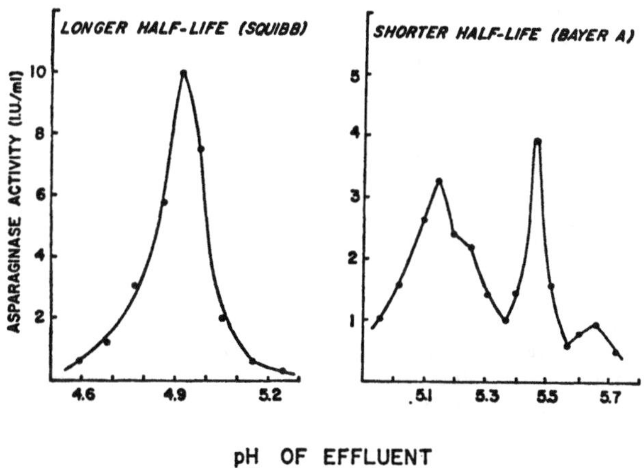

Fig. 4. The effect of preincubation with human serum on the isoelectric focusing pattern of L-asparaginase. Samples of EC-2 from Squibb and from Bayer were preincubated for 1 hour at 37° with fresh human serum (100 units in saline mixed with equal volume serum). The mixture was applied to the column after incubation and electrofocusing was carried out as described in legend of Fig. 1

A sample of each type (again one of Bayer A and one of Squibb) was preincubated for one hour at 37° with fresh human serum to determine if one type of enzyme or one of the peaks of the Bayer material was more stable to serum than another. The question was: Is there anything in serum which will cause a dramatic change? In Fig. 4, the first thing which strikes one is the change in the shape of the pattern obtained with the Bayer material. Although the position of Peak II did not change significantly, the first shoulder, usually seen at pH 5.05 has become a major peak at pH 5.1 and Peak I, usually at 5.32 is now a shoulder at pH 5.2. It seems therefore, that the material in the first shoulder is indeed a peak of activity which is unstable to electrofocusing and has been stabilized to a greater extent than the material in Peak I by the serum.

Since the serum had little or no effect on the position of the enzyme in Peak II, there probably was no interaction of any serum component with the enzyme in that peak. To determine if it would be selectively removed from the circulation of the animal, several mice were injected with a sample of the Bayer preparation. Normal mice were used in this experiment so that the LDH-elevating virus [6, 7] which is present in our tumor-bearing mice could be avoided. Some of these mice were bled (heart puncture) after two hours, the time found necessary to achieve a maximum of the enzyme in the circulation after an intraperitoneal injection, while others were bled 6 hours after injection. The sera collected from these bleedings were subjected to electrofocusing, the patterns of which are shown in Fig. 5.

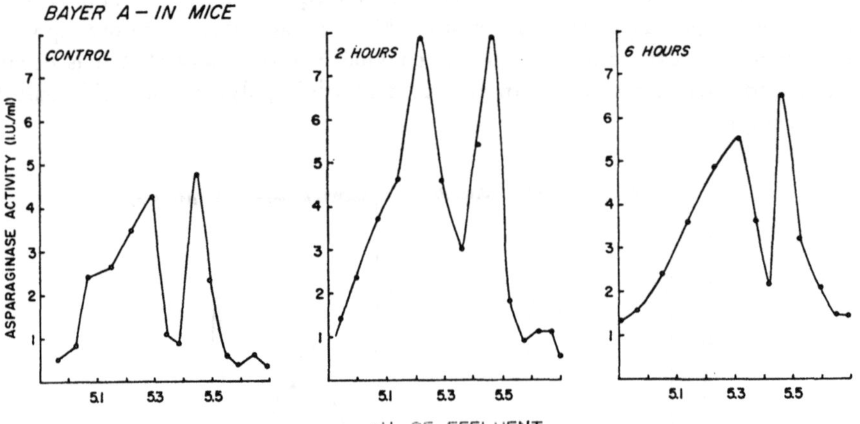

Fig. 5. Isoelectric focusing of asparaginase—Bayer A after circulating in the mouse. Mice were bled (heart puncture) two hours or six hours after intraperitoneal injection of the control Bayer A sample. Electrofocusing was carried out on the mouse sera or on the control enzyme as described in legend of Fig. 1

First, notice how much more stable to electrofocusing these enzymes are after they have been in the mouse. Of course, they are in the mouse serum during electrofocusing. Notice also that the front shoulder is at its usual position (pH 5.05) in the two hour sample, but is obscured in the pattern obtained from the six hour sample. Also in the two hour sample, Peak I moved from pH 5.3 to 5.2, but has returned to pH 5.3 in the six hour sample. All of the peaks are less stable to the procedure in the six hour sample, but it also appears that since Peak II is smaller relative to Peak I than is seen in the two hour sample, it has either become less stable than Peak I or has been selectively removed from the circulation.

In Fig. 6, it can be seen that the asparaginase from Lilly was considerably stabilized to the electrofocusing procedure after it had been in the mouse for ten hours. In this case, the shape of the pattern has not changed much but there has been a slight migration of the material in Peak I to a more acidic position. Also, as was the case with the Bayer material after six hours in the mouse, Peak I appears larger with respect to Peak II.

The isoelectric focusing patterns obtained from a sample of Bayer A which has been chemically modified in the Bayer laboratories, and designated Bayer X, is shown in Fig. 7. The isoelectric point of the principal peak of the control sample is at pH 4.63. A strong shoulder of activity is also present at pH 4.47. The material

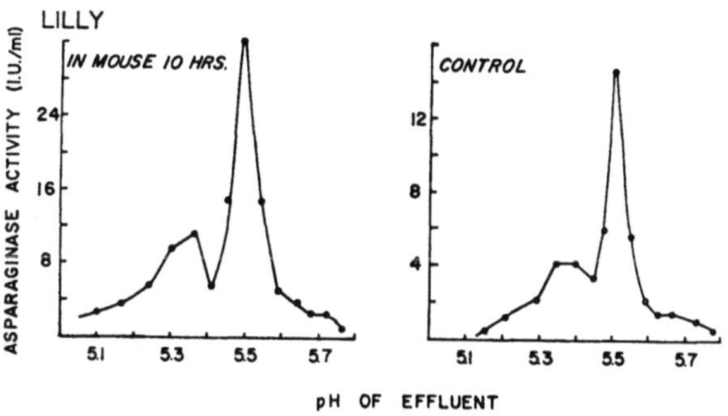

Fig. 6. Isoelectric focusing of asparaginase—Lilly after circulating in the mouse. Mice were bled (heart puncture) ten hours after intraperitoneal injection of the control Lilly sample. Electrofocusing was carried out on the mouse serum or on the control enzyme as described in legend of Fig. 1

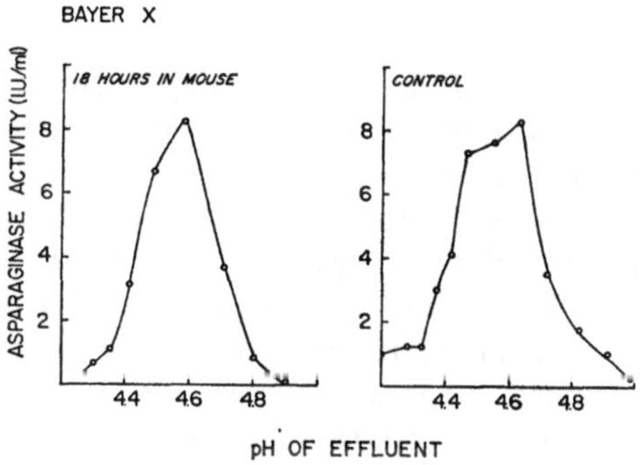

Fig. 7. Isoelectric focusing of asparaginase—Bayer-X (chemically modified Bayer A) after circulating in the mouse. Mice were bled (heart puncture) eighteen hours after intraperitoneal injection of the control Bayer X sample. Electrofocusing was carried out on the mouse serum or the control enzyme as described in legend of Fig. 1

which has been in the mouse for 18 hours, however, no longer has the definite shoulder, although it has retained the activity in the major peak which is now at pH 4.58, a pH slightly more acidic than the position of the control.

A sample of asparaginase from Erwinia carotovora was graciously provided by Dr. H. E. Wade of the Microbiological Research Establishment, England, so that a material from an entirely different source could be compared with materials prepared from E. coli (Fig. 8). The isoelectric points of the control sample are at pH

8.78 and 8.95, and very much more basic than any seen before. After the material had been in the mouse for six hours, Peak II has moved to a more basic position, pH 9.1, while Peak I was apparently only slightly changed at pH 8.8—8.85.

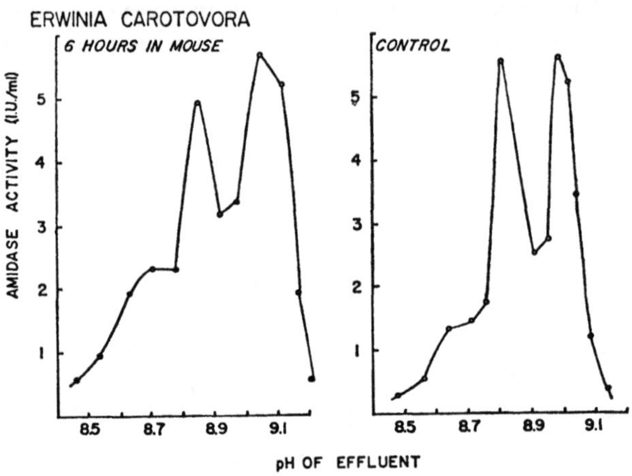

Fig. 8. Isoelectric focusing of asparaginase from Erwinia carotovora after circulating in the mouse. Mice were bled (heart puncture) six hours after intraperitoneal injection of the control Erwinia sample. (Personal communication from Dr. WADE informs us that the control pattern confirms data obtained by Mr. H. K. ROBINSON in his laboratory.) Electrofocusing was carried out on the mouse serum or the control enzyme as described in legend of Fig. 1

The rate of disappearance of the various samples from the circulation of the mouse was measured, since a correlation of isoelectric point to *in vivo* half life was suspected [8]. Normal mice were also used in all of these determinations in order to avoid the LDH-elevating virus. Animals were injected intraperitoneally with the preparation, bled from the tail at the specified intervals, and enzyme levels in the plasma were determined. Fig. 9 shows the data obtained from Bayer A (BA) and Bayer X (BX) plotted on semi-logarithmic paper. The slope of the resulting line represents the rate of enzyme disappearance from the blood. It can be seen that the *in vivo* half life of Bayer X is substantially longer (7.3 hours) than that of Bayer A (2.8 hours).

Figs. 1, 3 and 7, show that the isoelectric points of Bayer A are considerably higher (pH 5.3 and 5.5) than that of Bayer X (pH 4.63). This data supported the hypothesis that the isoelectric point was in some way related to the *in vivo* half life of these asparaginase preparations. The data summarized in Table 1 further supports that conclusion. All of the values in this table except those using the asparaginase from Kyowa Hakko were obtained from mice from a given supplier. We believe that the Kyowa Hakko value for *in vivo* half life is lower than it should be. Notice that the short half life was found with the samples which had an isoelectric point in the range pH 5.3—5.5. On the basis of the theory, the Lilly material was expected to have a slightly shorter half life than the Bayer A, but no significant difference could be detected. The lowest isoelectric point is that of Bayer X which has the longest *in vivo* half life.

The Merck material has a slightly longer half life than does the Squibb enzyme, even though the isoelectric points of the two samples are the same. The Merck sample exhibits an additional shoulder of activity at pH 4.85, however.

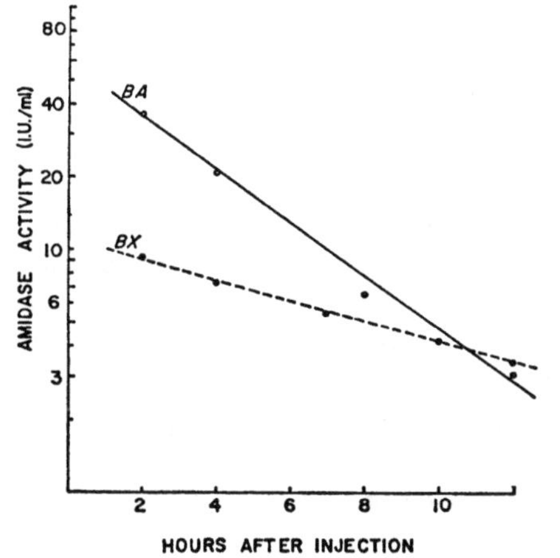

Fig. 9. Rate of disappearance of asparaginase activity from plasma of normal mice (Balb/c female). Mice were injected intraperitoneally with asparaginase—Bayer A (o———o) or with asparaginase—Bayer X (●———●) and bled from the tail vein at the specified intervals. Assays were carried out on aliquots of plasma as described in legend of Fig. 1

Table 1. *Correlation of isoelectric point with rate of disappearance of L-asparaginase from the blood of balb/c mice*

Sample	One-half life (hours)	pH of isoelectric point
Bayer A	2.8	5.32, 5.47
Bayer X	7.3	4.6
Kyowa Hakko	3.4 [a]	5.02
Lilly	2.9	5.39, 5.5
Merck	4.2	4.97
Squibb	4.0	4.97
Erwinia carotovora	4.1	8.79, 8.9

[a] Run in mice from a different supplier and is probably a low value. Note added in proof: The *in vivo* half-life of EC-2 from Kyowa Hakko has now been measured using mice from the same source as was used in the other experiments. The value obtained in those mice is 4.2 hours which is similar to that obtained with samples from Merck and Squibb.

The exception seen here is that of the Erwinia enzyme which should, according to the general correlation of the other samples, have disappeared extremely rapidly from the blood. Apparently, the generalization of the relation of the isoelectric point to the *in vivo* half life of asparaginase is valid only for the samples derived from E. coli; or alternatively, the correlation may be related to the distance of the isoelectric point from neutrality. Thus, the sample of isoelectric point pH 4.97 would be similar to that at pH 8.9: both being about 2 pH units away from neutrality.

We need more samples with an isoelectric point in the basic range to determine this.

Another factor to be considered in the use of asparaginase therapy is the concentration of glutaminase which is unavoidably being administered with the asparaginase. Evidence has recently been published [7] that this activity as well as the D-asparaginase activity is affected by the same enzyme. This glutaminase activity may in fact be the cause of much of the toxicity seen in patients and therefore be the limiting parameter in determining the optimum dosage to be used. All samples of asparaginase which have been investigated in this laboratory have a significant amount of glutaminase activity. Table 2 shows the amount of glutaminase activity given with each 1000 units of asparaginase. The amount of D-asparaginase in each sample is also given for reference. The level of glutaminase activity is between 4—6% of the asparaginase activity. The variation in the ratio of the three activities (L-asparaginase; L-glutaminase; D-asparaginase) of these enzymes indicates that the enzymic site, while similar in each of these asparaginases, is indeed distinct.

Table 2. *Other amidase activities in 1000 I.U. of L-asparaginase*

	L-glutaminase (units)	D-asparaginase (units)
Bayer A	39.5 ± 1.6 [a]	63.6 ± 3.0
Bayer X	40.9 ± 1.8	65.0 ± 2.8
Behring	44.1 ± 2.3	89.9 ± 4.6
Kyowa Hakko	49.6 ± 0.2	93.4 ± 4.2
Lilly	40.3 ± 2.0	76.1 ± 1.9
Merck	55.3 ± 3.0	89.1 ± 5.0
Squibb	49.4 ± 1.6	77.2 ± 2.9
Erwinia carotovora	152.4 ± 7.1	51.2 ± 1.2

[a] Mean ± standard error.

Fig. 10 shows a Lineweaver-Burk plot of the kinetic data obtained with material from Kyowa Hakko. It shows competitive inhibition by both D-asparagine and L-glutamine on the hydrolysis of L-asparagine. This, coupled with the fact that in all E. coli samples studied, the ratios of L-asparaginase activity to L-glutaminase activity and to D-asparaginase activity remain constant in the activity peaks obtained following electrofocusing as well as in the rate of disappearance from the circulation of the mouse [7], makes the serious consideration of this glutaminase activity in therapy compelling.

If one surveys the literature on glutaminase activities, one is struck by the realization that this enzyme is the most efficient for hydrolysis of glutamine under physiological conditions. Therefore, perhaps patients should be supplemented with glutamine between asparaginase injections.

In summary, efforts to detect reasons for some samples of L-asparaginase EC-2 to have shorter half life in patients than other samples of that enzyme have shown a diffuse nature with respect to the isoelectric points. The shorter half life materials contain enzymic species of 3—4 different isoelectric points while those shown to have longer lived circulation are focused as a more homogenous species with an isoelectric point near pH 4.95. The isoelectric point of the longest *in vivo* half life material (Bayer X) so far measured is at pH 4.63, while the shortest half life materials (Bayer A and Lilly) have isoelectric points near pH 5.5. This leads to a conclusion that a low isoelectric point is advantageous for increasing the time the enzyme will remain in the circulation of the patient. Evidence has also been presented that all of the asparaginase samples tested have a significant L-glutaminase activity, affected by the same enzymic site, which must be taken into account when considering asparaginase therapy.

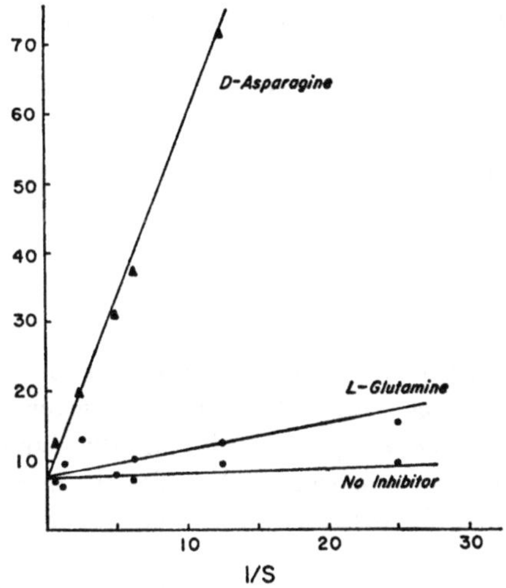

Fig. 10. Lineweaver-Burk Plot of the effect of D-asparagine and L-glutamine on the hydrolysis of L-asparagine. L-asparaginase from Kyowa Hakko (3.2×10^{-4} units) was incubated with varying amounts of ^{14}C-L-asparagine in the presence and absence of inhibitor in a final volume of 0.3 ml for 5 min. at 37°. The reaction was stopped by addition of 50 µl 1.5 M trichloroacetic acid. The entire reaction mixture was applied to a chromatographic column (Beckman Sperical Resin UR-30) with nitrogen pressure and eluted with 0.2 N sodium citrate buffer (19.6 g sodium citrate; 12.3 ml HCl; 5 ml Thiodiglycol; 2 ml detergent-Brig 35/liter) pH 3.22 at a flow rate of 62 ml/hr. Radioactivity in aspartic acid and asparagine was determined in a Packard Tri Carb liquid scintillation counter using BBOT: Naphthalene scintillator solution. Inhibitor added was 7.5 µmoles of L-glutamine or 4.0 µmoles of D-asparagine

References

1. Oettgen, H. F., Old, L. J., Boyse, E. A., Campbell, H. A., Philips, F. S., Clarkson, B. D., Tallal, L., Leeper, R. D., Schwartz, M. K., Kim, J. H.: Cancer Res. **27**, 2619 (1967).
2. Hill, J. M., Roberts, J., Loeb, E., Khan, A., MacLellan, A., Hill, R. W.: J. Amer. med. Ass. **202**, 116 (1967).
3. Tallal, L., Tan, C., Oettgen, H., McCarthy, M., Helson, L., Murphy, L.: Proc. Amer. Ass. Cancer Res. **10**, 364 (1969).
4. Haskell, C. M., Canellos, G. P., Leventhal, B. G., Carbone, P. P., Sperpick, A. A., Hansen, H. H.: Cancer Res. **29**, 974 (1969).
5. Oettgen, H. F., Schalten, K.: Klin. Wschr. **47**, 65 (1969).
6. Riley, V.: Nature **220**, 1245 (1968).
7. Campbell, H. A., Mashburn, L. T.: Biochemistry **8**, 3768 (1969).
8. Mashburn, L. T.: Proc. Amer. Ass. Cancer Res. **10**, 217 (1969).

Part III
Pharmacokinetics

The Distribution and Clearance of L-Asparaginase*

MORTON K. SCHWARTZ

From the Division of Biochemistry, Sloan-Kettering Institute for Cancer Research, New York, New York

With 1 Figure

The role of L-asparaginase in the chemotherapy of cancer and the possible mechanism of action of this enzyme in the control of growth of lymphomatous cells has been the subject of numerous presentations at this symposium. The purpose of this report is to describe an automated method for the assay of L-asparaginase and to present data concerning the distribution and clearance of administered L-asparaginase.

As shown in Equation 1, L-asparaginase catalyzes the hydrolysis of L-asparagine to form aspartate and NH_3. This reaction is not reversible and the synthesis of L-asparagine is mediated by the enzyme asparagine synthetase [1].

$$\text{L-asparagine} \xrightarrow{\text{L-asparaginase}} \text{Aspartic acid} + NH_3 \tag{1}$$

The manual methods for the determination of L-asparaginase activity involve incubation of enzyme and buffered 10 mM L-asparagine for an appropriate period and then measurement of the enzymatically liberated NH_3 by direct Nesslerization or aeration and titration [2]. When clinical trials of L-asparaginase were started at Memorial Hospital in the spring of 1967, it became apparent that it was not possible to perform all of the needed assays by the manual procedure. In order to meet the demands for L-asparaginase assays, a continuous flow automated procedure using an Autoanalyzer was developed [3].

Since Nesslerization does not lend itself to automation, the Berthelot reaction was used to measure liberated NH_3 [4]. The basis of this reaction is shown in Equation 2 and 3.

$$\underset{}{NH_3} + \underset{\text{Hypochlorite}}{HOCl} \longrightarrow \underset{\text{Chloramine}}{NH_2Cl} \tag{2}$$

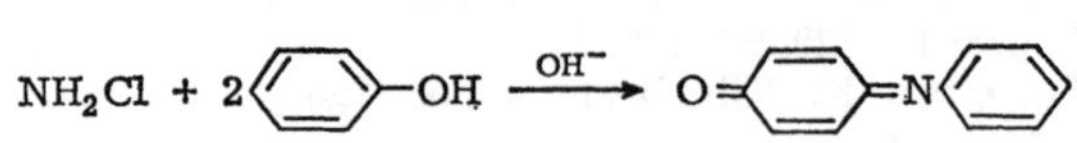

(3)

Phenol Indophenol (blue)

* Supported in part by Grant CA-08748 from the National Cancer Institute, National Institutes of Health and Grant T-431J from the American Cancer Society.

In this reaction NH_3 is reacted with hypochlorite to form chloramine and then with phenol to form an indophenol which in alkaline solution has a blue color. The Autoanalyzer modules, plastic tubes and reagents needed for the assay are listed in Table 1. Sample is aspirated from cups on the sampler turntable at a rate of 60 specimens per hour, mixed with L-asparagine and veronal buffer or buffer alone for the blanks and then passed into a 37° heating bath where the enzyme reaction proceeds. The reaction mixture is interspersed with bubbles of air to segregate the sample and to act as a squegee to clean the system. The final concentration of reactants are

Table 1. *Automated L-asparaginase*

Assay portion	Autoanalyzer modules	Plastic tubes	Reagents
1. Preparation Reaction Mixture	Sampler	a. Sample—0.25 ml/min b. Air—1.20 ml/min c. Buffer—2.00 ml/min d. Substrate—0.80 ml/min	 0.1 M, Veronal, pH 8.6 0.04 M L-asparagine in 0.1 Veronal, pH 8.6
2. Enzyme Incubation	Incubation Bath—37° (Incubation time about 5 min)	—	—
3. Removal of protein	Dialyzer	a. Recipient—2.90 ml/min b. Air—1.60 ml/min	H_2O —
4. Preparation of color reaction	—	a. Hypochlorite—NaOH 1.20 ml/min b. Phenol—1.20 ml/min	1% NaOCl—0.18 N NaOH 2% phenol—0.02% Na nitroferricyanide
5. Color Development	Incubation Bath—60°	—	—
6. Color Detection	a. Colorimeter 550 mμ b. Recorder	a. Waste—2.50 ml/min	—

10.5 mM L-asparagine, 91.8 mM veronal buffer and 0.0815 ml of enzyme sample per ml of reaction mixture. These concentrations are similar to those in the previously used manual method [2], except that it was necessary to change from a borate or tris to a veronal buffer. After incubation for about five minutes, the reaction mixture flows through a dialysis unit, the liberated NH_3 dialyzes into a recipient flowing stream of water and the protein containing solution passes to waste. Alkaline hypochlorite and phenol are then added and the mixture heated at 60° to develop the color and the absorbancy recorded after passage of the solution through a colorimeter equipped with 550 mμ filters. $(NH_4)_2SO_4$ standards ranging from 1.0 μmole to 10 μmole of nitrogen per ml are assayed in a similar fashion. When serum is assayed it is necessary to run a blank with buffer substituted for substrate to correct for the endogenous NH_3. An additional set of standards must be included with the blank run because L-asparagine depresses the color reaction.

The reproductibility of the assay is excellent with a coefficient of variation of less than 3 per cent. The lowest amount of activity that can be measured accurately is 0.03 IU/ml. Activity is expressed as International Units or that amount of enzyme which catalyzes the hydrolysis of 1 μmole of L-asparagine per minute per ml of enzyme sample. Specimens with L-asparaginase activity of 1 unit or less are used undiluted. Those with greater activity are diluted with saline. With the automated method one person can easily assay 100 or more specimens in a day.

During the intravenous administration of L-asparaginase to patients, plasma levels reach plateau values at about the seventh day and then if therapy is stopped gradually fall and no measurable activity is observed dependent on dose and plasma level after 2 to 10 days. The height of the plasma level is a function of both the dose and the source of the E. coli L-asparaginase. In Table 2 is shown a summary of

Table 2. *Maximum Plasma L-asparaginase levels*

		L-asparaginase								
		Bayer			Squibb			Merck		
I.V. Dosage IU/kg/day	Age	No. Pts.	Mean IU/ml	S.D.	No. Pts.	Mean IU/ml	S.D.	No. Pts.	Mean IU/ml	S.D.
10	Child	—	—	—	9	0.40	0.10	—	—	—
	Adult	—	—	—	13	0.37	0.21	—	—	—
200	Child	11	2.7	2.1	21	5.8	2.6	—	—	—
	Adult	19	2.6	1.6	9	5.8	2.5	—	—	—
1000	Child	21	6.5	4.0	5	22.7	3.4	5	14.5	2.2
	Adult	30	8.8	5.4	1	21.8	—	12	26.7	9.8
5000	Child	14	21.6	13.3	—	—	—	12	57.0	18.1
	Adult	8	25.5	8.8	—	—	—	6	70.1	38.9

the plasma levels in the patients receiving L-asparaginase obtained from Squibb Institute for Medical Research[2], Farbenfabrik Bayer, or Merck, Sharpe and Dohme Research Laboratories. The table lists means and standard deviations of the peak plasma value observed during each course of treatment. The bloods were collected just before injection of the next dose and therefore reflect plasma levels 24 hours after the last administered enzyme. There is no significant difference in the blood levels of adults and children given Squibb enzyme. A blood level of 0.40 IU/ml was obtained with a 10 IU/kg dose, 5.8 IU/ml at 200 IU/kg and 22.7 IU/ml at 1000 IU/kg. With the Bayer preparation the blood levels on comparable dosages were $^1/_2$ to $^1/_3$ those seen with the Squibb enzyme. Thus, at the 1000 IU/kg dose in children the mean plasma level with Squibb enzyme was 22.7 IU/ml and the Bayer preparation, 6.5 IU/ml. When Merck E. coli L-asparaginase was introduced, plasma levels were similar or higher than those obtained with the Squibb enzyme. The

[2] The majority of the material from Squibb was kindly supplied under a contract from the Cancer Chemotherapy National Service Center of the National Cancer Institute of the U.S.P.H.S.

highest levels were observed at a dose of 5000 IU/kg/day of Merck preparation. However, there was extreme variation from patient to patient and as seen, the mean level in six adults at the dosage was 70.1 IU/ml with a standard deviation of 38.9 IU/ml. The mean values obtained in the children and adults were not statistically significant.

The reason for differences in plasma levels with different commercial preparations of E. coli L-asparaginase became apparent when half-life studies were carried out. Animal studies had indicated that the half-life of L-asparaginase injected into various animals differed. Thus, in the normal mouse, the half-life was about 6 hours, in the rat about 1.5 hours, in the guinea pig 4.5 hours and in dog about 18 hours. In the patient half-life studies, L-asparaginase was dissolved in a minimal amount of sterile saline and either 200 IU or 1000 IU injected intravenously. Heparinized blood was collected before the administration of enzyme and at 0.5, 1, 1.5, 2, 4, 8, 12, 16, 20, 24, 36, 40 and 48 hours after the injection.

Either a monophasic or a biphasic curve is observed. The presence or absence of the biphasic curve is not necessarily related to dose or the source of the E. coli enzyme. Plasma levels of all preparations at zero time are about the same and are those theoretically expected based on the unitage injected and a plasma volume equal to 5% of body weight. The half-lives are not related to the amount of injected L-asparaginase, but are a function of the enzyme source.

In all five patients receiving 200 IU of Bayer L-asparaginase, a monophasic curve was seen. In four of seven patients receiving 1000 IU/kg a biphasic curve was observed. The longer segment was similar to that of the monophasic curves. The mean value of the long segment for the 12 patients receiving the Bayer preparations was a half-life of 11.2 hours with a standard deviation of 2.7 hours. In three of four patients receiving 200 IU of Merck enzyme a biphasic curve was obtained, and all of the patients receiving 1000 IU/kg of this enzyme had a monophasic curve. The mean value of the long segment half-life of Merck L-asparaginase was 22.6 hours with a standard deviation of 4.7 hours. There was a highly significant difference between the Bayer and Merck enzyme. Half-life studies with Squibb L-asparaginase were conducted in only two patients. In one case the half-life was 22 hours and in the second, 14 hours. Recent studies of the rate of disappearance of crystalline E. coli L-asparaginase prepared by Eli Lilly has indicated a short half life of about 10 to 12 hours. For any of the preparations there appears to be no correlation between half life and therapeutic response.

Some patients have now received several courses of L-asparaginase therapy. In Fig. 1 is shown the plasma levels in a patient with melanoma during a second course of treatment nine months after the first. On a dose of 1000 IU/kg/day of Merck L-asparaginase, the plasma level reached 20 IU/ml. Then, despite continued therapy, the plasma level began to fall and reached 7 units. During the period of fall the patient developed a rash on his ankles and spiked a fever after each administration of enzyme. This fall in L-asparaginase plasma levels, despite continued therapy, presumably represents an immunochemical response and has been observed in a number of patients including 7 of 11 children who received 5000 IU/kg/day. These findings are in keeping with Roberts findings that incubation at 37° for 20 minutes of E. coli L-asparaginase with immune C3H mouse serum decreased enzyme activity up to 50 percent [5].

The mechanism of clearance of L-asparaginase is not known. It is not found in urine of patients with high blood levels. Only a small amount is passed into the cerebrospinal fluid. Assays in bile or lymph have not been made. At dosages less than 5000 IU/kg no measurable activity is found in CSF. In 5 of 7 patients receiving 5000 IU/kg of Bayer enzyme there was no measurable activity. In one patient with a plasma level of 50.2 IU/ml, the CSF activity was 0.23 IU/ml; and in a second patient at a blood level of 15.3 IU/kg, 0.05 IU/ml was measured in the CSF. In four patients receiving 5000 IU/kg Merck enzyme, the blood levels were higher and the CSF activity ranged from 0.05 at a blood level of 15.3 to 0.23 IU/ml at a blood level of 50.2 IU/kg.

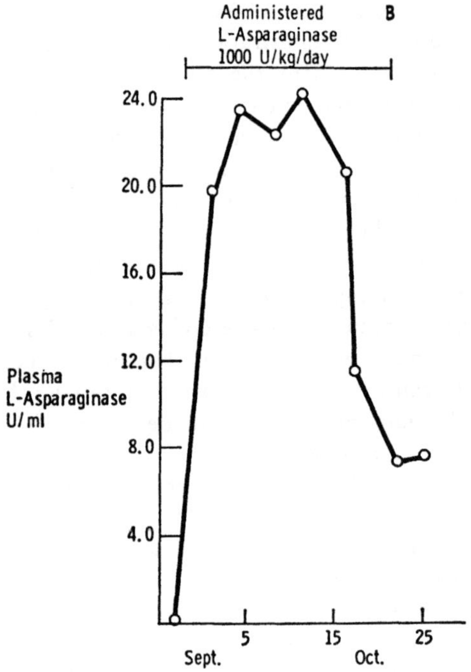

Fig. 1. Plasma L-asparaginase activity in a patient during a second course of L-asparaginase therapy

When enzyme is administered intrathecally there is a rapid clearance of L-asparapinase from the spinal fluid into the blood. When 200 IU was injected into each lateral ventricle of a patient, the CSF activity was 1.5 IU/ml immediately after injection. The next day no activity was measurable in the CSF and the plasma level was 0.5 IU/ml.

We have not found L-asparaginase in erythrocytes or significant increases in post mortem tissues despite substantial plasma levels. L-asparaginase is rapidly absorbed into the blood stream when administered intramuscularly. Plasma levels in a 13 year old receiving 1000 IU/kg intramuscularly at first three times a week, then 1500 IU/kg twice a week and then 3000 IU/kg once a week indicated rapid absorption. The blood specimens for analysis were drawn before the injection and thus represent blood levels 2 days after administration, 3 to 4 days after administration and finally 7 days after the enzyme was given. Even on the 3000 IU/kg/week dose, the plasma level was 0.8 IU/ml. Thus, on all the regimens plasma levels known to produce remissions are maintained.

References

1. Patterson, M. K., Orrand, J. Orr, G.: Biochem. biophys. Res. Commun. **26**, 228 (1967).
2. Meister, A.: Methods in Enzymology, Vol. II. New York: Academic Press 1954, p. 383.
3. Schwartz, M. K., Lash, E. D., Oettgen, H. F., Tomao, F. A.: Cancer **25**, 244 (1970).
4. Berthelot, M. P. E.: Repert. Chim. Appl. **1**, 284 (1859).
5. Roberts, J., Prager, M. O., Bachynsky, N.: Cancer Res. **26**, 2213 (1966).

Pharmacokinetic Behavior of L-Asparaginase in Men and in Animals

J. Pütter

Institute of Experimental Pathology of Farbenfabriken Bayer A.G., Wuppertal-Elberfeld, Germany

With 9 Figures

In modern therapeutic research it is a generally accepted that the knowledge of the qualitative and quantitative effects of a new drug is not sufficient for its characterization, but that as much as possible should be known about its fate in the body—i. e. absorption, blood levels, distribution, elimination, and biotransformation. In the case of Crasnitin [1] this is of special importance because therapy with enzymes is a rather new field of modern medicine, and the experience gained with other drugs may well be worthless with respect to asparaginase (Asnase) therapy. For this reason we made some efforts—like several other investigators [2, 3, 6, 7, 8]—to explore the fate of Asnase in the body, and I shall show in this paper that in our experiments Asnase has indeed some pharmacokinetic properties by which it differs considerably from other drugs.

In each pharmacological investigation we have the problem of whether results obtained in different species can be compared. This question is also important in pharmacokinetics of course. In Fig. 1 the Asnase-activity in the blood-plasma of three different animal species after intravenous injection of 500 IU/kg bodyweight is shown. Asnase activity was measured by incubating the heparinised diluted blood-plasma at pH 7.2 with asparagine (Asn) and by estimating the liberated ammonia by a modified Nessler-reaction. The elimination from the blood followed approximately—but not exactly—first order kinetics. From the calculated value at zero-time it can be concluded that the volume of the blood-plasma is the primary distribution volume. The half-life time (HLT) in the plasma was 23 hours in dogs, 4 hours in rabbits and 90 min in rats. From these results it seems that in smaller animals exogenous Asnase is more rapidly eliminated from the blood. Also smaller dogs eliminate it at a higher rate than big ones; e. g. in the relatively small beagle-dogs we find HLT-values of 14 hours only.

Nevertheless in mice Asnase is eliminated more slowly than in rats. We found a HLT of four hours. But this value is only an approximation because of the irregular elimination kinetics. Furthermore one finds different elimination rates in healthy and tumor-bearing mice, respectively [2, 10]. As Dr. Riley will cover this topic, I will not discuss the pharmacokinetis of Asnase in mice in this paper.

[1] Registered trade mark; Bayer-Leverkusen, Germany.

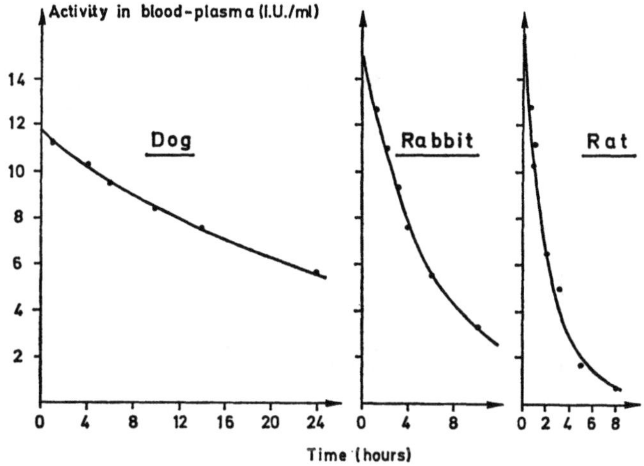

Fig. 1. Activity of Asnase in blood-plasma after i. v. injection of 500 IU of Crasnitin per kg bodyweight into dogs, rabbits, and rats; mean values of seven animals each

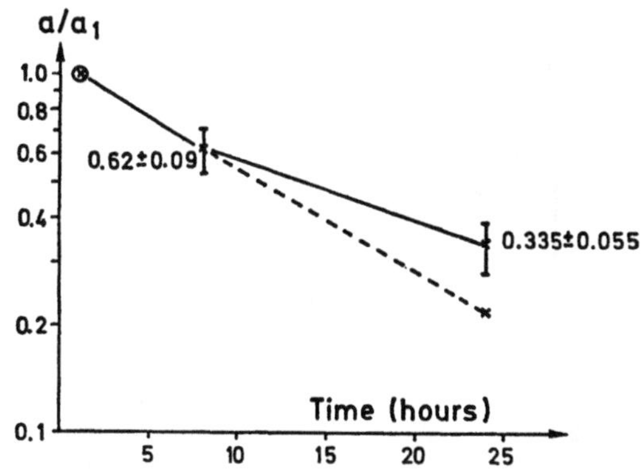

Fig. 2. Plasma-activities (a) of 10 beagle-dogs after i. v. administration of 250 IU/kg. Relative values in comparison to the mean 1 hour-value ($a_1 \equiv 1$). Semilogarithmic plot. Extrapolation of the 8 hours-value by assuming first order kinetics

Fig. 2 shows the kinetics of elimination of injected Crasnitin from the blood-plasma. 10 beagle-dogs were injected with 250 IU/kg. The plasma levels were expressed as relative values in comparison to the average 1 hour-value. The activities found at 1, 8, and 24 hours are plotted against time in a semilogarithmic system; the blood-level for 24 hours was calculated from the 8 hours value by assuming first order kinetics. The difference between the calculated and the experimental blood-levels is significant. Thus the kinetics of elimination do not exactly follow the mathematics of first order reactions. Therefore it is not justified to calculate HLTs of Crasnitin by extrapolation from early elimination rates. Better results are found by logarithmic interpolation between two adjacent experimental values as is demonstrated in the scheme of Fig. 3. By this way we found the HLTs which are referred to in this paper.

Usually we related all values to the 1 hour value because this was the earliest available in most cases.

Among our laboratory animals dogs were those which—as to elimination rate—were most similar to humans. In cooperation with Professor GEHRMANN (Wuppertal-

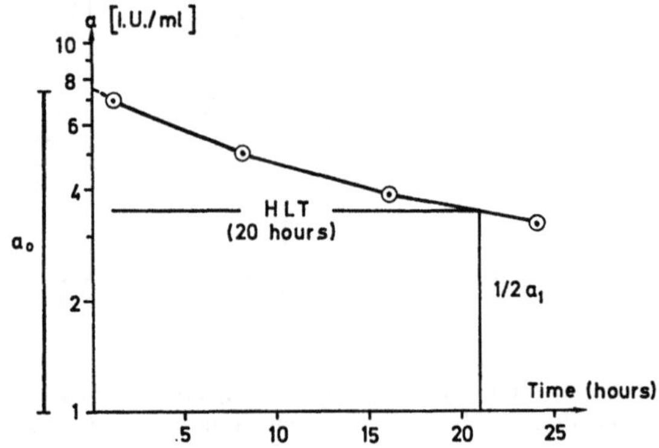

Fig. 3. Scheme for the calculation of half-life time (HLT) by interpolating between two values

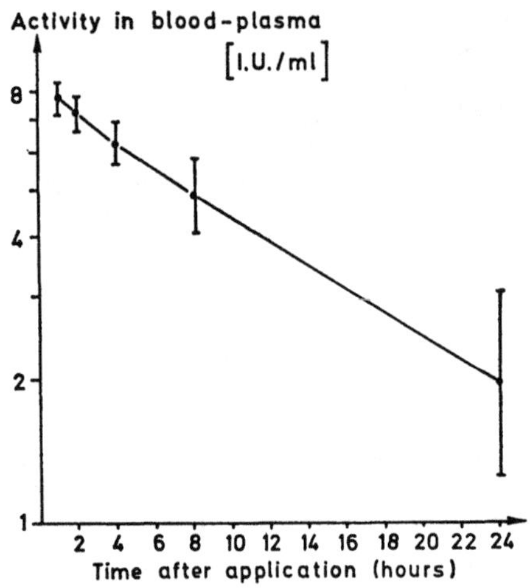

Fig. 4. Activity in human blood-plasma after i. v. injection of 200 IU Crasnitin per kg; geometric mean values from 10 patients; logarithmically calculated standard deviation

Barmen) we determined plasma levels in patients [9]. In Fig. 4 the plasma Asnase levels of 10 humans given 200 IU of Crasnitin (i. e. Asnase A [1]) per kg are plotted semilogarithmically against time. The vertical lines are the logarithmical standard-deviations [9]. The mean HLT is approximately 12 hours, whereas that of beagle-dogs was 14 hours.

With Asnase X [11] we found HLTs of 24 hours in humans [9]; the difference against Crasnitin is highly significant with $p < 0.001$. In contrast to this we found no significant differences in elimination rates of A and X, respectively, in dogs and mice. In humans a further difference between A and X is the cumulation during repeated daily administration; only X gives substantial cumulation (Fig. 5). On each day the differences between A and X determined before every new injection are significant.

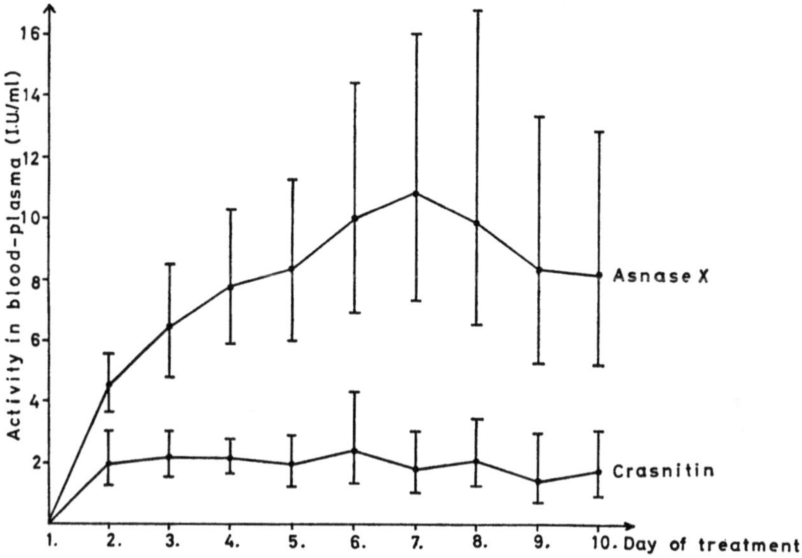

Fig. 5. Activity in blood-plasma (mean levels from 10 patients) in the course of treatment (once daily) with 200 IU/kg of Crasnitin and Asnase X respectively. The activities were determined immediately before each injection

For experimental and clinical purposes it is of interest by what route Asnase may be given. As we had expected it cannot be absorbed from the intestine; in rabbits even high doses of Crasnitin, instilled into a ligated intestinal loop, did not produce measurable blood-levels.

In further experiments rats were given 300 IU of Crasnitin intravenously, intraperitoneally, and intramuscularly. The individual curves are registered in figure 6. The highest and most constant values were always found after i. v. injection. On the other hand, 8 hours after i. p. injection the mean values in blood-plasma were higher than those after intravenous injection. Maximum levels after i. p. injection were reached after 2 hours. The intramuscular injection resulted in very low blood-levels. Also in experiments with rabbits we did not get favourable results by the intramuscular route. Nevertheless it cannot be completely excluded that in humans—by treatment with sufficient high doses—an intramuscular Asnase therapy might be possible.

The blood-levels shown until now only indicated the disappearance of asparaginase from blood. Nothing could be said about the fate of the disappearing enzyme activity. The question of whether all of the enzyme was destroyed without leaving the blood vessels or whether a part of it was distributed through the extracellular fluid remained to be elucidated. In dogs we found one third of the activity of the blood-plasma in the thoracic duct or in the cisterna chyli 24 hours after administration. From this result it can be concluded that Crasnitin can be distributed through the whole extravascular space; that means that Asnase activity must be found in tissues. In order to find reasonable measurable activity we first made a preliminary investigation into the time dependence of asparaginase content of several organs. In Fig. 7 we plotted the activity of Asnase in several organs against the time after i. p. injection of 500 IU/kg into C3H/HEJ-mice [12]. Each point of the graph represents one value from three pooled organs. From these results it was concluded that the highest activity in organs could be found approximately 90 min after the injection and that this time would therefore be the best time for comparing several organs.

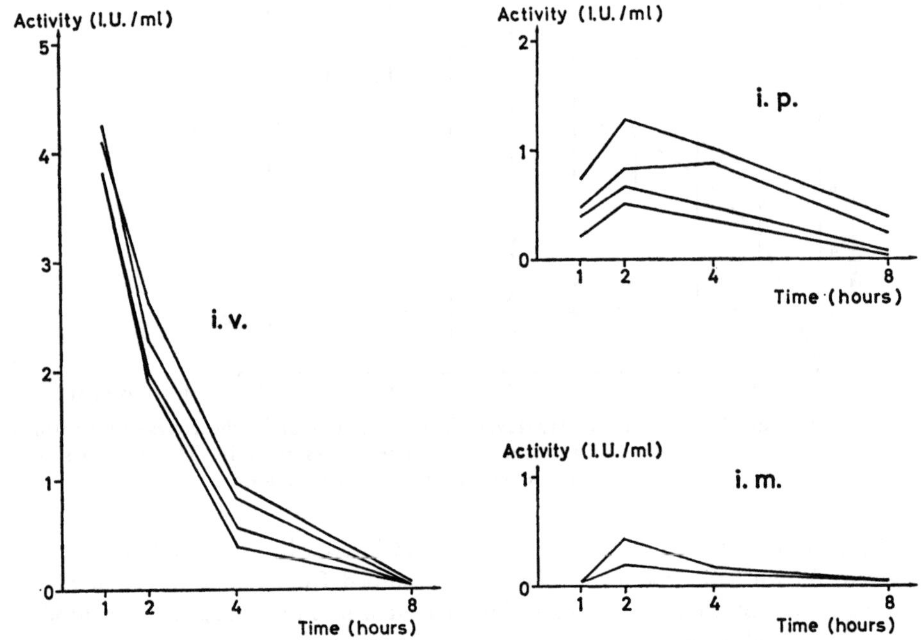

Fig. 6. Blood-levels after intravenous, intraperitoneal, and intramuscular injection of 300 IU of Crasnitin per kg into rats; individual curves

In Table 1 we have registered the content of Asnase in several organs after i. p. injection of 500 IU/kg [12]. We are obliged to Dr. BIERLING for giving us the tumor-bearing mice. In accordance with other authors [2, 4] we found substantial Asnase activity in untreated animals in most of the tissues investigated; these values of endogenous asparaginase were statistically evaluated and subtracted from the whole activity. A second correction was made by measuring the blood content of the organs and by subtracting the Asnase activity of this blood. Table 1 demonstrates that with the exception of the brain we found Asnase in all organs. The absence of Asnase from the brain is due, of course, to the blood-brain barrier. Low activity was found in the skeletal muscle, median activity in tumor and relatively high activitiy in liver, spleen and kidney. Apart from the spleen no great differences between healthy and tumor-bearing animals were detected; but it seems possible that we would find appreciable differences if we determined the Asnase level at later times after application.

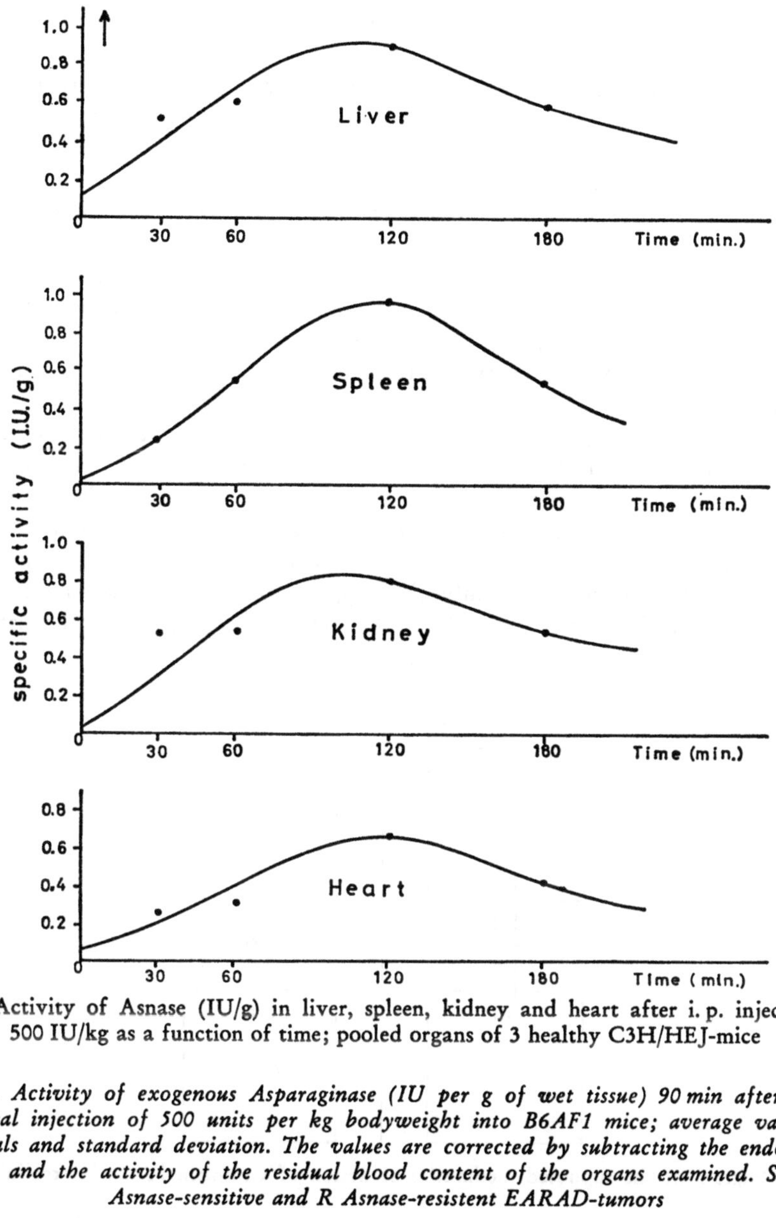

Fig. 7. Activity of Asnase (IU/g) in liver, spleen, kidney and heart after i. p. injection of 500 IU/kg as a function of time; pooled organs of 3 healthy C3H/HEJ-mice

Table 1. *Activity of exogenous Asparaginase (IU per g of wet tissue) 90 min after intraperitoneal injection of 500 units per kg bodyweight into B6AF1 mice; average values of 8 animals and standard deviation. The values are corrected by subtracting the endogenous activity and the activity of the residual blood content of the organs examined. S means Asnase-sensitive and R Asnase-resistent EARAD-tumors*

Animals	Blood-plasma	Liver	Spleen	Kidney	Heart-muscle	Sceletal muscle	Brain	Tumor
Healthy mice	1.74 ±0.57	0.42 ±0.19	0.66 ±0.26	0.45 ±0.23	0.22 ±0.10	0.08 ±0.02	0.02 ±0.02	
EARAD-S mice	3.17 ±0.49	0.45 ±0.14	0.37 ±0.08	0.45 ±0.23	0.22 ±0.1	0.08 ±0.03	—	0.24 ±0.08
EARAD-R mice	2.04 ±0.74	0.43	0.36	0.52	0.28	0.05	0.02 ±0.01	0.19 ±0.07

The difference in Asnase-activity between resistent and sensitive tumors is not significant.

When measuring the activity of exogenous Asnase in the Gardner-lymphoma we found significantly higher values in abdominal metastases of the ascites form (0.6 IU/g) than in the subcutaneously transplanted tumor (0.2 IU/g); probably this difference is the result of a different blood-supply. In the solid Ehrlich tumor we found 0.5 IU/g. Thus it can be concluded that the cause of resistance cannot be not the inaccessibility of a tumor to Asnase.

In other experiments we found well measurable activity of exogenous Asnase in the ascitic fluid of the Gardner lymphoma and of the Ehrlich carcinoma; however we did not find measurable activity in the cells of these ascites tumors. Thus we are sure that Crasnitin is able to exert its effects in the intercellular space, but not in the tumor cells themselves.

From some results of various investigators it can be concluded that the degradation of Asn in the blood-plasma is not the only mechanism of action of Asnase. How for example is it possible that lymphomas which are not Asn-dependent in vitro are Asnase-sensitive? The mechanism suggested in Fig. 8 gives an explanation for this apparent discrepancy. Asnase prevents the interchange of Asn diffusing from one cell into another. In this way not only the supply from outside the tumor tissue is disturbed, but furthermore a part of the Asn which is synthesised in the tissue may be lost.

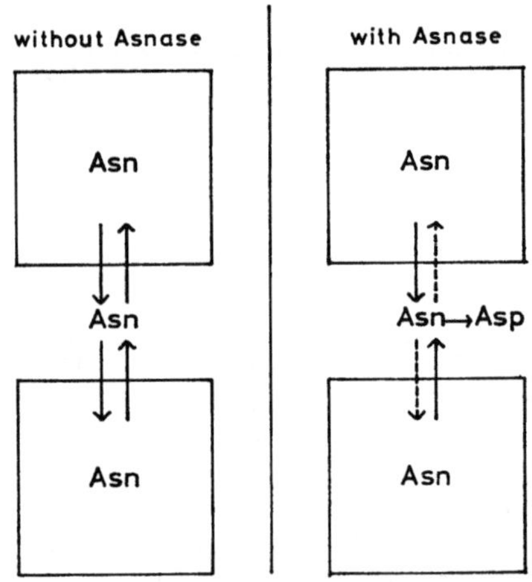

Fig. 8. Diagram of the supposed mechanism of action of Crasnitin in the intercellular space

From the last mentioned experiments we know that the disappearance of Asnase activity from the blood is at least partly due to the emigration of this enzyme into the extravascular fluid. But this cannot be the only route of Asnase elimination; for Crasnitin does not accumulate in the body, and therefore there must be some mechanism of eliminating Asnase from the body as a whole. In the urine of Crasnitin-treated dogs we did not find Asnase; it may be concluded that, if Asnase is excreted, it must be degraded or inactivated before excretion. One possible mechanism that we could find is the proteolytic degradation by kathepsin (Table 2). The kathepsin used was kindly supplied to us by Professor OTTO in Bonn; it is a partially purified extract from beef spleen. The degradation seems to be rather rapid, but it must be noted (see the right column of Table 2) that the addition of human blood-plasma results in a remarkable retardation of this inactivation process.

Table 2. *Influence of 0.17 mg kathepsin (0.0027 BAPNA-Units) on the activity of Crasnitin with and without addition of human plasma; 37° C; pH 6.5; activity expressed as % of the control at zero-time*

Time (min.)	Control	Kathepsin	Kathepsin +Plasma
0	100	100	100
60	100	78	97
120	100	54	95

Table 3. *Half-life times (hours) in 10 beagle-dogs after the 1st and 2nd injection of 300 IU per kg bodyweight in the same animals. The 2nd injection was given 7 days after the 1st injection*

Dog Nr.	1	2	3	4	5	6	7	8	9	10	mean	s. d.
1st inj.	12.3	13.8	15.5	13.5	15.5	13.1	18.5	13.0	13.6	18.0	14.7	±2.0
2nd inj.	10.5	9.3	12.5	—	11.0	13.5	10.2	13.3	11.0	9.0	11.1	±1.6

$p < 0.001$

Finally we have to deal with one additional mechanism of elimination of enzyme activity. The characteristic of this process is that it is accelerated by repeated injections of Crasnitin. In the experiment of Table 3 we gave ten beagle-dogs 300 IU of Crasnitin twice at an interval of 7 days. When Crasnitin was given to the dogs for the second time, the HLT had decreased in almost every animal. In dog 4 we could not determine the HLT because there were no measurable quantities of Asnase in the blood. In the other dogs the effect was not very marked, but nevertheless statistically highly significant. After a third and fourth injection of Crasnitin into the same dogs at an interval of 8 days each we found, one hour after the last injection, not more than one IU/ml in the plasma, that means less then one fifth of the normal blood-level after this dose. Using the gradient plate technique [5], our colleague Dr. LAUENSTEIN found antibodies against Asnase in all of these dogs after the third and fourth injection, but not after the second one. After the last injection the dogs were in a very poor condition and showed vomiting and signs of shock. On the other hand beagledogs which were given high doses of Crasnitin daily for several weeks did not show these allergic symptoms and had normal elimination rates. Based on these results we strongly recommend that Asnase should be given to patients daily without interruption.

For some purposes beagle-dogs have the disadvantage that they react too uniformly. Therefore, in order to find a correlation between blood-levels and antibody formation, we performed a similar experiment with 5 mongrel dogs (Table 4). They were given three times 300 IU of Crasnitin at an interval of 7 days each. Plasma activity was determined one hour and 8 hours after the first and after the last injection. In two of the five dogs the plasma levels were very low after the last injection; the elimination rate, as expressed by the quotient q of the 1 hour value divided by the 8 hours value, was very high. A third dog showed similar, but smaller changes. The two remaining dogs had nearly normal blood-levels and nearly unchanged elimination rates after the third injection. In the blood of these two dogs no antibodies against Asnase (estimated by precipitation techniques) were found whereas the other dogs with an accelerated elimination had antibody titres of one to sixteen, and the antibodies could be identified as directed against asparaginase by means of immunoelectrophoresis.

Table 4. *Effect of repeated administration of Crasnitin (300 IU/kg) on plasma-levels (IU/ml), elimination rate, and antibody-titre in 5 mongrel dogs. Injections were performed on the 1st, 8th, and 15th day. The relative elimination rate q is the quotient of the 1-hour-value divided by the 8-hour-value. Antibody-titre is indicated by the values obtained by the gradient-plate technique*

Weight of the dogs (kg)	Asnase activity in plasma						Antibody-titre 25th day
	1st day			15th day			
	1 h	8 h	q	1 h	8 h	q	
8.4	5.21	3.66	1.42	1.44	0.45	3.2	1 : 16
9.8	4.58	3.42	1.34	3.54	2.26	1.56	∅
14.1	5.00	3.30	1.52	3.27	1.71	1.91	1 : 16
17.9	7.09	4.98	1.42	5.93	3.38	1.75	∅
12.1	4.58	3.32	1.43	1.56	0.39	4.00	1 : 16

A similar experiment with 12 rabbits gave the same result in principle. The rabbits were given 300 IU/kg at an interval from 6 to 8 days. Blood levels were determined 4 and 8 hours after the intravenous injection. In Fig. 9 the decrease in blood-levels in one rabbit is demonstrated as a typical example. Beginning with the fourth injection, a rapid decrease in plasma activity could be observed. Only one rabbit had normal Asnase levels in the blood after the sixth injection. All the other rabbits developed high antibody titres (over 1 : 64) in the course of treatment.

Thus we are certain that the formation of antibodies is associated with an accelerated elimination of Asnase from the blood-plasma [3].

We did not carry out investigations using Asnase labeled with radioactive iodine. But based on enzyme determinations we consider it likely that in the case of Asnase we are dealing with a typical case of "immune-elimination". A decrease of activity based solely on direct blocking of the enzyme by antibodies seems impossible since the plasma of dogs with very low Asnase levels after normal dosage did not exhibit marked inhibition in vitro. We think that the interdependence between antibody-formation and elimination of Asnase is a very important problem and that further work must be done for its final elucidation.

Summing up our results we can establish the following facts:

1. In different species of animals the elimination rates of Crasnitin from the blood-plasma differ widely.
2. The elimination of Asnase from the blood-plasma follows approximately but not exactly first order kinetics.
3. Crasnitin injected into humans was eliminated from the blood with a half-life time (HLT) of 12 hours, whereas the HLT of Asnase X was twice as long.
4. Crasnitin may be injected with favorable results by the intravenous or intraperitoneal routes.
5. Immediately after i. v. injection Crasnitin is distributed only in the blood-plasma. Later it can also be detected in the lymph and in some organs.
6. In healthy and tumor-bearing mice exogenous Asnase could be demonstrated in all organs investigated (including tumor) except for the brain.
7. Endogenous Asnase was found in most of the mouse tissues examined.
8. Intravenously injected Crasnitin could be detected in the fluid but not in the cells of ascites tumors.
9. A katheptic fraction from beef spleen was able to degrade Asnase.
10. After repeated injections of Crasnitin into dogs and rabbits at intervals of several days its elimination is highly accelerated, probably because of antibody formation.

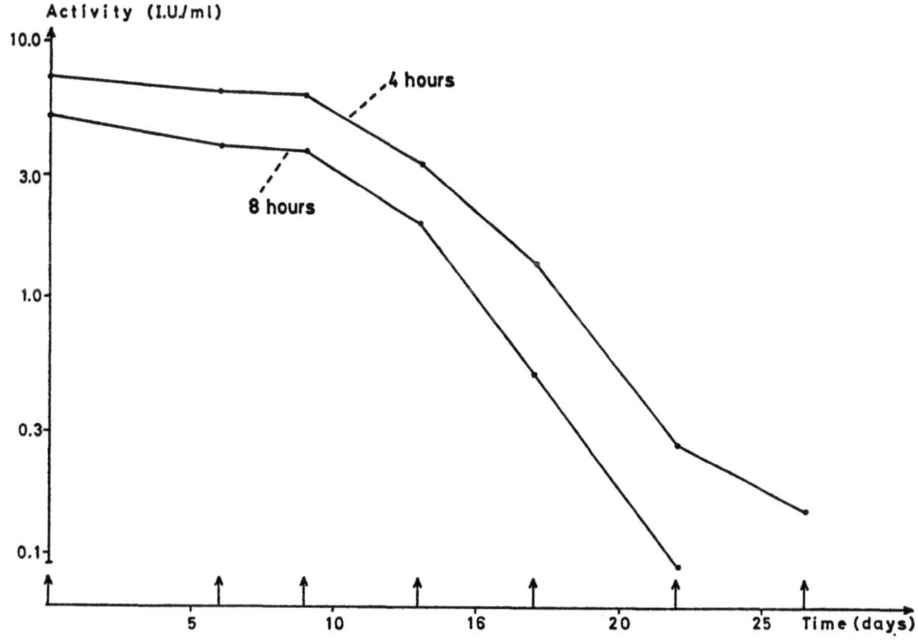

Fig. 9. Decrease in blood-levels in one rabbit (example of 12 rabbits) following repeated injections of Crasnitin (300 IU/kg) in an interval of several days; the injection days are marked by ↑; semilogarithmic plot

References

1. ARENS, A., RAUENBUSCH, E., IRION, E., WAGNER, O., BAUER, K., KAUFMAN, W.: Z. Physiol. Chem. **351**, 197 (1970).
2. BROOME, J. D.: Brit. J. Cancer **22**, 595 (1968).
3. CAPIZZI, R. L., PETERSON, R., COONEY, D. A., CREASEY, W. A., HANDSCHUMACHER, R. E.: Proc. Amer. Ass. Cancer Res. **10**, 12 (1969).
4. CLEMENTI, A.: Arch. intern. Physiol. **19**, 369 (1922).
5. FEINBERG, J. G.: Int. Arch. Allergy **11**, 129 (1957).
6. HANDSCHUMACHER, R. E.: unpublished results.
7. LASH, E. D., SCHWARTZ, M. K.: Clin. Chem. **14**, 798 (1968).
8. OHNUMA, T., HOLLAND, J. F., FREEMAN, A., SINKS, L.: Proc. Amer. Ass. Cancer Res. **10**, 66 (1969).
9. PÜTTER, J., GEHRMANN, G.: Klin. Wschr. **47**, 1324 (1969).
10. RILEY, V.: Proc. Amer. Ass. Cancer Res. **10** (1969), Abstr. 288.
11. WAGNER, O., IRION, E., ARENS, A., BAUER, K.: Biochem. biophys. Res. Commun. **37**, 383 (1969).
12. WIERER, U.: Thesis; Univ. of Erlangen (1970).

The Partitioning of L-Asparaginase between Blood and Lymph

J. G. Hall

Chester Beatty Research Institute, Institute of Cancer Research, Royal Cancer Hospital, Clifton Avenue, Belmont, Sutton, Surrey, England

With 4 Figures

Introduction

Although some details of the precise mode of action of L-asparaginase on malignant cells *in vivo* are unclear it seems reasonable to assume that the asparaginase must penetrate into the micro-environment of the tumor cells if it is have significant effect. Since, even in leukemias, it is likely that many of the tumor cells are in the extravascular compartment and since asparaginase is usually administered intravenously it follows that the ability of the asparaginase molecule to traverse capillary endothelium and gain access to the extravascular compartment may be a limiting factor in the ultimate anti-tumour effect of this enzyme. The purpose of this paper is to consider this problem in terms of what is already known about the extravasation of macro-molecules and also on the basis of experimental results obtained by observing the distribution of various samples of bacterial L-asparaginase in rats and sheep.

General Principles

The high arterial pressure of the mammalian circulatory system forces colloids, crystalloids and water through the permeable capillary walls into the extravascular space. However, when the blood reaches the venular portion of the capillary system the gradient of hydrostatic pressure is less and the colloid osmotic pressure of the blood brings about the reabsorption of some water and crystalloids. Large colloid molecules such as the plasma proteins cannot be reabsorbed and they remain in the tissue spaces and by virtue of their osmotic pressure some water and crystalloids remain with them. Thus the tissue fluid is formed by the excess of filtration over reabsorption. However, this is a continuous process and if oedema is to be prevented the tissue fluid must be drained away by the lymphatic system at a rate proportional to its rate of formation, and returned to the blood via the main lymph trunks. A simple demonstration of the recirculation of plasma proteins can be achieved by injecting radioactively labelled, isologous serum albumen intravenously into an animal in which a chronic lymphatic fistula has been established. The idealized results of such an experiment are shown graphically in Fig. 1. Almost immediately after the injection radioactive protein starts to appear in the lymph and the level of activity in the blood declines as more and more protein leaves the blood and enters the extravascular protein pool and thus the lymph. After a few hours "equilibration" occurs and a steady state is reached so that the specific radio activity of the plasma proteins in the blood and lymph are equal. In absolute terms, of course, there will always be less radioactivity in the lymph than in the blood since the concentration of total protein in the lymph is usually only 20—30% of that of the blood. The exact equilibration time will depend on a number of factors such as the function and degree of activity of the particular capillary bed from which the lymph is derived and the colloid osmotic pressure and arterial pressure of the blood.

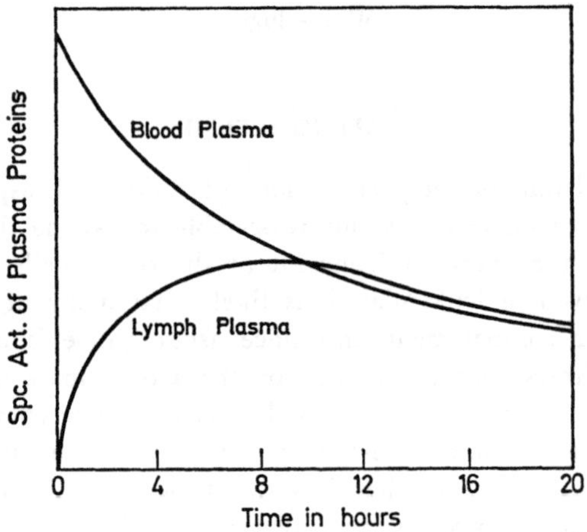

Fig. 1. The idealized results of an experiment in which radioactivity-labelled isologous serum albumin was injected intravenously into an animal in which a lymphatic fistula had been established

Although all fractions of the plasma proteins are present in the lymph they are not present in the same proportions as in the blood plasma. There is no doubt that the molecular size is the most important factor in determining the ease with which a plasma protein will escape through the capillary wall, enter the interstitial fluid and thus the lymph. Thus, the smallest plasma protein molecule, albumen (Mol. wt. approx. 7×10^4), escapes most easily and accounts for a greater percentage of the plasma proteins in lymph than it does in blood [1]. Conversely, the large macroglobulin antibodies (Mol. wt. approx. 10^6) do not leave the blood at all readily and although they account for up to 12% of the globulins in the blood they only account for about 4% of the globulins in lymph, so that the actual concentration of macroglobulins in the interstitial fluid is only about 6% of that in the blood [2]. This is shown graphically in Fig. 2 where the titres of 19 S macroglobulin antibodies in the blood and interstitial fluid (peripheral lymph) measured throughout the course of an immune response in a sheep, are compared.

Of course, such observations relate directly only to plasma proteins, i. e., native protein molecules which are "designed" to exist as circulating entities for long periods of time. Some totally foreign molecules, such as the dextrans, seem to obey roughly the same rules, i. e. they remain as circulating entities for several days after they have been injected and partition between blood and lymph according to their molecular size. However, it cannot be over-emphasized that this does not apply necessarily to all or even most totally foreign molecules. Such material may be cleared rapidly from the blood stream by the phagocytic cells of the reticulo-endothelial system, predominantly in the liver and spleen. Two sets of factors probably contribute to the rapidity of this clearance. The first concerns the antigenicity of the molecule, or in colloquial terms, the strength of its "non-self" marker. The second concerns the physicochemical properties of the molecule; these cannot be defined, as yet, in detail but there seems little doubt that quite subtle differences in electro-

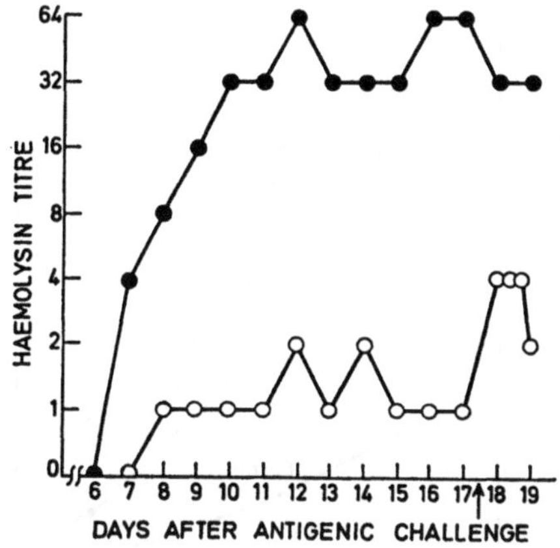

Fig. 2. The titres of 19 S macroglobulin antibodies in the blood plasma (●——●) and peripheral lymph plasma (o——o) of a sheep, following antigenic challenge with goat red-cells. The arrow denotes the time at which inflammation was induced in the area of skin drained by the lymphatic fistula by applying a solution of fluorodinitrobenzene in acetone

static charge and spatial configuration that are not necessarily related to the antigenic determinant, can make protein molecules highly attractive fodder for the phagocytic cells. For example, even mildly denatured isologous serum albumen is rapidly cleared from the circulation by the phagocytic cells of the reticuloendothelium system.

Experimental

In order to determine the behaviour of bacterial L-asparaginase as a circulating molecule it was injected into experimental animals and thereafter serial samples of body fluids were collected and assayed for asparaginase activity.

Preliminary experiments were carried out in rats. Male Wistar rats weighing approx. 200 g received a single intravenous dose of various samples of asparaginase at a modulus of 8000 units/kg BW. The rates of disappearance of asparaginase from the blood are shown graphically in Fig. 3. It can be seen that asparaginase derived from E. coli (Bayer, Eli-Lilly or Squibb) behaved in much the same way. An initial blood level of about 4 units/mg serum protein (i. e. 50—60 units/ml) was attained but this declined rapidly, the circulating half life being about 3 hrs. Asparaginase derived from Erwinia caratovora (M. R. E. Porton), given in the same dose range achieved an initial blood level only half that of the E. coli product and had a circulating half-life of only 1.5 hrs.

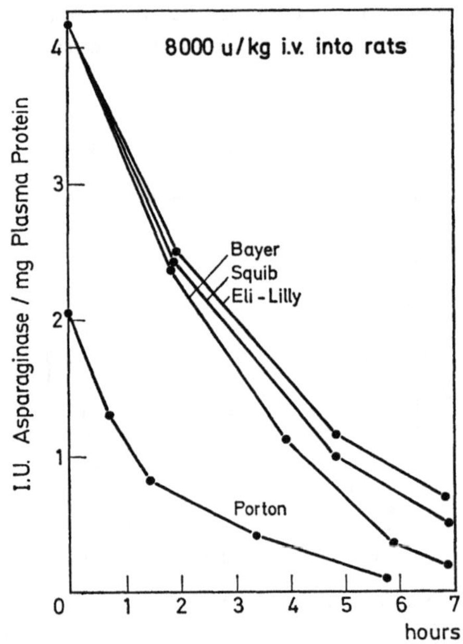

Fig. 3. The rates of fall of asparaginase activity in the blood of rats that had been given a single intravenous dose of bacterial asparaginase from various sources

The ability of bacterial asparaginase to traverse the capillary endothelium and thus enter the lymph was tested by injecting it intravenously into sheep which had a chronic lymphatic fistula in the efferent duct of either the prescapular or prefemoral lymph node. Again, E. coli asparaginase behaved reproducibly whatever the commercial source and the results obtained with the Bayer asparaginase (Fig. 4) are typical. The sheep received a single dose of 12,000 units, intravenously; there were no obvious toxic effects apart from a minor and transient increase in respiration rate. An initial blood plasma value of nearly 12 u/ml was obtained and the circulating half-life of the enzyme was 5 hrs. Asparaginase activity appeared in the first lymph plasma sample which was collected throughout the first 30 min after the intravenous injection. The asparaginase activity reached a maximum level in the lymph of nearly 1 unit/ml (i. e. about 10% of the blood plasma maximum) 2—3 hrs. after the injection and thereafter declined as shown in the graph.

One sheep was tested with asparaginase derived from Erwinia caratovora. Although this sheep was of approximately the same body weight as the others the initial blood level was 9 units/ml, even though a dose of 17,000 units had been given. The circulating half-life of the enzyme was only 2 hrs. i. e. less than half that of the E. coli asparaginase. Furthermore, only traces of enzyme activity appeared in the lymph (less than 0.3 units/ml).

In none of the experiments on sheep were there any significant changes in the lymphocyte counts in the blood or lymph.

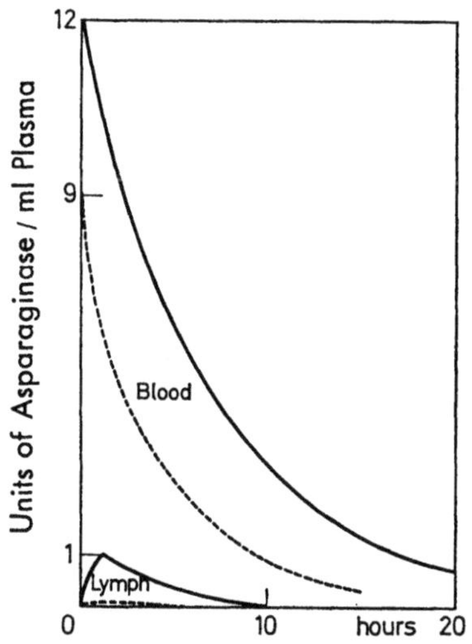

Fig. 4. The results of experiments in which either E. coli (Bayer) or Erwinia caratovora (M.R.E. Porton) asparaginase was injected intravenously into sheep in which the efferent duct of a single lymph node had been cannulated. ——— Bayer 12,000 u.i.v., half-life ≙ 5 hr. – – – – Porton 17,000 u.i.v., half-life ≙ 2 hr.

Conclusion

In both rats and sheep asparaginase from E. coli has a longer circulating half-life than that derived from Erwinia caratovora, but both enzymes were cleared rapidly from the blood and only small amounts appeared in the lymph. It must therefore be concluded that much of the material was removed from the circulation by the reticuloendothelial system. Because of this, a steady-state situation was not achieved and it is thus impossible to comment in detail on the kinetics of the appearance of the enzyme in lymph. However in the case of the E. coli asparaginase it is clear that the enzyme molecule can penetrate capillary endothelium reasonably well and if high blood levels could be maintained a significant amount of the enzyme could be expected to enter the tissue spaces. In this respect the behaviour of asparaginase derived from Erwinia caratovora seems to be different, for in spite of the fact that a comparable blood level was achieved initially only very small amounts appeared in the lymph and there is thus a prima facie case for believing that this type of asparaginase may be less able to traverse capillary endothelium than the E. coli enzyme. This result was not entirely unexpected. Erwinia asparaginase is known to have a tendency to aggregate spontaneously and this property, or associated phenomena, may account for its less "physiological" behaviour.

Acknowledgment

I would like to thank Mr. M. W. WEG of the Chemical Pathology Department, Royal Marsden Hospital, Fulham Road, S.W. 1, for carrying out the asparaginase assays.

References

1. YOFFEY, J. M., COURTICE, F. C.: Lymphatics, Lymph and Lymphoid Tissue. London: Edward Arnold Ltd. 1956.
2. HALL, J. G., SMITH, M. E., EDWARDS, P. A., SHOOTER, K. V.: Immunology 16, 773 (1969).

Critical Influence of an Enzyme-Elevating Virus upon Long-Term Remissions of Mouse Leukemia Following Asparaginase Therapy

Vernon Riley, Darrel H. Spackman, M. A. Fitzmaurice

Department of Microbiology
Pacific Northwest Research Foundation, Seattle, Washington 98104, U.S.A.

With 13 Figures

Introduction

Although the possibility of a carcinolytic virus as a potential therapeutic agent against cancer is not a new concept, the observed beneficial influence of a non-cytopathic, and otherwise benign replicating agent as an adjunct in asparaginase therapy was somewhat unexpected and to our knowledge has no theoretical antecedent. This virus is variously known as the lactate dehydrogenase-elevating virus, the LDH-virus, the enzymes-elevating virus and by other designations [65, 67].

The LDH-virus induces no overt pathology in the mouse host. Its most remarkable feature, which is used as a diagnostic test for its presence and a basis for its quantitative assay, is the induction of a tenfold increase in the level of the host plasma lactate dehydrogenase (LDH). This enzyme elevation has been shown to be the combined result of a twofold impairment in the clearance, or rate of disappearance of the enzyme from the plasma, and of a five-fold increase in the endogenous influx of LDH into the plasma from cellular sources [62, 63, 65, 68, 69]. Other plasma enzymes showing lesser, but similar elevations are: isocitrate dehydrogenase, malate dehydrogenase, glutamic-oxaloacetic-transaminase (aspartate amino-transferase), phosphohexose isomerase, and glutathione reductase [48, 49, 65]. Asparaginase is not elevated in the plasma of mice infected with this virus, except in the case of exogenously administered enzyme which will be discussed later.

The physiological mechanism underlying the therapeutic action of L-asparaginase against some leukemias and tumors appears on the surface to be clear [1, 2, 4, 6—16, 29—31, 38—40, 43, 44, 56, 57, 73—75, 77, 79]. We have utilized the generally accepted and reasonable working hypothesis that asparaginase-sensitive leukemia cells require an extracellular source of asparagine, presumably because of a metabolic defect which lessens the capacity of these cells to synthesize their own asparagine [7—9, 13—15, 19—21, 25—28, 36—38, 43, 47, 53]. It has further been shown that asparaginase-sensitive tumors have a lower rate of asparagine synthesis than do resistant sublines [16], which is consistent with this concept. In further corroboration, a relative deficiency in the enzyme asparagine synthetase has also been found in asparaginase-sensitive leukemia cells when compared with non-sensitive leukemias [34, 35, 57—59, 70, 71].

Impressive remissions have been obtained with sensitive leukemias and lymphomas in mice by the administration of L-asparaginase [5, 19, 42, 43, 44, 51, 60]. These experimental results have led to extensive clinical evaluation of asparaginase therapy in patients with leukemia and other forms of cancer [21, 29, 30, 50, 54]. Unfortunately, the results obtained so far in man have not compared favorably with those realized in the experimental mouse models. The significant discrepancy in therapeutic results observed in mouse and human leukemia has induced us to examine the mechanism of asparaginase action, and more specifically, to investigate the extent and character of the benefits which the LDH-virus appears to provide in conjunction with asparaginase. The following report suggests that the nature of the beneficial influence which the virus mediates is not as simple as was originally assumed [63—66].

Materials and Methods

Tumor

The EARAD-1 asparaginase-sensitive leukemia employed in these experiments was obtained from Dr. L. J. OLD of the Sloan Kettering Institute. Tissue culture passage was utilized to free the tumor of the LDH-virus since tumor cells do not support this virus under *in vitro* conditions [64, 65]. This leukemia may be transplanted in an ascites form by intraperitoneal injections or subcutaneously to yield lymphomatous tumors which can be readily measured. Standard three-dimensional measurements of tumor growth or regressions were made with calipers to provide the tumor volumes reported here.

Mice

Hybrid (C57BL/6$\times$A)F_1 mice were implanted subcutaneously in the hip with tumor cell suspensions in physiological saline containing between 10^5 and 10^6 cells in a 0.1 ml volume. Female mice between 6 and 10 weeks of age, weighing 18 to 22 grams at the time of tumor implantation were generally employed.

Virus

The lactate dehydrogenase-elevating virus (LDH-virus) was administered intraperitoneally to appropriate experimental groups, usually three days prior to asparaginase administration. A 1 to 100 dilution of pooled mouse plasma having an original titer of $10^{10}ID_{50}$ infectious units was used [65].

Asparaginase

Commercially prepared (Squibb) Escherichia coli (EC-2) L-asparaginase (L-asparagine amido hydrolase) having approximately 300 International Units per mg of protein was injected intraperitoneally (i. p.) in a 0.2 ml volume of saline solution per 20 grams of mouse body weight [17, 18, 32, 44]. Asparaginase concentrations were determined by standard methods [18, 45].

Blood Sampling Techniques

Inasmuch as the circulating amino acid pool *in vivo* represents a host equilibrium between influx, clearance, enzymic alterations, and perhaps other physiological events, it is apparent that losses of certain amino acids will occur in blood removed from the host if the samples are not obtained, processed, and stored under conditions designed specifically to prevent such losses. Rapid changes would be expected to occur in asparagine concentration following the administration of asparaginase, which has a specific effect on this amino acid. Appropriate sampling procedures have therefore been employed to minimize amino acid alterations during bleeding and the processing of plasma samples for amino acid analysis.

Essential principles of these procedures include keeping the blood samples cold during processing, reducing sample preparation time to a minimum, and precipitation of plasma proteins, including all enzymes, as rapidly as possible after the withdrawal of the blood sample.

Blood samples of about 0.2 ml per mouse were removed by the orbital bleeding technique [61] using pre-chilled, disposable, heparinized bleeding tubes. The actual bleeding procedure requires only a few seconds; the tubes are then quickly stoppered and plunged into an ice bath, chilling the blood immediately to 0° C. The blood samples are centrifuged at 0° C, and the cold plasmas are transferred directly into pre-weighed, disposable tubes containing the protein precipitating agent which inactivates all enzyme activity and stabilizes the amino acid pattern.

Amino Acid Determinations

Amino acid assays were carried out on a Beckman Model 120B amino acid analyzer modified to provide accelerated, semi-automatic runs. Recently revised and improved methods of analysis [76] were employed using sodium citrate buffers for the basic amino acids and lithium citrate buffers for the acidic and neutral amino acids [3]. The latter buffer system is essential for the satisfactory separation of asparagine, glutamic acid and glutamine.

Results

Asparaginase Clearance: Influence of the LDH-Virus

An apparent basis for this viral adjunct to drug therapy is illustrated by Fig. 1. These data demonstrate the differential rates of disappearance of an exogenous dose of EC-2 L-asparaginase from the blood of normal mice, compared with those either acutely or chronically infected with the LDH-virus [66]. The clearance rates shown are equivalent to an asparaginase half-life ($T_{1/2}$) of about four hours for normal mice and 25 hours for mice infected with the LDH-virus. It may be noted from the two upper super-imposed enzyme disappearance curves of Fig. 1 that the experimental results were similar for both acutely and chronically infected mice. The former had carried the virus for 18 hours, while the chronically infected mice had been inoculated with authentic LDH-virus 55 days prior to asparaginase administration. The minimum time, following infection, for inducing host clearance impairment is relevant in understanding the paradoxical observations reported by others of seeming differences in asparaginase action against newly implanted tumors treated with asparaginase one hour following implantation, as compared with the surprisingly better therapeutic effects against established 7-day-old tumors [5, 42, 55, 66]. The LDH-virus must be present in the host for a minimum of about 12 hours before it induces the beneficial drug clearance impairment [65].

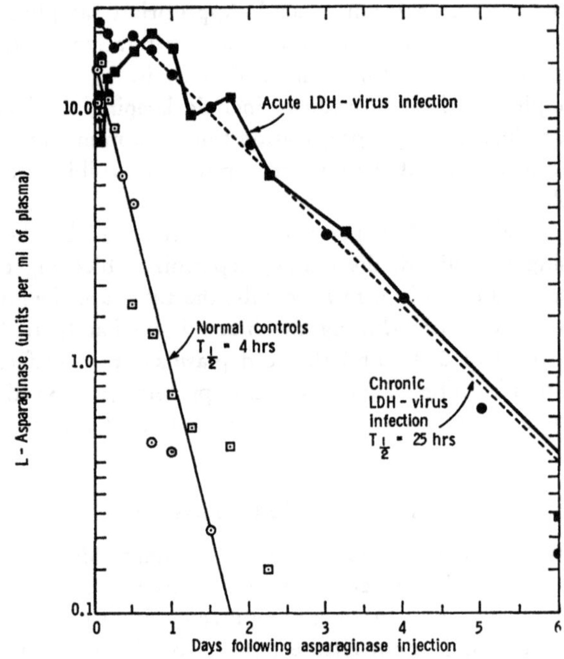

Fig. 1. Comparison of EC-2 L-asparaginase disappearance or clearance in normal mice with that of mice infected with the LDH-elevating virus

Presence of the LDH-Virus in Tumor-bearing Mice

It is now reasonably certain that the LDH-virus was present, but not recognized in most, and probably all, of the transplanted mouse tumors employed in the early, as well as the current, asparaginase experimental models. A summary of the LDH-virus status of various mouse leukemias and related tumors employed by investigators for asparaginase therapy studies is shown in Table 1. Although the majority of the tumors listed here were obtained through the cooperation of colleagues at the Sloan Kettering Institute, it has been established through separate studies, both by us and other investigators, that this virus is present in most transplanted mouse tumors in widely separated laboratories [49]. Over 50 neoplastic varieties have been shown to carry the infection [65]. Particularly pertinent to asparaginase studies is the LDH-virus status of the various EARAD tumors, and the Gardner 6C3HED lymphosarcoma [33, 37]. The experimental leukemias, EL-4, ERLD, K-36, P1534, P1798 and L1210 have all exhibited the presence of the virus. The LDH-virus was also shown to be present in the non-asparaginase-sensitive Friend and Rauscher leukemias when tested at various times between 1961 and 1969.

Table 1. *Assay of normal and tumor-bearing mice for plasma LDH levels and for the presence or absence of the LDH-elevating virus*

Mice and tumors tested	Mouse strain	Plasma LDH values	LDH-virus (PIT) [c]
Normal mice	BAF_1 [b]	300 to 400	(—)
EARAD-1	BAF_1	4,000 to 95,000	(+)
EARAD-1 (resistant)	BAF_1	229,000	(+)
EL-4	C57BL/6	19,900	(+)
ERLD	C57BL/6	58,400	(+)
K-36	BKF_1 [b]	28,700	(+)
RAD Al	A	6,700	(+)
ASL1 (from bank) [a]	A	66,000 to 70,000	(+)
EARAD-1 (tissue culture)	BAF_1	11,000 to 37,200	(—)
Gardner 6C3HED	C3H	Elevated	(+)
P1534 Leukemia	DBA/2	Elevated	(+)
P1798 Leukemia	Balb/C	Elevated	(+)

[a] Deep-frozen tumor bank storage.
[b] $BAF_1 = (C57BL/6 \times A)F_1$; $BKF_1 = (C57ML/6 \times AKR)F_1$.
[c] PIT: Plasma infectivity test for LDH-virus.

The plasma LDH values of the leukemia-bearing hosts, shown in Table 1, all exhibit a typical virus-tumor synergistic LDH elevation indicative of the presence of the LDH-virus. However, to determine whether this plasma LDH elevation is specifically caused by the LDH-virus, a plasma infectivity test (PIT) was performed by injecting whole blood or plasma from the tumor-bearing animals into pre-tested LDH-virus-free normal mice and then re-testing their plasma after 72 to 96 hours for a five to tenfold elevation of LDH. The PIT data in Table 1 indicate that all tumors tested by this unequivocal method carried the virus, with the exception of one tumor line which was obtained from tissue culture.

Influence of the LDH-Virus upon Asparaginase Therapy

The question naturally occurs as to what experimental consequences may result from the presence or absence of the LDH-virus, particularly when asparaginase is employed for therapeutic purposes. Does this demonstrated ability of the virus to alter the enzyme clearance capacity of the host have any influence on asparaginase therapy?

The effects of the LDH-virus and asparaginase upon leukemia remission and survival time of mice implanted with EARAD-1 tumors are shown in Table 2.

It may be noted that 95 per cent of the virus-infected mice treated with asparaginase were tumor-free at 40 days following tumor implantation in contrast to no survivals of mice treated with asparaginase only.

Table 2. *Asparaginase therapy in the presence and absence of the LDH-virus. Mice dead with leukemia at various times following tumor inoculation*

No. of days post-tumor inoculation	Tumor controls [a]		Tumor + Asparaginase [b]		Tumor + Asparaginase + LDH-virus [c]	
	No.	%	No.	%	No.	%
20 days	3/21	14.0	2/19	10.5	0/20	0
30 days	21/21	100	18/19	94.7	0/20	0
40 days	21/21	100	19/19	100	1/20 [d]	5

[a] Tumor: Asparagine-dependent EARAD-1 leukemia injected subcutaneously.
[b] 5,000 IU/kg of EC-2 L-asparaginase injected i. p. on the seventh or ninth day following tumor inoculation.
[c] LDH-virus ($10^6 ID_{50}$) injected i. p. on the fourth day following tumor inoculation.
[d] Surviving mice were free of detectable tumors.

A graphic presentation of typical time-course experimental results observed with asparaginase therapy in the presence and absence of the LDH-virus is given in Fig. 2. This illustrates the difference in therapeutic response of the asparaginase-sensitive EARAD-1 mouse leukemia following administration of single or multiple doses of asparaginase. Each dose consisted of 5,000 IU per kilogram. In the virus-infected mice receiving a single dose of asparaginase, the established lymphomatous

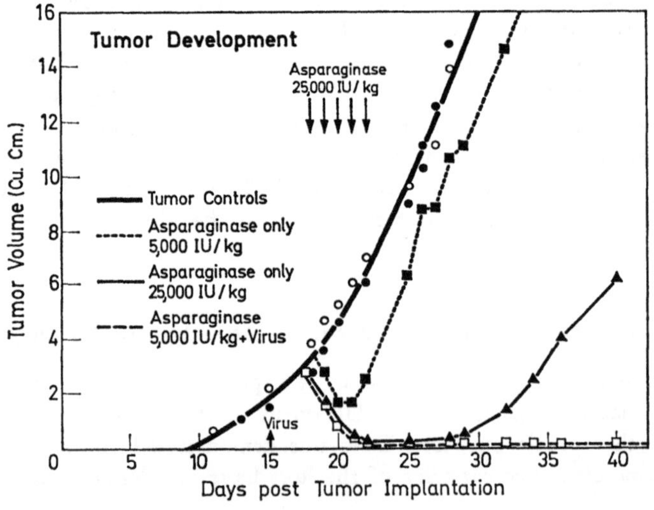

Fig. 2. Tumor response to asparaginase therapy in the presence and absence of the LDH-elevating virus. The LDH-virus-free mice receiving 25,000 IU/kg were given 5 consecutive daily doses of 5,000 IU/kg, as indicated by the arrows at the top margin

mass, as well as the accompanying disseminated leukemic disease, regressed and the animals remained in remission during the entire observation period. In contrast, non-infected mice receiving an identical 5,000 IU/kg dose of asparaginase exhibited early relapse and death, while those receiving five similar daily consecutive doses, totalling 25,000 IU/kg, survived longer but also suffered leukemia recurrence and death.

Influence of the LDH-Virus upon Asparaginase Dose

Fig. 3 shows the results of further analysis of the difference in asparaginase clearance occurring between normal mice and comparable animals infected with LDH-virus. The two straight lines, resulting from logarithmic plots, illustrate the comparative enzyme disappearance curves. The steep line depicts the enzyme disappearance rate of 100 IU of asparaginase (5,000 IU/kg) from the plasma of a normal mouse; whereas the broken line shows the disappearance or clearance curve of 10 units of asparaginase (500 IU/kg) from the plasma of virus-infected animals. It is apparent that after an elapsed period of approximately 16 hours, that the virus-infected mice, having an original plasma concentration of only 10 units, have a higher level of circulating asparaginase than the non-virus animals which had an initial plasma concentration of 100 units. This results from the six-fold difference in enzyme half-life.

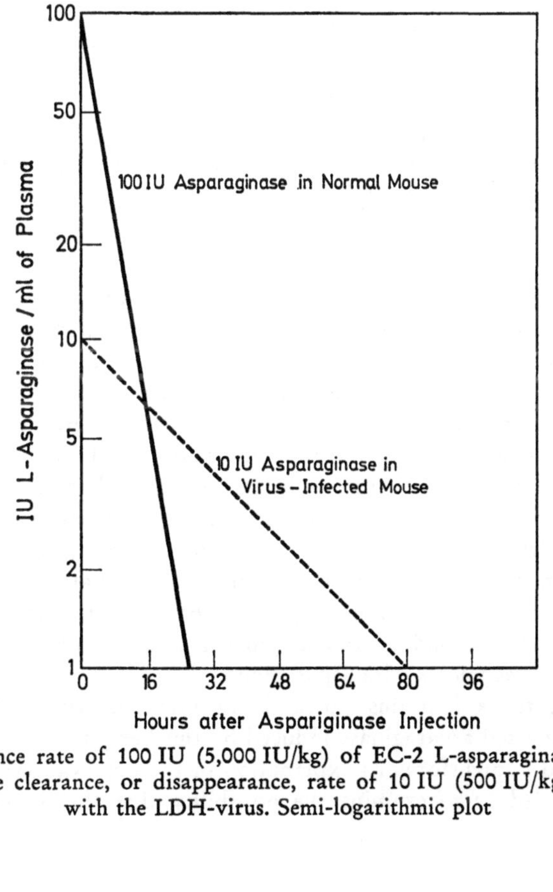

Fig. 3. Disappearance rate of 100 IU (5,000 IU/kg) of EC-2 L-asparaginase in normal mice compared with the clearance, or disappearance, rate of 10 IU (500 IU/kg) in mice infected with the LDH-virus. Semi-logarithmic plot

Since this asparaginase clearance is plotted on a semi-log scale, the exact quantitative aspects are graphically distorted. To place this phenomenon in a more realistic asparaginase dose perspective, Fig. 4 shows the arithmetic relationships. It may be seen that during the first 16 hours the tumor cells of the non-virus animals with the larger asparaginase dose are exposed to a higher concentration; however, after this initial time period, the virus-infected animals injected with only 1/10 of the higher dose have the advantage of a higher persisting drug level.

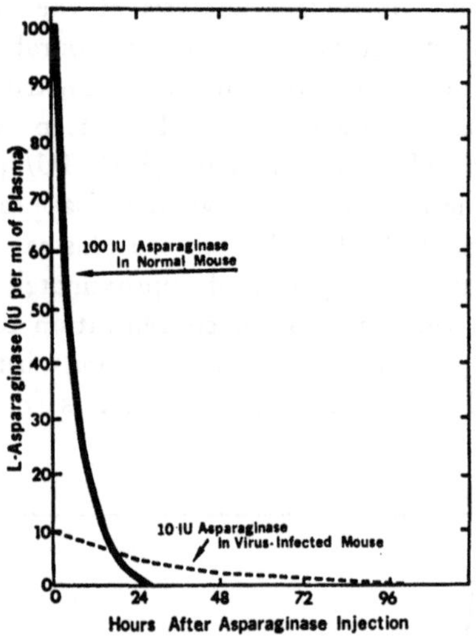

Fig. 4. Asparaginase clearance.
Arithmetic plot of EC-2 L-asparaginase disappearance in the presence and absence of the LDH-elevating virus. Ten and 100 IU of asparaginase per 20 gm mouse equals 500 and 5,000 IU per kg

The practical therapeutic consequences of this are illustrated in Fig. 5. In this experiment, all animals were injected at weekly intervals with asparaginase. In the absence of the LDH-virus, a dose of 5,000 IU/kg was employed; whereas a comparable group infected with the LDH-virus received only 500 IU/kg at the weekly intervals. In the absence of the virus it may be seen that regression of the tumors is incomplete following asparaginase injection and that growth of the tumor is resumed early. Repeated doses of 5,000 IU/kg induced only partial tumor regression, and in each instance growth quickly recurred leading to the eventual death of the animals. In contrast, the virus-infected animals which had received 1/10 of the above dose, namely 500 IU/kg, on the same schedule, exhibited an initial complete regression of the tumor and a prolonged remission, until an asparaginase-resistant cell population started to grow. This secondary tumor growth was relatively non-responsive to repeated 500 IU/kg treatments with asparaginase.

It is tempting to explain this entire therapeutic potentiation by the impaired clearance of the injected asparaginase induced by this benign virus, since this appears to be a simple and straightforward explanation of the observations. However, other experiments have led us to examine the possibility that the presence of the virus may be providing auxiliary therapeutic mechanisms over and beyond the simple asparaginase clearance phenomenon and its associated dose enhancement.

For example, Fig. 6 illustrates an experiment in which we attempted to simulate in virus-free mice the asparaginase level that would have resulted from impaired clearance if the animals had been infected with the LDH-virus. This was accomplished by injecting asparaginase every four hours. The heavy central line shows the

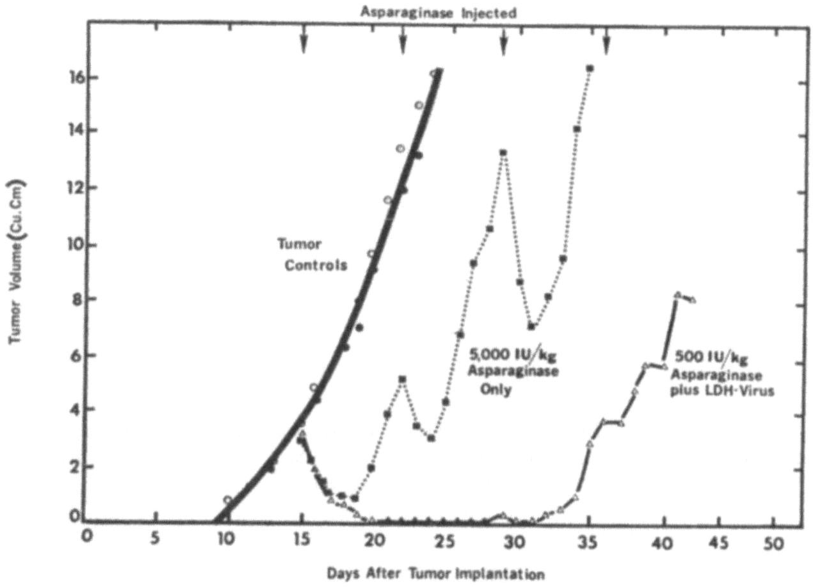

Fig. 5. Tumor development.
Tumor regression and recurrence following weekly injections of asparaginase in the presence and absence of the LDH-elevating virus. The non-infected mice received weekly doses of 5,000 IU/kg, while the virus-infected mice received only 500 IU/kg on the same weekly schedule

calculated clearance curve of 100 IU of asparaginase (5,000 IU/kg) expected in a virus-infected animal. The saw-tooth dotted lines indicate the levels of asparaginase maintained in the normal animals by repeated injections of the enzyme. For reasons that are not yet entirely clear, we did not obtain the expected therapeutic effect that was observed with the virus-infected animals. There is now additional evidence, which suggests that the virus may be inducing beneficial therapeutic effects other than its established influence on the asparaginase-mediated blood levels of asparagine.

Regression of Asparaginase-Treated Tumors in the Presence and Absence of the Virus

The regression of asparaginase-sensitive tumors in the presence of LDH-virus infection was independent of the dose of asparaginase within the range employed in our experiments. This is illustrated by Fig. 7. Weekly doses of 500, 1,000 and 5,000

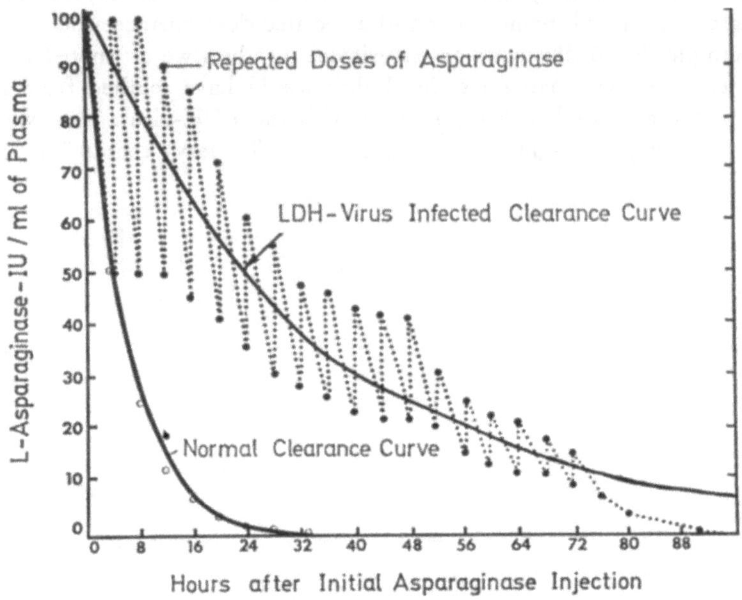

Fig. 6. Simulation of the LDH-virus-mediated asparaginase clearance curve, by injecting repeated doses of asparaginase into non-infected mice. See text for discussion of the comparative therapeutic effects

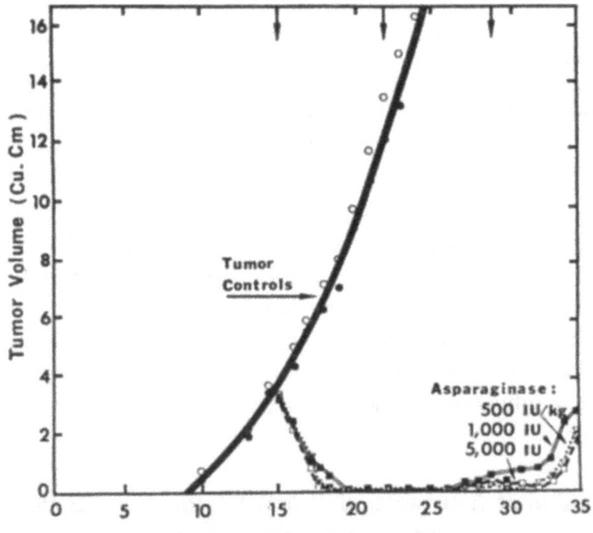

Fig. 7. Tumor response (with virus).
Regression and recurrence of tumors in mice infected with the LDH-elevating virus, following weekly injections of various doses of EC-2 L-asparaginase

IU per kg produced essentially the same tumor regression rates and duration of remission in virus-infected mice. Complete regression of the subcutaneous tumors, relatively long remission periods, and the eventual recurrence of asparaginase-resistant tumors was observed in all groups infected with the LDH-virus, regardless of the asparaginase dose, within this range. Unlike the tumor response in earlier experiments, the serially transplanted EARAD-1 has apparently acquired a higher population of asparaginase-resistant cells, since the original permanent remissions observed with single doses are no longer obtained.

In contrast to the uniform initial regression of the lymphomas in the LDH-virus-infected mice, tumors in non-infected mice exhibited a differential response to the various doses of asparaginase, as shown in Fig. 8. Without the LDH-virus, regression of the tumors was partial at all dose levels, with only a short delay before tumor growth resumed. All the mice in these groups died relatively early, in contrast to the virus-infected groups shown in Fig. 7.

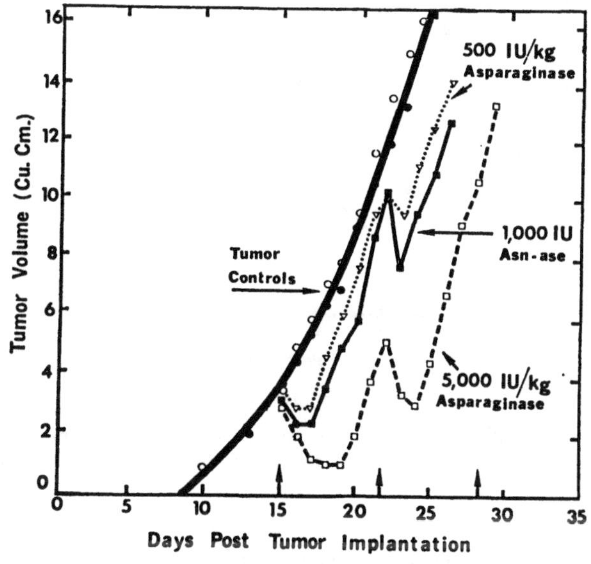

Fig. 8. Tumor response (no virus).
Regression and recurrence of tumors in non-infected mice, following weekly injections of various doses of asparaginase

Asparaginase-LDH-Virus Synergism

Fig. 9 is a time-course plot of mouse body weights which illustrates that undeciphered events take place in the combined presence of the LDH-virus and asparaginase which are not seen in non-infected animals that received repeated doses of asparaginase. A significant temporary decrease in mouse body weight occurred shortly after a single dose of asparaginase was administered to mice previously infected with the LDH-virus. The control animals, and those which received virus only or asparaginase only, had relatively normal body weights. Untreated tumor-bearing mice also showed no decrease in body weight.

These observations may be pertinent in examining the possibility that the role of the LDH-elevating virus in augmenting asparaginase therapy may be more complicated than a simple time-course improvement in the asparaginase blood level. It is also appropriate to remember that several enzymes, in addition to LDH, are elevated as a consequence of this virus infection. It would not be inconsistent therefore, if the concentration of other amino acids or other metabolic substates were altered in the plasma of such mice.

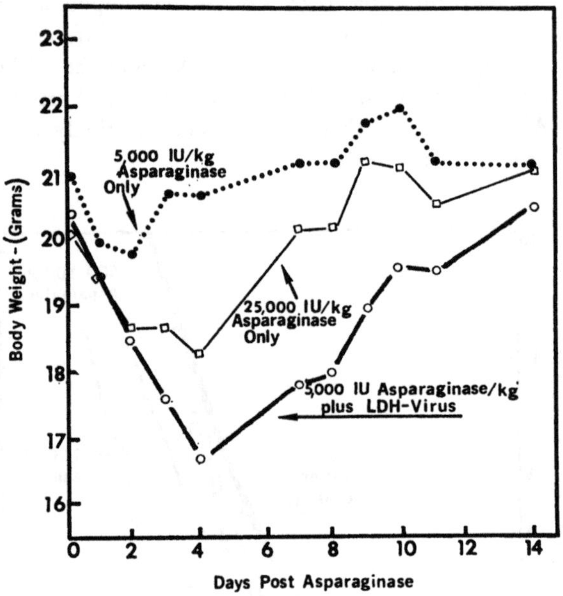

Fig. 9. Body weight.
Comparative effects of EC-2 L-asparaginase upon the body weights of normal mice and those infected with the LDH-elevating virus

In an effort to better understand this weight loss phenomenon, the food consumption of these animals was also measured. As illustrated in Fig. 10, it was noted that the food intake of mice receiving a combination of asparaginase and virus was reduced. Consistent with the differential weight loss, there was also a smaller food consumption following the administration of only 5,000 IU/kg of asparaginase to virus-infected mice than with 25,000 IU/kg of asparaginase without the virus. The usual dose of 5,000 IU/kg of asparaginase in the absence of the virus caused no appreciable reduction in food consumption.

Enhanced tumor therapy associated with food reduction and weight loss naturally raises the question of the effect of reduced caloric intake. This could explain improved therapeutic effects since it is known that under some conditions caloric restriction has an influence upon tumor incidence and tumor growth rates [78]. Experiments were, therefore, undertaken to test this possibility by starving the animals under controlled conditions so that their caloric intake and subsequent weight loss simulated that induced by the combination of asparaginase and virus. When this was done and tumor measurements were compared, it was found that the starvation-induced weight loss had no appreciable effect upon the growth rate of the implanted asparagine-sensitive tumors or upon the survival of the hosts. Thus, it appears that the improvement in asparaginase therapy associated with LDH-virus infection is not a consequence of caloric reduction.

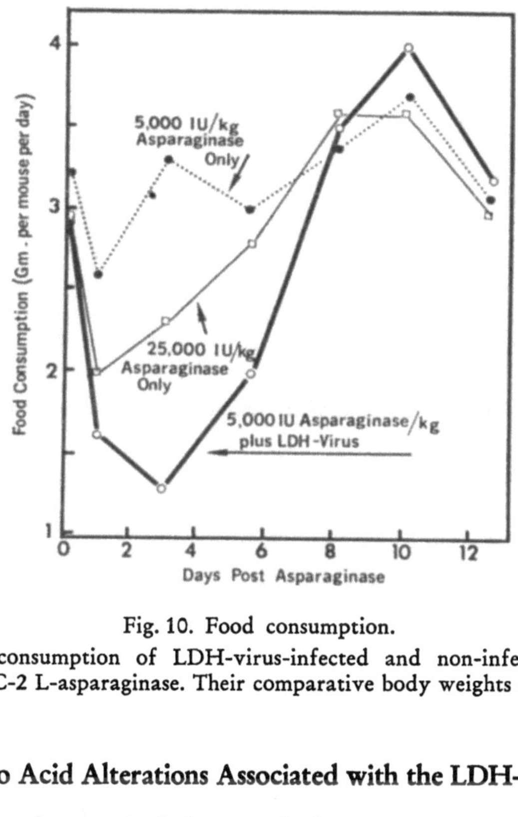

Fig. 10. Food consumption.
Comparative food consumption of LDH-virus-infected and non-infected mice receiving various doses of EC-2 L-asparaginase. Their comparative body weights are shown in Fig. 9

Amino Acid Alterations Associated with the LDH-Virus

Inasmuch as the therapeutic influence of the LDH-virus appears to be greater than can be explained solely in terms of asparaginase dose increase, the question arises as to what additional effects the virus might have on the asparaginase-treated tumor-bearing mouse.

Fig. 11 shows a restricted portion of an amino acid chromatogram obtained with normal mouse plasma. There are four peaks of primary interest in this chromatogram; namely, aspartic acid, asparagine, glutamic acid, and glutamine. This is a typical chromatogram showing the seven amino acid peaks which are eluted between aspartic acid and glutamine. A cogent question which we have explored is what happens to the concentration of these various amino acids following asparaginase administration in the presence and absence of the LDH-elevating virus.

Fig. 12 provides a partial answer to these questions by illustrating the consequences of asparaginase administration in normal mice known to be free of the

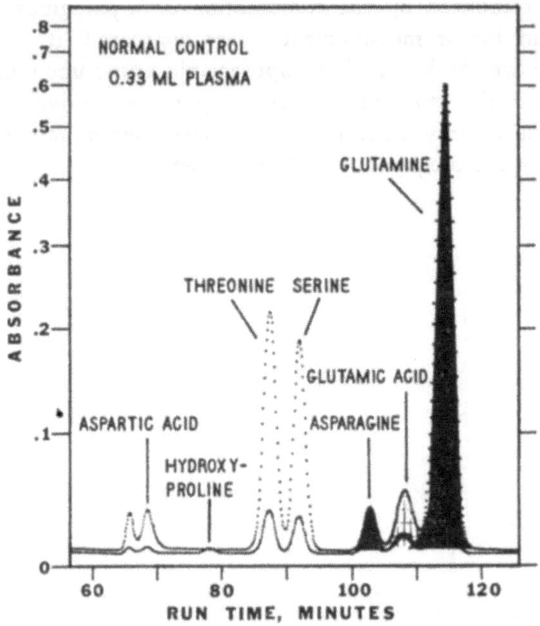

Fig. 11. Portion of a chromatogram of the amino acids found in normal mouse plasma

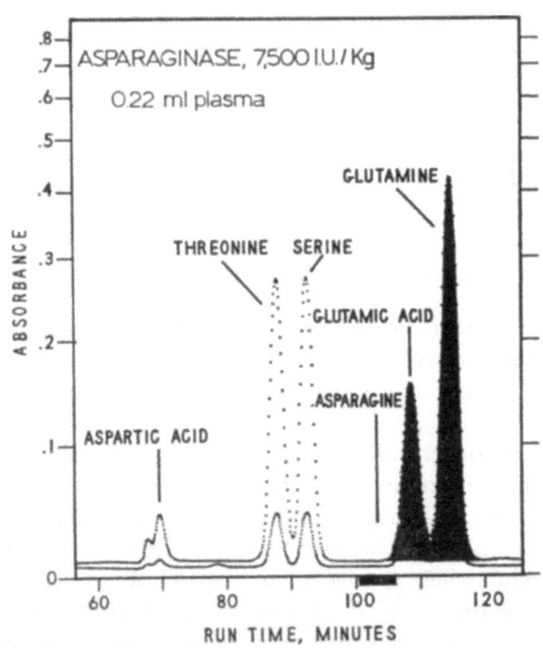

Fig. 12. Portion of a chromatogram of the amino acids found in mouse plasma 48 hours following administration of 7,500 IU/kg of EC-2 L-asparaginase to normal mice

LDH-virus. It may be noted that at 48 hours following injection of 7,500 IU/kg of L-asparaginase, the aspartic acid peak is approximately the same size as it was in the normal untreated controls; the glutamine peak has been reduced slightly and the glutamic acid peak has been correspondingly increased, whereas the asparagine peak, as anticipated, has disappeared entirely, as may be noted by the perfectly flat base line. This represents a reduction in the plasma asparagine concentration to less than one nanomole per milliliter. It would thus seem that tumor-bearing animals appropriately treated with asparaginase at this dosage are effectively deprived of blood-borne asparagine.

Since circulating asparagine is readily reduced to essentially zero by asparaginase only, how does the presence of the LDH-virus add any further benefits that would influence asparaginase therapy? Attention is drawn particularly to the minor reduction in the size of the glutamine peak in this chromatogram. Although 3 to 6 per cent glutaminase activity is known to be present in the EC-2 L-asparaginase preparations [17], its capacity to significantly deplete circulating plasma glutamine under ordinary circumstances has not been observed.

Fig. 13 illustrates the relative concentrations of these amino acids following analysis of blood plasma obtained from animals receiving the same amount of asparaginase as those whose chromatogram is depicted in Fig. 12, but, in addition, were infected intentionally with the LDH-elevating virus prior to asparaginase administration. It may be seen that the most striking alterations due to the presence of the virus are the complete disappearance of both the plasma asparagine and glutamine

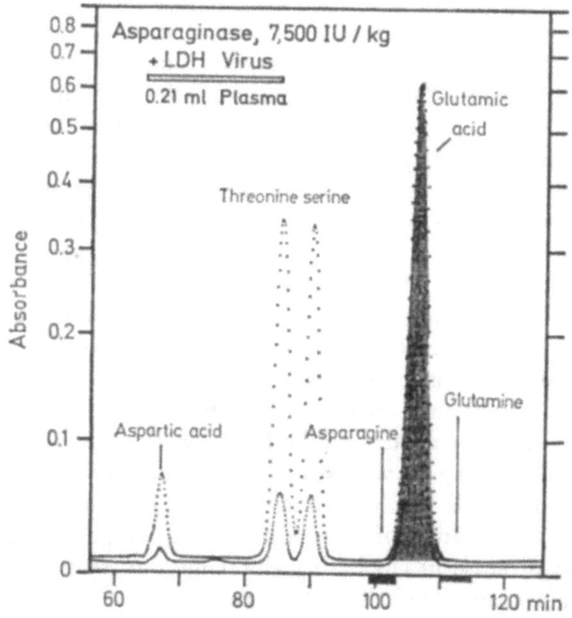

Fig. 13. Portion of a chromatogram of the amino acids found in mouse plasma 48 hours following administration of 7,500 IU/kg of EC-2 L-asparaginase to mice infected with the LDH-elevating virus

peaks, together with a corresponding increase in plasma aspartic acid and glutamic acid. Hence, the effects of the administered asparaginase in the presence of the LDH-virus has been the hydrolysis of both asparagine and glutamine, with resulting increases in aspartic acid and glutamic acid in the peripheral circulation. Since glutamine serves as a nitrogen donor in the synthesis of asparagine [41, 57], and glutamic acid is relatively impermeable to the cell membrane, this conversion of plasma glutamine to glutamic acid following asparaginase administration in the presence of the LDH-virus may effectively deprive the leukemia cells of asparagine in more ways than one. The effectiveness of glutamine removal in the presence of the LDH-virus, and the length of time that glutamine is absent or low in concentration in the plasma depend on the amount of asparaginase administered per dose and the number and frequency of doses. Following a single injection of 5,000 IU/kg of EC-2 asparaginase, asparagine is completely absent from the blood of all mice, infected and non-infected, at two hours after asparaginase injection. In the absence of the LDH-virus, asparagine was found again in the plasma on the sixth day following the injection. With the LDH-virus present, no asparagine was detected in the plasma until the 14th day following asparaginase injection.

Discussion

In studies with the E. coli-derived enzyme, EC-2 L-asparaginase, Campbell and Mashburn [17] have reported evidence that the deamination of both L-asparagine and L-glutamine is accomplished by the same enzyme molecule and probably at the same enzymic site. Under simulated physiological conditions the relative enzymic rates found for the hydrolysis of L-asparagine compared with L-glutamine were 1.0 and 0.03 respectively. This corresponds with the various reports cited in this monograph that EC-2 L-asparaginase preparations contain from 3 to 6 per cent glutaminase activity. Campbell and Mashburn have shown that the rates of disappearance or clearance from the peripheral blood for L-asparagine and L-glutamine were identical, the half-life being 3 hours in normal mice and 28 hours in mice infected with the LDH-virus. This is consistent with the values reported here and elsewhere [64, 66].

Apparently, in normal mice, the disappearance rate of the injected enzyme is sufficiently rapid that glutamine is not significantly depleted from the circulating blood in the absence of the LDH-virus, at least with the asparaginase dosages employed in most experiments. However, in LDH-virus-infected mice there is sufficient retention of the enzyme, due to the impaired clearance, to permit substantial hydrolysis of the circulating glutamine, as well as all of the circulating asparagine.

It is pertinent to recall that the virus, by itself, does not have any measurable influence on the concentration of plasma asparagine or glutamine. It thus appears that the observed decrease in circulating glutamine represents a combined effect of asparaginase administration and the LDH-virus infection. Since the EC-2 L-asparaginase molecule has a small percentage of glutaminase activity, it follows that the LDH-virus has a proportionate ability to impair the clearance of such glutaminase activity as well as impairing the clearance of asparaginase. This has the effect of increasing and extending the glutaminase activity much in the same way that the virus augments the asparaginase activity of the EC-2 enzyme.

Irrespective of speculation on the details of the mechanism [63, 64, 65], the observed facts to consider are that in the combined presence of the LDH-virus and asparaginase, two amino acids are removed from the circulation, rather than one, and the therapeutic effects against mouse leukemia are greatly improved.

It may be pertinent that glutamine is a versatile amino acid and is also the immediate biochemical precursor of asparagine [41]. Thus the presence of high concentrations of circulating glutamine may provide a vital source of essential nutrient for a residual population of leukemia cells [22, 23, 24, 47, 72].

The multiple effects of the LDH-virus upon asparaginase therapy against murine leukemia and lymphomas provides experimental opportunities for elucidating some of the mechanisms involved in the action of asparaginase against asparagine-dependent tumors. It should also now be quite clear that the presence or absence of this virus should be controlled in asparaginase studies employing mouse systems.

Various side effects, immunological reactions, and miscellaneous toxicities associated with asparaginase administration naturally concern clinical investigators, as is adequately documented in other chapters of this monograph. The data reported here suggest that enhancement of the minor glutaminase activity of a given dose of EC-2 L-asparaginase through the influence of the LDH-virus, may be directly or indirectly involved in causing the reduced food consumption, weight loss, and other unmeasured toxicities. It is uncertain at this point whether these toxic manifestations are associated with glutamine deprivation or increased concentrations of glutamic and aspartic acid. Increased generation of ammonia resulting from the deamination of asparagine and glutamine, or other factors may also be implicated. The synergistic reaction observed between asparaginase treatment and the LDH-virus infection, however, provides obvious leads for examining these various possibilities.

Although adverse immunological reactions have not been a conspicuous problem in animal studies, it may be useful to draw attention to the recent report which indicates that the LDH-virus acts as an immunological adjuvant [46]. Although no specific evidence has been observed in our studies that implicates this characteristic of the LDH-virus, its possible role in benefically supporting long-term leukemia remissions should be considered.

Summary

A striking difference has been observed in the therapeutic effectiveness of asparaginase against sensitive mouse leukemias when treated in the presence or absence of the benign LDH-elevating virus. When this virus is eliminated from the universally infected classical mouse tumors generally employed for experimental asparaginase studies, the therapeutic response of the tumor-bearing or leukemic host to asparaginase is markedly diminished.

In the absence of the virus, partial regression of the neoplastic disease can be obtained, but early recurrence is usually observed, analogous to that found in leukemia patients treated with asparaginase. Tumor-bearing mice which are intentionally infected with the LDH-virus exhibit long-term and, in some cases, permanent remissions following even single doses of asparaginase.

The mechanism of this phenomenon has been studied. Preliminary results suggest that two factors may be involved: (1) Impaired clearance of the administered asparaginase from the circulating blood of the host; and (2) potentiation of the minor glutaminase activity associated with EC-2 L-asparaginase, which permits a significant decrease in circulating glutamine. Thus the enhanced therapeutic effects obtained in the presence of the virus may be related to the more effective hydrolysis of the two amino acids rather than one. Standard clinical doses of asparaginase, in the absence of the virus, depleted asparagine only, whereas both asparagine and its precursor glutamine were depleted when the host was infected with the LDH-virus.

It is postulated that persisting high levels of plasma glutamine may compromise the effectiveness of asparaginase therapy, and that the apparent leukemia cures seen in LDH-virus-infected mice may be due to the effective hydrolysis of these two amino acids which are somehow critical to the survival of these particular neoplastic cells.

Acknowledgements

These studies were supported in part by research grants from the American Cancer Society (T-522), and the ACS, Washington State Division; the National Institute of Health (NIH Grant FR-5520); the Brown-Hazen Fund of the Research Corporation; and the Ledbetter Fund.

We are indebted to Dr. Lloyd J. Old, Sloan Kettering Institute, New York, for the EARAD-1 asparaginase-sensitive leukemia. The EC-2 L-asparaginase (Squibb) was provided by Dr. Saul A. Shepartz of the Cancer Chemotherapy National Service Center, National Cancer Institute, and Dr. Stephen K. Carter, of the Cancer Therapy Evaluation Branch, National Cancer Institute. Special research animals were supplied by S. M. Poiley, Mammalian Genetics and Animal Production Section, CCNSC, National Cancer Institute. Miscellaneous NCI support was possible through the kind interest of Charles G. Zubrod.

Some of the asparaginase clearance studies were done in collaboration with Drs. H. A. Campbell and C. Chester Stock. Counsel and support was provided by Dr. Gilbert Dalldorf and Dr. William B. Hutchinson. We are indebted to Clyde N. Lulham and Lester Teschner, Jr., for technical assistance.

References

1. Ainis, H., Kurtz, M., Kramer, P. I., Weimer, H. E., Ryan, R. M., Jameson, E.: *In vivo* and *in vitro* studies on the action of guinea pig serum against the ascites form of the Murphy-Sturm lymphosarcoma. Cancer Res. **18**, 1309 (1958).
2. Becker, F. F., Broome, J. D.: L-asparaginase: Inhibition of early mitosis in regenerating rat liver. Science **156**, 1602 (1967).
3. Benson, J. V., Jr., Gordon, M. J., Patterson, J. A.: Accelerated chromatographic analysis of amino acids in physiological fluids containing glutamine and asparagine. Anal. Biochem. **18**, 228 (1967).
4. Borella, L., Journey, L. J., Hiramoto, R.: *In vivo* and *in vitro* effects of the L-asparaginase fraction of guinea pig serum in the 6C3HED ascites lymphosarcoma. Cancer Res. **26**, 2451 (1966).
5. Boyse, E. A., Old, L. J., Campbell, H. A., Mashburn, L. T.: Suppression of murine leukemias by L-asparaginase. Incidence of sensitivity among leukemias of various types: Comparative inhibitory activities of guinea pig serum L-asparaginase and *Escherichia coli* L-asparaginase. J. exp. Med. **125**, 17 (1967).
6. Breuer, L. H., Jr., Warner, R. G., Benton, D. A., Loosli, J. K.: Dietary requirement for asparagine and its metabolism in rats. J. Nutr. **88**, 143 (1966).
7. Broome, J. D.: Evidence that the L-asparaginase activity of guinea pig serum is responsible for its antilymphoma effects. Nature **191**, 1114 (1961).
8. — Evidence that the L-asparaginase of guinea pig serum is responsible for its antilymphoma effects. I. Properties of the L-asparaginase of guinea pig serum in relation to those of the antilymphoma substance. J. exp. Med. 118, 99 (1963).
9. — Evidence that the L-asparaginase of guinea pig serum is responsible for its antilymphoma effects. II. Lymphoma 6C3HED cells cultured in a medium devoid of L-asparagine lose their susceptibility to the effects of guinea pig serum *in vivo*. J. exp. Med. **118**, 121 (1963).

10. BROOME, J. D.: Antilymphoma activity of L-asparaginase *in vivo:* Clearance rates of enzme preparations from guinea pig serum and yeast in relation to their effect on tumor growth. J. nat. Cancer Inst. **35**, 967 (1965).
11. — A method for estimating free asparagine and glutamine in biological fluids as trinitrophenyl derivatives. Nature **211**, 602 (1966).
12. BROOME, J. D.: Studies of the tumor inhibitory action of L-asparaginase. Ninth International Cancer Congress, Tokyo, Japan. Abstracts of papers, p. 335 (1966).
13. — Factors which may influence the effectiveness of L-asparaginase as tumor inhibitors. Brit. J. Cancer **22**, 595 (1968).
14. — L-asparaginase: The evolution of a new tumor inhibitory agent. Trans. N. Y. Acad. Sci. **30**, 690 (1968).
15. — Studies on the mechanism of tumor inhibition by L-asparaginase. Effects of the enzyme on asparagine levels in the blood, normal tissues and 6C3HED lymphomas of mice. Differences in asparagine formation in asparaginase-sensitive and resistant lymphoma cells. J. exp. Med. **127**, 1055 (1968).
16. — SCHWARTZ, J. H.: Differences in the production of L-asparagine in asparaginase-sensitive and resistant lymphoma cells. Biochim. biophys. Acta (Amst. **138**, 637 (1967).
17. CAMPBELL, H. A., MASHBURN, L. T.: L-asparaginase EC-2 from *E. coli.* Some substrate specificity characteristics. Biochemistry **8**, 3768 (1969).
18. — — BOYSE, E. A., OLD, L. J.: Two L-asparaginases from *E. coli* B. Their separation, purification and antitumor activity. Biochemistry **6**, 721 (1967).
19. — OLD, L. J., BOYSE, E. A.: Leukemia inhibitory and L-asparaginase activities of guinea pig serum. Proc. Amer. Ass. Cancer Res. **5**, 10 (1964).
20. DOLOWY, W. C., CORNET, J., HENSEN, D., AMMERALL, R.: Response of intracerebral Gardner lymphoma to guinea pig L-asparaginase and *Escherichia coli* L-asparaginase. Proc. Soc. exp. Biol. (N. Y.) **123**, 133 (1966).
21. — HENSEN, D., CORNET, J., SELLIN, H.: Toxic and antineoplastic effects of L-asparaginase. Study of mice with lymphoma and normal monkeys and report on a child with leukemia. Cancer **19**, 1813 (1966).
22. EAGLE, H., WASHINGTON, D. L., LEVY, M., COHEN, L.: The population-dependent requirement by cultured mammalian cells for metabolites which they can synthesize. II. Glutamic acid and glutamine; aspartic acid and asparagine. J. Biol. Chem. **241**, 4994 (1966).
23. HAGER, S. E., JONES, M. E.: Initial steps in pyrimidine synthesis in Ehrlich ascites carcinoma *in vitro.* The synthesis of carbamyl phosphate by a soluble glutamine-dependent carbamyl phosphate synthetase. J. Biol. Chem. **242**, 5667 (1967).
24. — — A glutamine-dependent enzyme for the synthesis of carbamyl phosphate for pyrimidine biosynthesis in fetal rat liver. J. Biol. Chem. **242**, 5674 (1967).
25. HALEY, E. E., FISCHER, G. A., WELCH, A. D.: The requirements of L-asparagine of mouse leukemia cells L5178 in culture. Cancer Res. **21**, 542 (1961).
26. HANDSCHUMACHER, R. E., BATES, C. J., CHANG, P. K., ANDREWS, A. T., FISCHER, G. A.: 5-diazo-4-oxo-L-norvaline: reactive asparagine analog with biological specificity. Science **161**, 62 (1968).
27. — Mechanisms of control of tumor growth: asparaginase and asparagine analogs. In: Exploitable Molecular Mechanisms and Neoplasia. Baltimore: Williams and Wilkins Co. 1969, p. 565.
28. HEYMANN, H., GINSBERG, T., GULICK, Z. R., KONOPKA, E. A., MAYER, R. L.: The preparation and some biological properties of the asparagine analog L-2-amino-2-carboxyethanesulfonamide. J. Amer. Chem. Soc. **81**, 5125 (1959).
29. HILL, J. M., ROBERTS, J., LOEB, E., KHAN, A., MACLELLAN, A., HILL, R. W.: L-asparaginase therapy for leukemia and other malignant neoplasms: Remission in human leukemia. J. Amer. med. Ass. **202**, 882 (1967).
30. — LOEB, E., MACLELLAN, A., KHAN, A., ROBERTS, J., SHIELDS, W. F., HILL, N. O.: Response to highly purified L-asparaginase during therapy of acute leukemia. Cancer Res. **29**, 1574 (1969).
31. HIRAMOTO, R., TATE, C., HAMLIN, M.: Guinea pig serum inhibitory factor and asparaginase activity. Proc. Soc. exp. Biol. (N. Y.) **121**, 597 (1966).

32. Ho, P. P. K., Frank, B. H., Burck, P. J.: Crystalline asparaginase from *E. coli*. Science **165**, 510 (1969).
33. Holmquist, N. D.: Effect of normal sera of several related rodents on 6C3HED lymphoma *in vivo*. Proc. Soc. exp. Biol. (N. Y.) **113**, 444 (1963).
34. Horowitz, B., Madras, B. K., Meister, A., Old, L. J., Boyse, E. A.: Asparagine synthetase activity of mouse leukemias. Proc. Amer. Ass. Cancer Res. **9**, 33 (1968).
35. — — — — — Stockert, E.: Asparagine synthetase activity of mouse leukemias. Science **160**, 533 (1968).
36. Kidd, J. G.: Regression of transplanted lymphomas induced *in vivo* by means of normal guinea pig serum. I. Course of transplanted cancers of various kinds in mice and rats given guinea pig serum, horse serum, or rabbit serum. J. exp. Med. **98**, 565 (1953).
37. — Sobin, L. H.: The incorporation of L-asparagine-^{14}C by lymphoma 6C3HED cells; its inhibition by guinea pig serum. Cancer Res. **26**, 208 (1966).
38. Kim, J. H., Boyse, E. A., Old, L. J., Campbell, H. A.: Inhibition of HeLa cultures by preparations of *E. coli* L-asparaginase. Biochim. biophys. Acta (Amst.) **158**, 478 (1968).
39. Kwak, K. S., Jameson, E., Ryan, R. M., Kurtz, H. M.: The effect of varying implant cell numbers on the inhibitory activity of guinea pig serum on Walker carcinosarcoma 256 in the rat. Cancer Res. **21**, 44 (1961).
40. Lerman, M. I., Verevkina, I. V.: The inhibition of asparaginase from the blood serum of guinea pigs. Biokhimiia **27**, 526 (1962).
41. Levintow, L.: Evidence that glutamine is a precursor of asparagine in a human cell in tissue culture. Science **126**, 611 (1957).
42. Mashburn, L. T., Boyse, E. A., Campbell, H. A., Old, L. J.: A comparison of concurrent and delayed tests for antitumor activity of L-asparaginase. Proc. Soc. exp. Biol. (N. Y.) **124**, 568 (1967).
43. — Wriston, J. C., Jr.: Tumor inhibitory effect of L-asparaginase. Biochem. Biophys. Res. Comm. **12**, 50 (1963).
44. — — Tumor inhibitory effect of L-asparaginase from *Escherichia coli*. Arch. Biochem. Biophys. **105**, 450 (1964).
45. Meister, A.: Glutaminase, asparaginase and alpha-keto acid-ω-amidase. In: Methods in Enzymology, Vol. II. Eds.: S. P. Colowick and N. O. Kaplan. New York: Acad. Press Inc. 1955, p. 380.
46. Mergenhagen, S. E., Notkins, A. L., Doughterty, S. F.: Adjuvanticity of lactic dehydrogenase virus; influence of virus infection on the establishment of immunologic tolerance to a protein antigen in adult mice. J. Immun. **99**, 578 (1967).
47. Neuman, R. A., McCoy, T. A.: Requirement of Walker carcinosarcoma 256 *in vitro* for asparagine and glutamine. Science **124**, 24 (1956).
48. Notkins, A. L., Scheele, C.: Impaired clearance of enzymes in mice infected with the lactic dehydrogenase agent. J. Nat. Cancer Inst. **33**, 741 (1964).
49. — The lactic dehydrogenase virus. Bacteriol. Rev. **29**, 143 (1965).
50. Oettgen, H. F., Old, L. J., Boyse, E. A., Campbell, H. A., Phillips, F. S., Clarkson, B. D., Tallal, L., Leeper, R. D., Schwartz, M. K., Kim, J. H.: Inhibition of leukemias in man by L-asparaginase. Cancer Res. **27**, 2619 (1967).
51. Old, L. J., Boyse, E. A., Campbell, H. A., Daria, G. M.: Leukaemia inhibiting properties and L-asparaginase activity of sera from certain South American rodents. Nature **198**, 801 (1963).
52. — — — Brodey, R. S., Fidler, J., Teller, J. D.: Treatment of lymphosarcoma in the dog with L-asparaginase. Cancer **20**, 1066 (1967).
53. — — — L-asparaginase and leukemia. Sci. Amer. **219**, 34 (1968).
54. — — — Brodey, R. S., Fidler, J., Teller, J. D.: Treatment of lymphosarcoma in the dog with L-asparaginase. Lancet **1967 I**, 447.
55. — Iritani, C., Stockert, E., Boyse, E. A., Campbell, H. A.: Increased anti-leukaemia activity of *E. coli* asparaginase in mice infected with LDH-elevating virus. Lancet **1968 II**, 684.
56. Patterson, M. K., Jr., Conway, E., Whittle, W., McCoy, T. A.: *In vitro* effects of guinea pig serum on the Jensen JA-1 and JA-2 sarcomas. Proc. Soc. exp. Biol. (N. Y.) **119**, 5 (1965).

57. PATTERSON, M. K., ORR, G.: L-asparaginase biosynthesis by nutritional variants of the Jensen sacroma. Biochem. Biophys. Res. Comm. **26**, 228 (1967).
58. PRAGER, M. D., BACHYNSKY, N.: Asparagine synthetase in asparaginase resistant and susceptible mouse lymphomas. Biochem. Biophys. Res. Comm. **31**, 43 (1968).
59. — — Asparagine synthetase in normal and malignant tissues; correlation with tumor sensitivity to asparaginase. Arch. Biochem. Biophys. **127**, 645 (1968).
60. — ROBERTS, J., BACHYNSKY, N.: Immunity to the 6C3HED ascites tumor following treatment of tumor-bearing mice with *E. coli* L-asparaginase. J. Immun. **98**, 1045 (1967).
61. RILEY, V.: Adaptation of orbital bleeding technic to rapid serial blood studies. Proc. Soc. exp. Biol. (N. Y.) **104**, 751 (1960).
62. — Transmissable agents and anemia of mouse cancer. N. Y. State J. Med. **63**, 1523 (1963).
63. — Asparaginase therapy: influence of the LDH-virus. Proc. Amer. Ass. Cancer Res. **10**, 73 (1969).
64. — Role of the LDH-elevating virus in leukaemia therapy by asparaginase. Nature **220**, 1246 (1968).
65. — Lactate dehydrogenase in the normal and malignant state: In: Methods in Cancer Research, Vol. Ed.: H. BUSCH. New York: Acad. Press. Inc. 1968, p. 493.
66. — CAMPBELL, H. A., STOCK, C. C.: Influence of the LDH-elevating virus upon the clearance of asparaginase in the mouse. Proc. Soc. exp. Biol. (N. Y.) **133**, 38 (1970).
67. — LILLY, F., HUERTO, E., BARDELL, D.: Transmissable agent associated with 26 types of experimental mouse neoplasms. Science **132**, 545 (1960).
68. — LOVELESS, J. D., FITZMAURICE, M. A.: Comparison of a lactate dehydrogenase-elevating virus-like agent and *Eperythrozoon coccoides*. Proc. Soc. exp. Biol. (N. Y.) **116**, 486 (1964).
69. — — — SILER, W. M.: Mechanism of lactate dehydrogenase (LDH) elevation in virus-infected hosts. Life Sci. **4**, 487 (1965).
70. ROBERTS, J., BURSON, G., HILL, J. M.: New procedures for purification of L-asparaginase with high yield from *E. coli*. J. Bacteriol. **95**, 2117 (1968).
71. — PRAGER, M. D., BACHYNSKY, N.: The antitumor activity of *Escherichia coli* L-asparaginase. Cancer Res. **26**, 2213 (1966).
72. SANSOM, B. F., BARRY, J. M.: The use of asparagine and glutamine for the biosynthesis of casein and plasma proteins. Biochem. J. **68**, 487 (1958).
73. SCHREK, R., DOLOWY, W. C., AMMERAAL, R. N.: L-asparaginase: Toxicity to normal and leukemic human lymphocytes. Science **155**, 329 (1967).
74. SCHWARTZ, J. H., REEVES, J. Y., BROOME, J. D.: Two L-asparaginases from *E. coli* and their action against tumors. Proc. Nat. Acad. Sci. **56**, 1516 (1966).
75. SOBIN, L. H., KIDD, J. G.: A metabolic difference between two lines of lymphoma 6C3HED cells in relation to asparagine. Proc. Soc. exp. Biol. (N. Y.) **119**, 325 (1965).
76. SPACKMAN, D. H.: (Unpublished data, 1969).
77. SULD, H. M., HERBUT, P. A.: Guinea pig serum and liver asparaginases: Purification and antitumor activity. J. Biol. Chem. **240**, 2234 (1965).
78. TANNENBAUM, A., SILVERSTONE, H.: The influence of the degree of caloric restriction on the formation of skin tumors and hepatomas in mice. Cancer Res. **9**, 724 (1949).
79. YELLIN, T. O., WRISTON, J. C., JR.: Antagonism of purified asparaginase from guinea pig serum toward lymphoma. Science **151**, 998 (1966).

Part IV
Experimental Effects

Experimental Studies with L-Asparaginase in Mouse Leukemias*

JOSEPH H. BURCHENAL, DAN BENVENISTI **, and MALIN DOLLINGER ***

Division of Applied Therapy, Sloan-Kettering Institute for Cancer Research, and the Department of Medicine, Memorial Hospital for Cancer and Allied Diseases New York, New York 10021

With 13 Figures

The classic experimental studies of KIDD [1, 2], BROOME [3—5], and others [6—14] in mice on the enzyme L-asparaginase (A-ase), originally as guinea pig serum and later as preparations of varying degrees of purity from *E. coli,* showed it to be a unique agent with a very high chemotherapeutic index which is capable of curing some mouse leukemias and tumors at high doses without assistance from host immune mechanisms. Since the drug also has a similar chemotherapeutic index in man [15—23], the metabolism and the mechanism of action of the drug in various strains of mouse leukemia and in patients with acute leukemia have been compared in an attempt to understand why—unlike in mouse leukemia—it has not so far been possible to produce regularly with this agent long-term unmaintained remissions in human acute leukemia. To this end, the dependence of various mouse and human cell lines on asparagine *in vitro,* the reversibility of the antileukemic effect of A-ase *in vitro* and *in vivo,* the effects of dose and dosage schedule on early and advanced ascitic, subcutaneous, and intracerebral leukemia, and the effect of prior or concomitant treatment with other chemotherapeutic agents on both the half-life of the drug and the increase in survival time of the leukemic animals have been investigated.

We have confirmed the better effects of higher doses of A-ase [10—13]. Fig. 1 shows the survival time of BDF_1 mice inoculated with leukemia L5178Y/CA55 treated for 5 days starting on day 10 with varying dosage levels of A-ase. Increases in survival time were seen with 10 IU/kg and 40 IU/kg, but much better survival time and an appreciable number of 50-day survivors were noted with 1,000 IU/kg.

---

* These studies were supported in part by National Cancer Institute Grants CA-08748 and CA-05826 and American Cancer Society Grant T-45.

** David A. Gimbel Fellow.

*** Present address: Dept. of Medicine, University of California School of Medicine, Los Angeles.

This type of experiment has been repeated many times in leukemia EARAD1 and L5178Y/CA55, and the superiority of such high doses in producing not only greater increases in survival time but also a definite percentage of 50-day "cures" in EARAD1 and L5178Y/CA55 has been established. It has been suggested that in man the main effect of A-ase is to reduce the asparagine content of the plasma and extracellular fluids to zero, and that this can be done with very small doses of A-ase, such as 10 IU/kg daily, which suffice to produce remissions in patients with acute leukemia and increase the survival time in mice with transplanted leukemia. According to this theory, no further benefit should accrue from greatly increasing the dosage. The studies on mouse leukemia, however, suggest that there is probably a gradient in the various tissues and that in order to destroy all the leukemic cells, particularly in some of the more privileged locations it is necessary to give very high doses of A-ase. This suggests that the same situation might obtain in man and that, although 5 to 10 IU/kg daily will produce remissions, these might last longer if higher doses such as 1,000 to 5,000 IU/kg were employed. Preliminary clinical evidence seems to substantiate this. As shown in Fig. 2, the median duration of un-

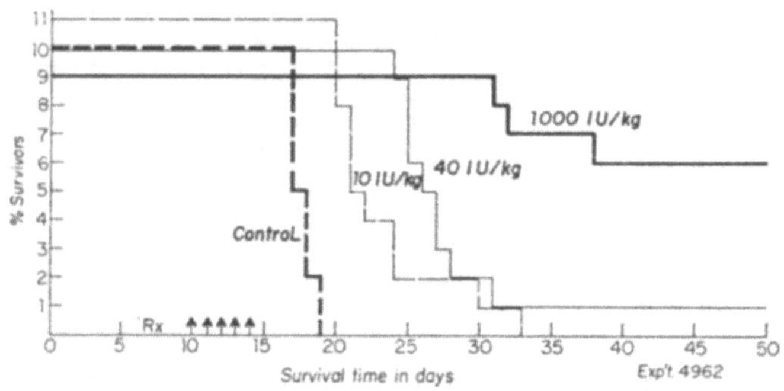

Fig. 1. Effect of dose of asparaginase on advanced leukemia L5178Y/CA55 i. p.

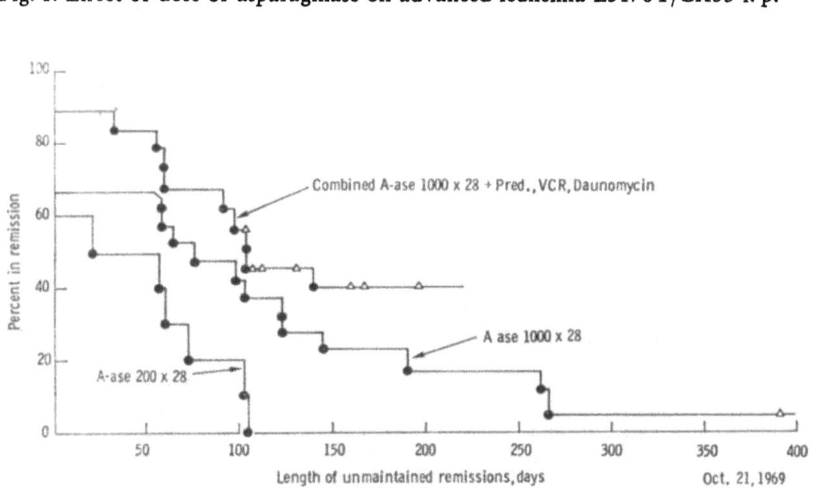

Fig. 2. Length of unmaintained remissions after A-ase 200 IU/ug, 1000 IU/ug or 100 IU/ug combined with pred., VCR, and Daunomycin △ = Pts. still in remission

maintained remission was longer in a small inhomogeneous series of children with acute lymphoblastic leukemia when treated with 1,000 IU/kg daily×28 as compared to 200 IU/kg daily×28.

It has been possible to block the inhibitory effect of A-ase in cell culture by stoichiometric amounts of L-asparagine (Table 1). *In vivo,* by using approximately the minimal effective dose of A-ase (20 IU/kg i. p. daily for 5 days) and giving L-asparagine 4% in 5% glucose solution as drinking water, the mice received large amounts of the amino acid and the inhibitory effect of A-ase was blocked (Fig. 3), confirming the findings of Ohnumo, et al. [24]. This occurred, however, only at minimal inhibitory doses of A-ase, and larger doses of A-ase could not be blocked.

Table 2 shows the incorporation of ^{3}H-valine into short-term cultures of A-ase sensitive and resistant mouse leukemias, compared with sensitive human lymphoblastic

Table 1. *H^{3} valine incorporation into protein of A-ase sensitive and resistant mouse and human leukemic cells*

Leukemia	In vivo sensitivity	CPM [a] +Asparagine	CPM [a] −Asparagine	CPM [a] +A-ase	Percentage inhibition −Asp	Percentage inhibition +A-ase
EARAD1	S	7,929	3,414	1,988	57	75
EARAD1	S	9,987	4,138	1,844	59	82
L5178Y	S	26,776	16,272	5,774	39	78
L5178Y/CA55	S	23,771	11,074	3,221	53	86
EARAD1/A-ase	R	12,528	10,864	12,609	13	0
L5178Y/CA55/A-ase	R	16,277	15,945	15,153	2	7
L1210	R	6,736	7,372	7,161	0	0
P815	R	8,903	8,478	9,557	5	0
Human A.L.L.:						
E.F.	S (CR [b] 4 mo.)	2,380	1,798	1,403	24	41
M.F.	S (CR 6 mo.)	7,940	7,860	5,461	1	31
L.E.	S (CR 3 mo., 6 mo.)	1,901	1,773	1,425	7	25
M.K.	S (CR 5 mo.)	11,178	9,872	8,612	12	23

[a] Average of three tubes.
[b] CR = complete remission.

Table 2. *Blocking of A-ase effect on L5178Y/CA55 cells by L- and D-asparagine*

Treatment at 48 hr. Incubation: A-ase (IU/ml)	L-asparagine (mg/ml)	D-asparagine (mg/ml)	Cell count (96 hr.)
—	—	—	1,479,710
0.01	—	—	88,580
0.01	2.4	—	1,405,220
0.01	—	2.4	1,290,560
0.01	—	2.4	1,448,490

Basal medium contained L-asparagine 15 µg/ml

leukemic cells. L1210 and L5178Y/CA55/A-ase, both of which were totally resistant even to doses of 5,000 IU/kg daily×5 *in vivo*, showed no difference in the incorporation of ^{3}H-valine into protein in the presence or absence of A-ase. Cells from the marrows of children with acute lymphoblastic leukemia whose disease subsequently proved to be sensitive to A-ase sometimes showed a definite effect of asparagine deprivation, but this effect was not so consistent nor so marked as with cells from the A-ase sensitive mouse leukemias L5178Y, L5178Y/CA55, and EARAD1.

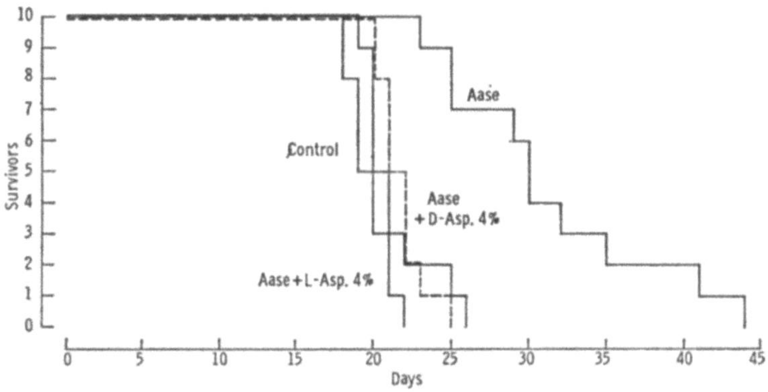

Fig. 3. Inhibition of antileukemic effect of A-ase 30 IU/kg q.d.×5×i.p. by L- or D-asparagine 4% in drinking water

The excellent correlation in mouse leukemia between *in vitro* dependence of cells on asparagine and their response to A-ase *in vivo* is better and more clear-cut than in the human leukemias. This may be partially ascribed, however, to the slower rate of metabolism of human cells and the lower percentage in the proliferative stage, and also to the fact that the leukemic cells from the mouse are a relatively pure culture, whereas the bone marrow from the patient usually has a certain admixture of normal cells. The degree of dependence on asparagine or sensitivity to A-ase in this test is greater in the sensitive mouse leukemias than in the human leukemias, even though in these particular patients unmaintained remissions of 2 to 6 months were achieved after 400 to 5,000 IU/kg of A-ase for 28 days.

It has previously been shown that a single dose of A-ase is much more effective in mouse leukemia if given on day 3 to day 7 after inoculation of the leukemic cells rather than on day 0 [10]. We have confirmed this, and studies of the half-life of A-ase in normal and in 3 to 5-day leukemic mice demonstrated the reason. As can be seen in Fig. 4, the half-life of the drug in normal BDF_1 mice is approximately 5 hours, whereas in BDF_1 mice inoculated 5 days previously either i. p. or i. c. with L5178Y/CA55 or even with EARAD1 (which does not take in these mice), it is greater than 24 hours. Further studies demonstrated that similar effects both on chemotherapeutic activity and half-life could be achieved by using filtrates of the leukemic cell suspensions. The increase in half-life caused by prior inoculation of the mice with leukemic cells either i. p. or i. c. or with filtrates strongly suggests that this effect is due not to the leukemic inoculum *per se* but rather to a filterable agent in the inoculum. The recent report by RILEY [25] of similar activity of the RILEY LDH-elevating virus suggests that this may be the explanation of our results.

Unlike most chemotherapeutic agents, A-ase by i. p. injection is effective against advanced as well as early leukemia (Fig. 1) and is also effective against leukemia inoculated intracerebrally (Fig. 5), as shown previously by DOLOWY [8, 11], although a somewhat higher dose is generally required. This chemotherapeutic effect is potentiated by bis-β-chloroethyl-nitrosourea (BCNU) (Fig. 5) and is apparently achieved without the penetration of A-ase itself into the brain or tumor since assays on brains from these mice show negligible quantities of A-ase (Fig. 6).

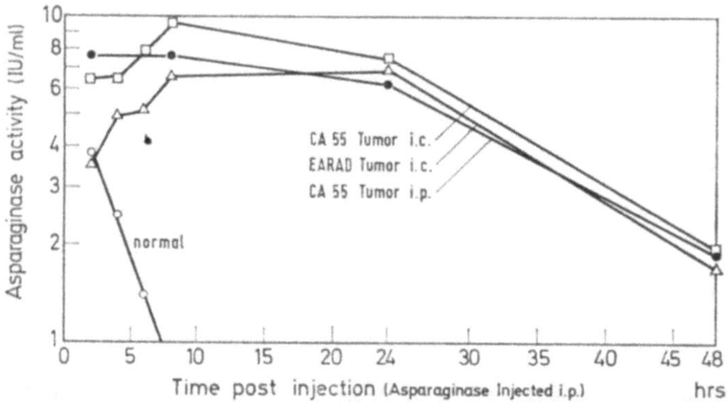

Fig. 4. Asparaginase half-life in plasma of normal and tumor-bearing BDF_1 mice

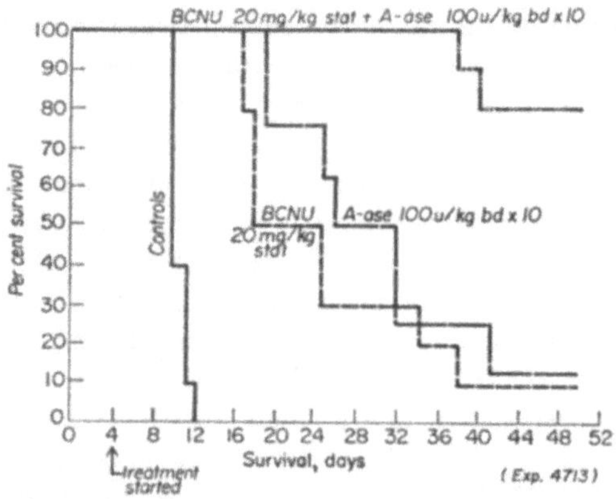

Fig. 5. Effects of L-asparaginase and BCNU on intracerebrally inoculated leukemia L5178Y clone CA55

A-ase was totally ineffective in prolonging survival time of mice withs asparagine-independent transplanted leukemias L1210 and P815 or sublines of originally dependent leukemias in which resistance to A-ase had developed (L5178Y/CA55/A-ase, EARAD1/A-ase) after passage through treated hosts.

Recently BENVENISTI, et al. in our laboratory [26—28] have studied the inhibition by A-ase of valine and thymidine incorporation in a line of resistant leukemic cells (L5178Y/CA55/A-ase) not dependent on asparagine for growth. They found that high levels (1 to 10 IU/ml) would cause 50% or greater inhibition, and that this inhibition could be completely reversed by the addition of 0.9 mg/ml of arginine or glutamine as well as by asparagine. This inhibitory effect is similar regardless of whether the A-ase is derived from agouti serum or *E. coli*, or is crystalline or amorphous, thus presumably removing the possibility that this inhibition could be due to endotoxin from *E. coli* or an associated glutaminase.

Since the combination of 1-β-D-arabinofuranosyl cytosine (Ara-C) and a purine antagonist such as mercaptopurine (6-MP) or thioguanine (TG) has been more effective than either drug alone against L1210 leukemia in mice [29] and in acute myeloblastic leukemia in man [30, 31], these drugs were studied in combination with A-ase [12, 23, 32]. Prior treatment with Ara-C or with Ara-C and TG potentiated the effect of a single dose of A-ase in a line of mouse leukemia (EARAD1) sensitive to Ara-C [32] (Fig. 7). It was considered possible that such prior therapy might in

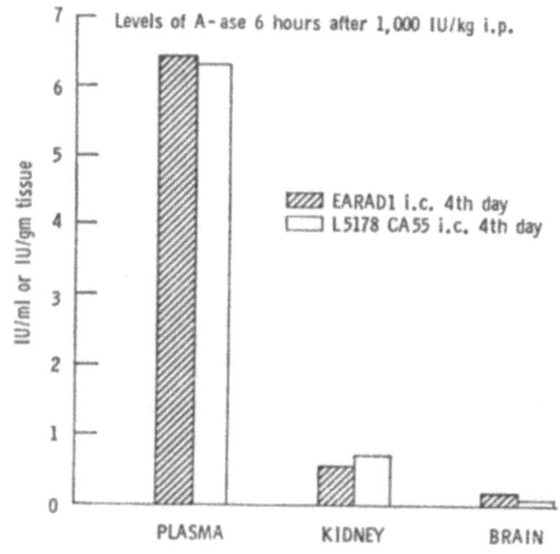

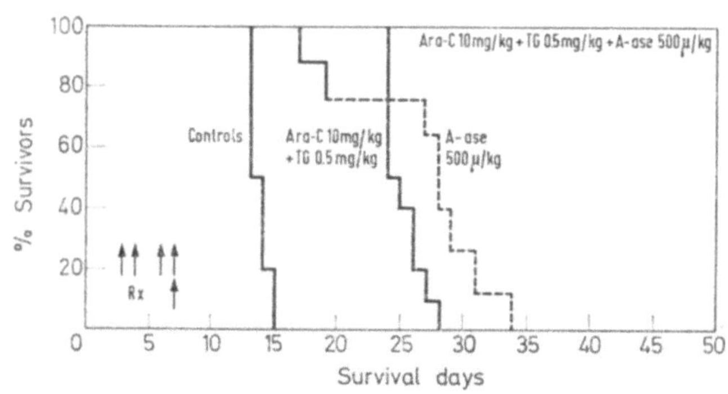

Fig. 7. Effect of prior treatment with Ara-C and TG (d3—7) on antileukemic activity of a single dose of A-ase 500 µ/kg (d.7) on leukemia EARAD1 i.p.

some way have increased the half-life of A-ase, but blood levels at various times after a single dose of 1,000 IU/kg of A-ase were similar in mice which had or had not had pre-treatment with Ara-C and TG (Fig. 8). This combination of Ara-C and A-ase was not additive in a subline of leukemia resistant to Ara-C (L5178Y/CA55),

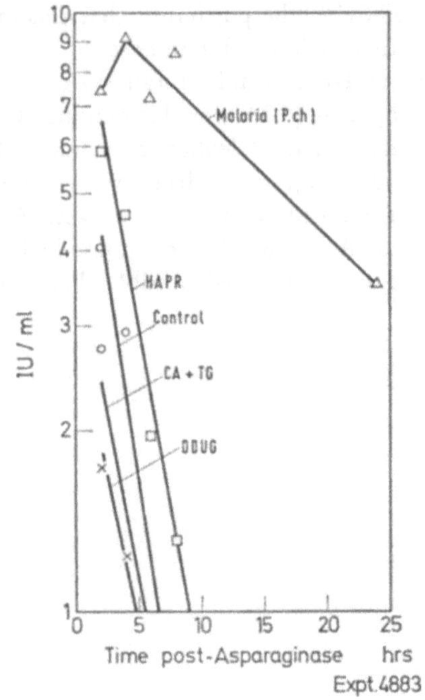

Fig. 8. Effect of prior therapy (for 5 days) or Malaria on half-life of Asparaginase (1000 IU/kg i.p.) in BDF_1 mice

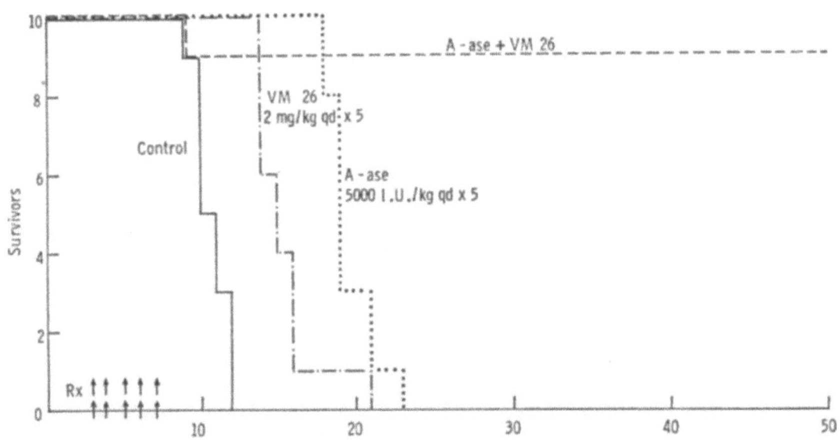

Fig. 9. Potentiation of effect of A-ase by 4′-Demethyl-epipodophyllotoxin-β-D-thenylidene-glucoside (VM-26) against leukemia L5178Y

although another inhibitor of ribonucleotide reductase, 5-hydroxy-2-formylpyridine thiosemicarbazone (5-HP) did potentiate A-ase in this leukemia.

In leukemia L5178Y, a line somephat less sensitive to A-ase than EARAD1, even large doses of A-ase (5,000 IU/kg qdx5) will only increase survival time and will not produce cures. When this dose of A-ase is given in combination, however, with a variety of antileukemic agents, most only slightly to moderately active alone, a high percentage of cures is achieved [32]. The Vinca alkaloids, vincristine (VCR) [32] and vinblastine (VLB), 4-demethyl-epipodophyllotoxin-β-D-thenyliden glucoside (VM-26) (Fig. 9), the antibiotics, Actinomycin D (Fig. 10), Daunomycin [32] and Adriamycin (Fig. 11), and the antimetabolites, Methotrexate, 5-HP (Fig. 12), 6-hydroxylaminopurine [12] and diacetyldiphenylurea-bis-guanyl-hydrazone

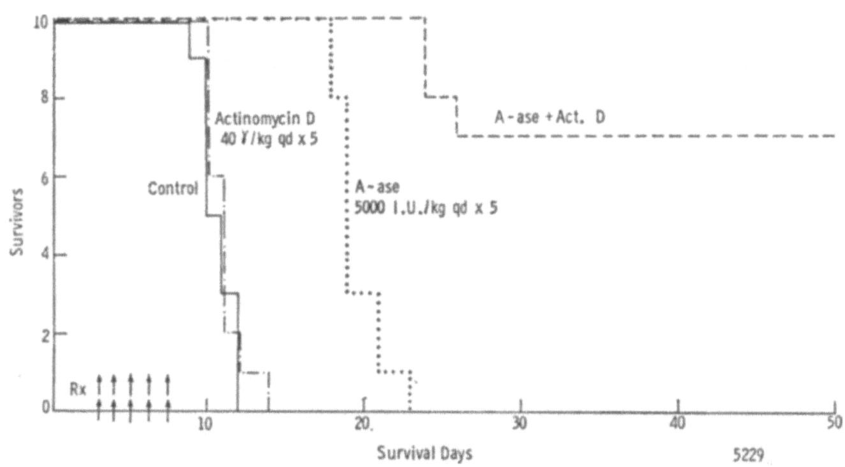

Fig. 10. Potentiation of effect of A-ase by Actinomycin D against leukemia L5178Y

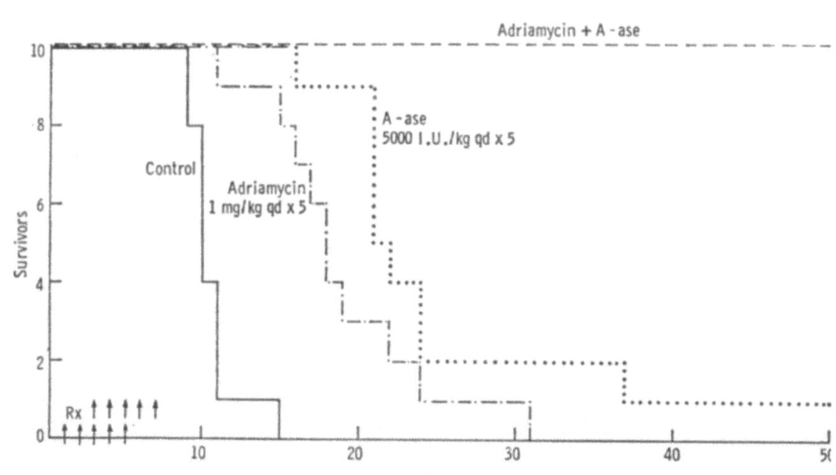

Fig. 11. Potentiation of effect of A-ase by Adriamycin against leukemia L5178Y

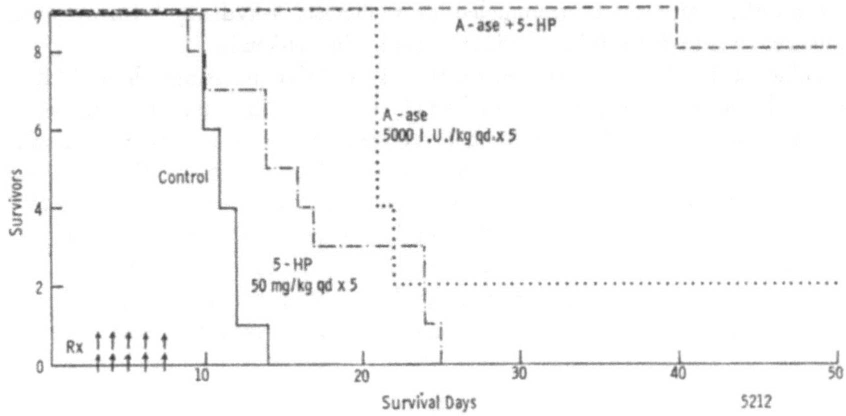

Fig. 12. Potentiation of effect of A-ase by 5-Hydroxy-2-formylpyridine thiosemicarbazone (5-HP) against leukemia L5178Y

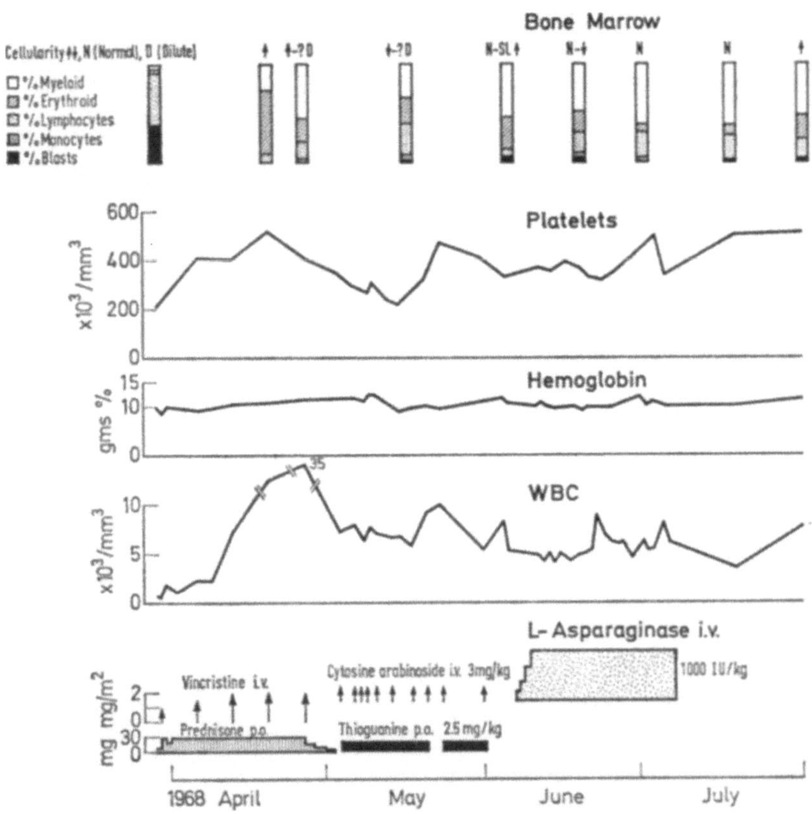

Fig. 13. D.I. 3 1/12 ♀ acute lymphoblastic leukemia

(DDUG) [12] are all monotonously active in potentiating the antileukemic effects of A-ase, although no common denominator in their mechanism of action has become apparent as yet. In most cases these compounds seem to be more effective when given before or simultaneously with the first dose of A-ase rather than afterwards. Increased toxicity on simultaneous daily administration has been noted with some combinations, particularly in mice with leukemia EARAD1.

These combinations are now being studied clinically [23], and it has become apparent that the simultaneous administration of A-ase, VCR, and Daunomycin is associated with increased manifestations of VCR and Daunomycin toxicity. A possible explanation of this may be that the impairment in liver function due to the A-ase may delay the metabolism or excretion of VCR and Daunomycin by the liver. It is too early to tell whether therapeutic benefit in the form of long-term unmaintained remissions will result from this regimen.

Because of the somewhat increased toxicity following simultaneous administration, these drugs are being given sequentially in some patients. Thus a course of VCR and prednisone would be given for 4 weeks, followed by Ara-C and TG for 4 weeks, followed by A-ase 1,000 IU/kg daily, again for 4 weeks, after which no maintenance therapy would be given. Two patients who have received such treatment are still in unmaintained remission for over 13 and 15 months, respectively, since the discontinuation of therapy (Fig. 13).

The 50-day cures in mice achieved by A-ase in combination suggest that it might be possible in this manner to destroy more leukemic cells than with either drug alone, and thus, perhaps in some patients by the combination of these drugs with A-ase simultaneously or sequentially, the eradication of all leukemic cells might be achieved [23, 32].

References

1. Kidd, J. G.: Regression of transplanted lymphomas induced *in vivo* by means of normal guinea pig serum. I. Course of transplanted cancers of various kinds in mice and rats given guinea pig serum, horse serum, or rabbit serum. J. Exper. Med. **98**, 565 (1953).
2. — Regression of transplanted lymphomas induced *in vivo* by means of normal guinea pig serum. II. Studies on the nature of the active serum constituent: Histological mechanism of the regression: Tests for effects of guinea pig serum on lymphoma cells *in vitro:* Discussion. J. Exper. Med. **98**, 583 (1953).
3. Broome, J. D.: Evidence that the L-asparaginase activity of guinea pig serum is responsible for its antilymphoma effects. Nature **191**, 1114 (1961).
4. — Evidence that the L-asparaginase of guinea pig serum is responsible for its antilymphoma effects. I. Properties of the L-asparaginase of guinea pig serum in relation to those of the antilymphoma substance. J. Exper. Med. **118**, 99 (1963).
5. — Antilymphoma activity of L-asparaginase *in vivo:* Clearance rates of enzyme preparations from guinea pig serum and yeast in relation to their effect on tumor growth. J. Nat. Cancer Inst. **35**, 967 (1965).
6. Old, L. J., Boyse, E. A., Campbell, H. A., Aria, G. M.: Leukaemia-inhibiting properties and L-asparaginase activity of sera from certain South American rodents. Nature **198**, 801 (1963).
7. Mashburn, L. T., Wriston, J. C.: Tumor inhibitory effect of L-asparaginase from *Escherichia coli.* Arch. Biochem. Biophys. **105**, 450 (1964).
8. Dolowy, W. C., Cornet, J., Henson, D., Ammeraal, R.: Response of intracerebral Gardner lymphoma to guinea pig L-asparaginase and *Escherichia coli* L-asparaginase. Proc. Soc. exp. Biol. (N. Y.) **123**, 133 (1966).

9. CAMPBELL, H. A., MASHBURN, L. T., BOYSE, E. A., OLD, L. J.: Two L-asparaginases from *Escherichia coli* B. Their separation, purification, and antitumor activity. Biochemistry **6**, 721 (1967).
10. BOYSE, E. A., OLD, L. J., CAMPBELL, H. A., MASHBURN, L. T.: Suppression of murine leukemias by L-asparaginase. J. Exper. Med. **125**, 17 (1967).
11. BURCHENAL, J. H., LASH, E., SCHWARTZ, M., DOLLINGER, M.: Effects and concentrations of L-asparaginase in intracerebrally inoculated leukemia. Proc. Amer. Ass. Cancer Res. **9**, 10 (1968).
12. — DOLLINGER, M. R.: L-asparaginase in transplanted mouse leukemia. XIIth Congress, Internatl. Soc. Hematology, New York, 1968. Abstracts of the Simultaneous Sessions, p. 6 (1968).
13. ADAMSON, R. H., FABRO, S.: Antitumor activity and other biologic properties of L-asparaginase (NSC-109229). A. Review. Cancer Chemother. Rep. **52**, 617 (1968).
14. COONEY, D. A., HANDSCHUMACHER, R. E.: Investigation of L-asparagine metabolism in animals and human subjects. Proc. Amer. Ass. Cancer Res. **9**, 15 (1968).
15. HILL, J. M., ROBERTS, J., LOEB, E., KHAN, A., MACLELLAN, A., HILL, R. W.: L-asparaginase therapy for leukemia and other malignant neoplasms. J.A.M.A. **202**, 882 (1967).
16. OETTGEN, H. F., OLD, L. J., BOYSE, E. A., CAMPBELL, H. A., PHILLIPS, F. S., CLARKSON, B. D., TALLAL, L., LEEPER, R. D., SCHWARTZ, M. K., KIM, J. H.: Inhibition of leukemias in man by L-asparaginase. Cancer Res. **27**, 2619 (1967).
17. HASKELL, C. M., CANELLOS, G. P., LEVENTHAL, B. G., CARBONE, P. P., SERPICK, A. A., HANSEN, H. H.: L-asparaginase toxicity. Cancer Res. **29**, 974 (1969).
18. HILL, J. M., LOEB, E., MACLELLAN, A., KHAN, A., ROBERTS, J., SHIELDS, W. F., HILL, N. O.: Response to highly purified L-asparaginase during therapy of acute leukemia. Cancer Res. **29**, 1574 (1969).
19. SCHWARTZ, M. K., LASH, E. D., OETTGEN, H. F., TOMAO, F. A.: L-asparaginase activity in plasma and other biological fluids. Cancer **25**, 244 (1970).
20. OETTGEN, H. F., STEPHENSON, P. A., SCHWARTZ, M. K., LEEPER, R. D., TALLAL, L., TAN, C. C., CLARKSON, B. D., GOLBEY, R. B., KRAKOFF, I. H., KARNOFSKY, D. A., MURPHY, M. L., BURCHENAL, J. H.: The toxicity of *E. coli* L-asparaginase in man. Cancer **25**, 253 (1970).
21. CLARKSON, B. D., KRAKOFF, I., BURCHENAL, J., KARNOFSKY, D., GOLBEY, R., DOWLING, M., OETTGEN, H., LIPTON, A.: Clinical results of treatment with *E. coli* L-asparaginase in adults with leukemia, lymphoma and solid tumors. Cancer **25**, 279 (1970).
22. TALLAL, L., TAN, C., OETTGEN, H., WOLLNER, N., MCCARTHY, M., HELSON, L., BURCHENAL, J., KARNOFSKY, D., MURPHY, M. L.: *E. coli* L-asparaginase in the treatment of leukemia and solid tumors in 131 children. Cancer **25**, 306 (1970).
23. BURCHENAL, J. H.: Clinical evaluation and future prospects of asparaginase. Editor, please correct and/or complete: In: Mathé, G., ed.: Recent Results in Cancer Research, Vol. 30. Berlin-Heidelberg-New York: Springer 1970.
24. OHNUMA, T., BERGEL, F., BRAY, R. C.: Enzymes in Cancer. Asparaginase from chicken liver. Biochem. J. **103**, 238 (1967).
25. RILEY, V.: Role of the LDH-elevating virus in leukaemie therapy by asparaginase. Nature **220**, 1245 (1968).
26. BENVENISTI, D. S., BURCHENAL, J. H., VALLIER, J., HOROWITZ, H., MILLER, H. K., OCHOA, M., JR.: Inhibition of protein and nucleic acid syntheses in resistant mouse leukemias (L5178Y/CA55/A-ase, EARADl/A-ase, P815) and normal human lymphocytes ($SKLN_1$) by Agouti serum and *E. coli* L-asparaginase. Proc. 12th Ann. Meeting, Amer. Soc. Hematology, Cleveland, 1969.
27. BENVENISTI, D., BURCHENAL, J. H., OCHOA, M., JR.: Inhibition of protein and nucleic acid synthesis in cells of asparaginase-sensitive mouse and human leukemias by L-asparaginase *(in vitro)*. In preparation, to be submitted to Cancer Research.
28. — — HOROWITZ, B., MILLER, H. K., OCHOA, M., JR.: Inhibition of protein and nucleic acid synthesis in asparaginase-resistant mouse leukemia cells and human lymphocytes by L-asparaginase *(in vitro)*. In preparation, to be submitted to Cancer Research.

29. Burchenal, J. H., Dollinger, M. R.: Cytosine arabinoside (NSC-63878) in combination with 6-mercaptopurine (NSC-755), methotrexate (NSC-740), or 5-fluorouracil (NSC-19893) in L1210 mouse leukemia. Cancer Chemother. Rep. **51**, 435 (1967).
30. Gee, T. S., Yu, K. P., Augustin, B. T., Krakoff, I. H., Clarkson, B. D.: Combination therapy of adult acute leukemia with thioguanine (TG) and 1-β-D-arabinofuranosyl-cytosine (CA). Proc. Amer. Ass. Cancer Res. **9**, 23 (1968).
31. — — Clarkson, B. D.: Treatment of adult acute leukemia with arabinosylcytosine and thioguanine. Cancer **23**, 1019 (1969).
32. Burchenal, J. H.: Success and failure in present chemotherapy and the implications of asparaginase. Cancer Res. **29**, 2262 (1969).

Experimental Investigations on Problems of the Clinical Use of L-Asparaginase

R. Bierling

Institute of Experimental Pathology of Farbenfabriken Bayer A.G., Wuppertal-Elberfeld, Germany

With 10 Figures

Introduction

In 1968 sufficient L-asparaginase (Crasnitin) [1] became available from our own production to start clinical trials. At this time we thought it would be useful to study experimentally problems which arose from the clinical use of the enzyme. Consequently we investigated the influence of the following factors on tumor inhibition: dosage, duration of treatment, treatment schedules, treatment of Crasnitin resistant tumors, combined treatment with Crasnitin, and immunological factors in enzyme therapy.

Materials and Methods

The L-asparaginase used was produced in the Bayer factory and is designated as E.C. 3.5.1.1. from type 2 of Escherichia coli strain ATCC 9637.

Our experiments were performed on mouse leukemia EARAD 1 which we obtained by courtesy of Dr. Old from the Sloan-Kettering Institute.

In our laboratory this radiation-induced leukemia is maintained in its ascitic form in isogenic (C51BL/6×A)F1 mice. For experiments it is transplanted subcutaneously where local tumors develop initially.

Usually Crasnitin treatment was started on day 8 after inoculation when these tumors had a diameter of 5—8 mm. After effective doses of the enzyme the tumor totally regressed within 3—5 days. After small effective doses the remaining viable leukemia cells of the tumor spread into various organs, particularly into liver and kidney. Such animals died of generalized leukemia. After high effective doses the recurrence developed at the site of transplantation. These animals were killed by the recurring local tumors.

From the Crasnitin-susceptible leukemia EARAD 1 we developed a subline resistant to the enzyme. Its resistance to the effects of the enzyme is being maintained by treating the passage animals with 5×1000 U/kg.

[1] List of registered trade marks used in this paper on page 124.

The following tables contain the details of dose, frequency and route of administration. The parameters of evaluation are 1. the mean survival time (expressed as per cent of the survival time of the controls) and 2. the cure rate (percent of cured animals). In our figures black bars signify the survival time index, shaded bars the rate of cures.

Results

1. Dosage

The question of the optimal dose of Crasnitin has not yet been clearly answered.

The effect of the dose on survival time and cure rate in our test system is shown in Fig. 1. In these experiments the total dose consisted of 5 daily injections on 5 consecutive days. The upper curve demonstrates that the cure rate increased up to a total dose of about 10,000 U/kg or 5 daily doses of 2000 U/kg respectively. With higher doses the anti-tumor effect seemed to reach a plateau, and no significant

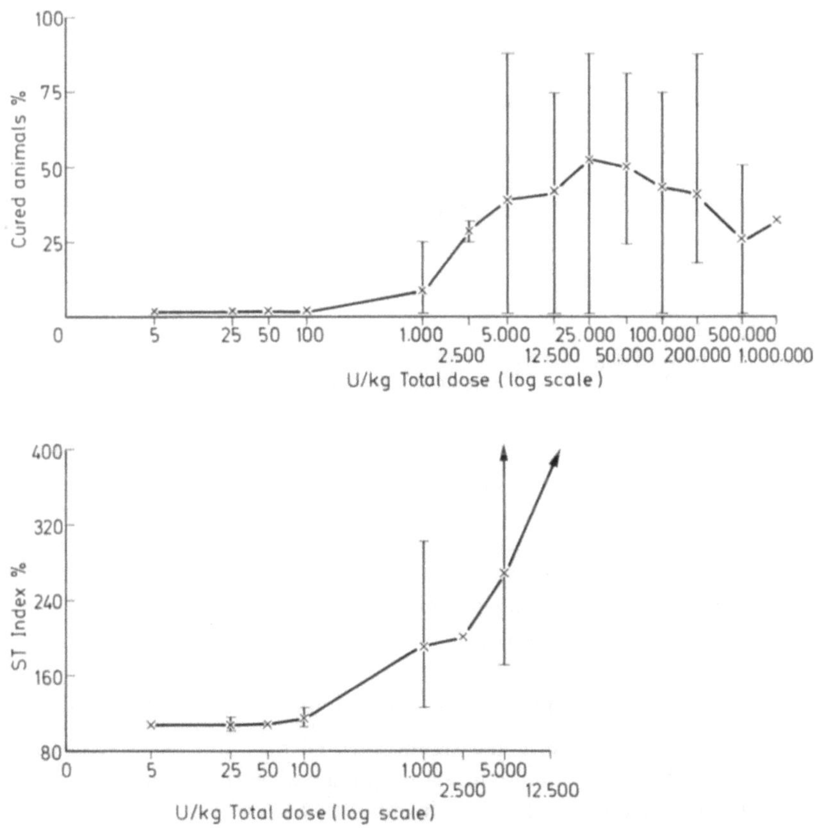

Fig. 1. Effect of increasing total doses of Crasnitin on cure rate (upper curve) and survival time (lower curve) of mice bearing EARAD 1-leukemia. Total doses consist of 5 daily injections on 5 consecutive days

increase of the cure rate was obtained. Doses higher than approximately 500,000 U/kg proved to be toxic. The lower curve shows the increase of the survival time index in the same dose range.

The increase of both parameters with daily doses of up to 40,000 U/kg is presented in Fig. 2.

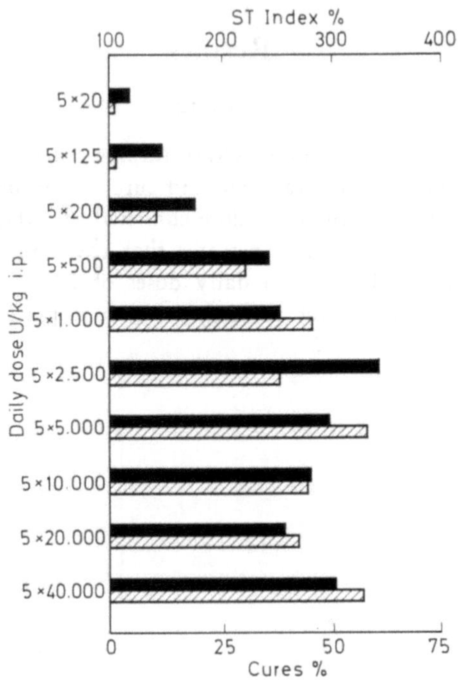

Fig. 2. Survival time and cure rate after 5 administrations of increasing daily doses of Crasnitin. Bars represent average values from at least 5 experiments. (Survival time: black bars, cure rate: hatched bars. These symbols have been used in all other figures.)

It is evident, that in the test system of leukemia EARAD 1 daily doses of 200 U/kg were at the lower border of antitumor activity.

In order to see whether there is a plateau of effectiveness we carried out an experiment where 20×500 or 20×5000 U Crasnitin/kg were administered within a period of 4 weeks. The result is shown in Fig. 3. Within the range of the plateau even a total dose of 100,000 U/kg obviously did not improve the rate of cures compared with cures after 10,000 U/kg.

2. Duration of Treatment, Frequency of Administration, Total Dose

Our next aim was to study the significance of the duration of treatment with Crasnitin. Fig. 4 shows the tumor inhibition obtained with an increasing number of injections of the same dose, in this experiment of 200 U/kg.

When Crasnitin was administered 1×daily (left graph) the survival time index significantly increased with an increasing number of daily doses. The trend of the cure rate was not as clear.

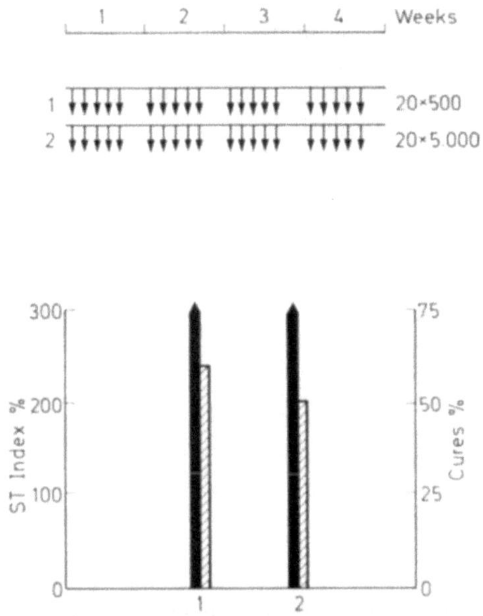

Fig. 3. Cure rate and survival time after the administration of 20×500 and 20×5000 U Crasnitin/kg respectively within a period of 4 weeks

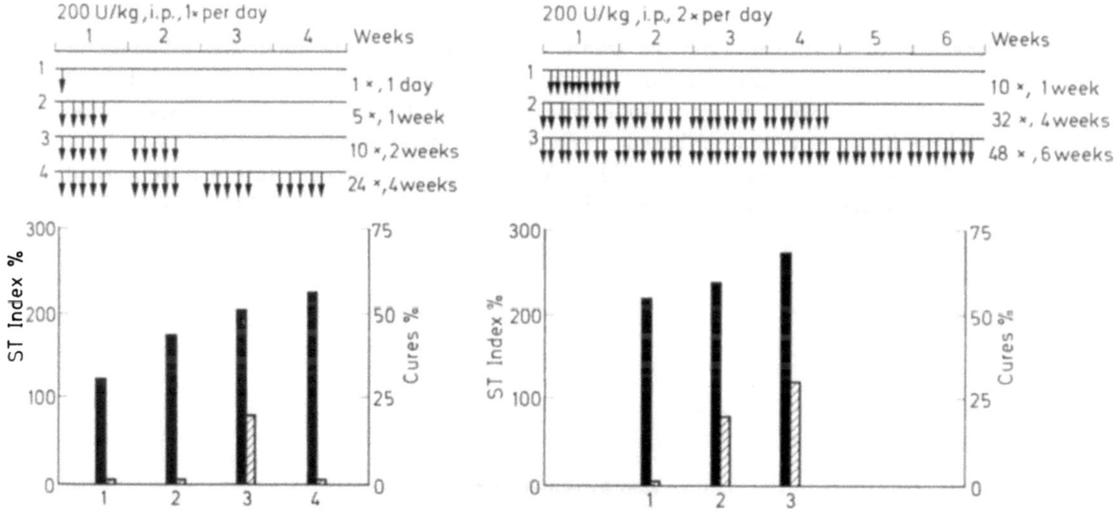

Fig. 4. Influence on survival time and cure rate of an increasing number of injections of 200 U Crasnitin/kg (longer duration of treatment). Left: 1× daily, right: 2× daily. (Bars are numbered according to treatment schedule.)

The right graph demonstrates, however, that, when 200 U/kg were administered 2× daily, the cure rate also increased with an increased number of injections.

Another question was what would happen if a constant total dose was split up into different daily doses which consequently would lead to a different duration of treatment. The results of this experimental series are presented in Fig. 5. Irrespective of the daily dose the effect increased corresponding to a longer duration of treatment.

Both these experiments demonstrate the significance of an adaequate duration of Crasnitin treatment for tumor inhibition.

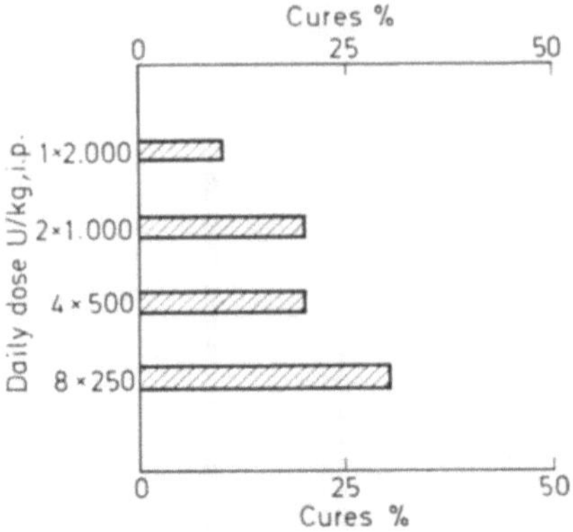

Fig. 5. Influence on cure rate of different numbers of injections adding up to the same total dose. A single dose of 2000 U Crasnitin/kg had been split up into partial doses

3. Schedules of Treatment

Our next investigation dealt with the therapeutic effectiveness of different schedules of treatment. First we wanted to know something about the influence of intervals between two injections of Crasnitin. For this study a constant total dose of 4800 U/kg was split up into single doses of 1200, 400 and 200 U/kg, respectively. These daily doses were distributed over a constant period of 4 weeks.

The results are presented in Fig. 6. With regard to the cure rate 4 injections of 1200 U/kg once weekly were less effective than 12 injections of 400 U/kg 3× per

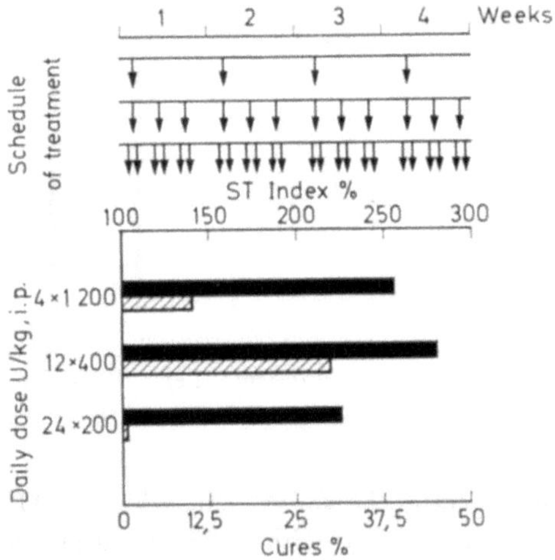

Fig. 6. Effect of intervals between different doses on leukemia inhibition. Different partial doses derived from a constant total dose were administered within a period of 4 weeks

week. The administration of 24×200 U/kg 6× weekly, however, just prolonged the survival time of the mice but did not result in cures.

The last results are related to the influence of dose and half life of Crasnitin on the tumor inhibition. Both factors are responsible for the duration and the degree of the tumor inhibiting asparagine depletion of blood and tissues. If with low doses the short half life of the enzyme reduces its effectiveness very early this reduction could be compensated for by shorter intervals of administration. This is shown in Fig. 7. When we administered 10×125 U/kg in intervals of only 8 instead of 24 hours the survival time increased considerably and the cure of a mouse was obtained which had not been observed in numerous previous experiments using the same dose.

Referring to the relation of dose, half life and tumor inhibition we wanted to correlate the asparagine deprivation induced by different doses of Crasnitin with its

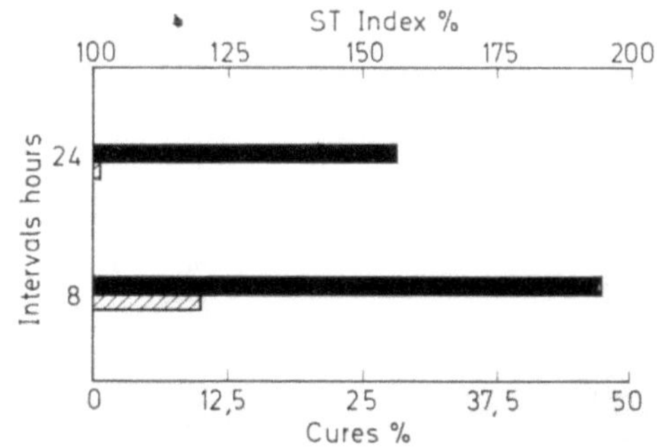

Fig. 7. Effect of intervals between similar doses on leukemia inhibition. 10×125 U Crasnitin/kg were administered at intervals of 24 and 8 hours, respectively

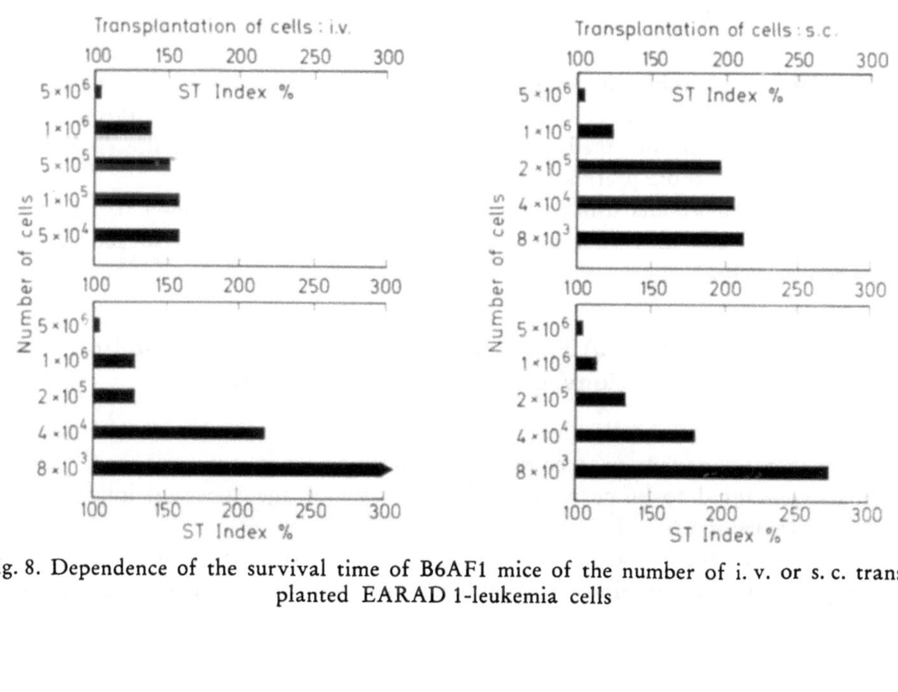

Fig. 8. Dependence of the survival time of B6AF1 mice of the number of i. v. or s. c. transplanted EARAD 1-leukemia cells

tumor inhibitory effect in blood and tissues. This work is based on the fact that the survival time of mice depends of the number of viable EARAD 1 cells left after the enzyme treatment (Fig. 8).

In this experiment mice free of leukemia were treated once i. p. with different doses of the enzyme. 4, 8, 16 and 24 hours later these animals were inoculated with 5×10^6 cells i. v. or s. c. These cells were transplanted into a more or less asparagine depleted environment. The results of these assays are presented in Fig. 9. In the left diagram cells were transplanted subcutaneously into i. p. pretreated mice. This graph shows clearly the dependence of the survival time and cures of the factors regulating asparagine depletion as existing in subcutaneous tissues.

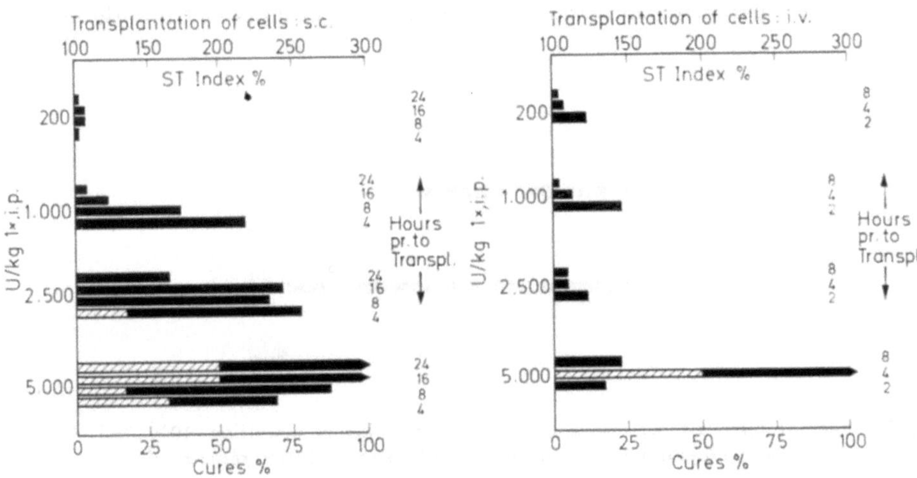

Fig. 9. Leukemia inhibition after a single dose of Crasnitin (i. p. or i. v.) prior to the transplantation (i. v. or s. c.) of EARAD 1-leukemia cells

The right graph represents similar experiments in which after the i. v. pretreatment of the animals tumor cells were transplanted intravenously. In this assay the i. v. transplanted cells survived and killed the animals within the life span of the controls, except for those pretreated with 5000 U/kg.

Comparing the results using the same doses and the same timing it may be of interest to state the difference of tumor inhibition in blood and in subcutaneous tissues respectively.

4. Treatment of EARAD 1-R Tumors Resistant to Crasnitin with Conventional Anti-Tumor Agents

The question of the following studies was how to overcome a serious limit of Crasnitin therapy, namely enzyme resistant recurrences.

First we wanted to know what kind of anti-tumor agents would influence such recurrent tumors of EARAD 1-leukemia.

The results of these trials are contained in Table 1. It shows that actinomycin C (Sanamycin), cytosine-arabinoside, Melphalan and Natulan are effective against such

Table 1. *Effect of anti-tumor agents in EARAD 1-R-tumors resistant against crasnitin*

Agent [a]	Dose mg/kg	Survival time index %	Cures %
Crasnitin	5×1000 U/kg	100.0	0
Actinomycin C	5×0.1	125.0	0
6-Azauracil	4×150	100.0	0
Cytosine-arabinoside	4×40	146.7	0
Endoxan	3×50	100.0	0
5-Fluorouracil	4×20	100.0	0
Melphalan	4×10	133.3	0
Myleran	4×40	106.7	0
6-Mercaptopurin	5×25	106.3	0
Methotrexat	5×2	112.5	0
Natulan	4×300	153.3	0
Proresid	4×100	106.7	0
Rubidomycin	4×3	106.7	0
6-Thioguanin	4×30	121.4	0
Trenimon	3×0.08	95.9	0
Vincristin	5×0.5	114.3	0

[a] List of registered trade marks on page 124.

resistant EARAD 1-R-tumors. With these agents a significant increase of survival time is obtained.

5. Combined Treatment of EARAD 1-Tumors with Crasnitin plus other Anti-Tumor Agents

In order to prevent the development of resistance, in the past years the chemotherapy of tumors has tended more and more towards the combination of various drugs. An optimal combination of drugs with Crasnitin is still being developed.

For this reason we tried to evaluate the effect of the combined treatment of Crasnitin plus various other anti-tumor agents. In these trials the order of administration of the substance varied: first the agent was administered prior to, then alternating with and finally after the enzyme.

Table 2 contains the results of these assays. The combination of Crasnitin with actinomycin C (Sanamycin), cytosine-arabinoside, Vincristin, Melphalan, Natulan and Proresid, considerably increased the survival time of mice. This enhancement was mostly observed if these drugs were administered after the treatment with the enzyme. Besides Natulan and Vincristin this enhancement of tumor inhibition could not be obtained with a reversed sequence of the drugs.

6. Immunological Factors of Enzyme Treatment

Besides the development of resistance immunological factors may be a further limit for enzyme therapy.

In the serum of asparaginase treated patients the occurrence of specific antibodies against the enzyme was ascertained by KHAN and coworkers. This finding raised the question as to whether the combination of immunosuppressive drugs with Crasnitin would inhibit the development of these antibodies.

Table 2. *Combined treatment with crasnitin plus other anti-tumor agents*

Agent	Dose mg/kg	Agent alone		Agent combined with 5×125 U Crasnitin/kg		
		ST Index %	Cures %	Sequence of agents	ST Index %	Cures %
Crasnitin	5×125 U/kg	140	0	—	—	—
Actinomycin C	3×0.1	125	0	2.	225	38
Cytosine-arabinoside	4×30	133	0	2.	207	0
Endoxan	3×80	114	0	2.	143	0
5-Fluorouracil	3×20	114	0	2.	143	0
Melphalan	4×7.5	127	0	1.	167	0
6-Mercaptopurin	3×50	107	0	2.	147	0
Methotrexat	3×4	114	0	2.	143	0
Natulan	4×300	167	0	1.+2.	187	0
Proresid	4×100	113	0	2.	160	0
Rubidomycin	3×2	100	0	2.	163	0
6-Thioguanin	4×20	139	0	2.	154	0
Trenimon	3×0.1	107	0	2.	136	0
Vincristin	5×0.5	125	0	1.	181	0

For this assay we designed a scheme which is outlined in Table 3. Group 6 of this schedule shows that prior to the transplantation of tumor cells antibody formation was to be induced by the treatment of mice with 7×1000 U/kg. One week later cells of EARAD 1-leukemia were transplanted subcutaneously. Another 8 days later Crasnitin treatment of the developing tumors with 5×1000 U/kg was started. In the experimental group 8 this Crasnitin tumor therapy was combined with actinomycin C known for its immunosuppressive properties. The other experimental groups just served as controls.

Fig. 10 shows the results of this assay. The bars are numbered according to the experimental groups in Table 3. The meaning of these different bars is as follows.

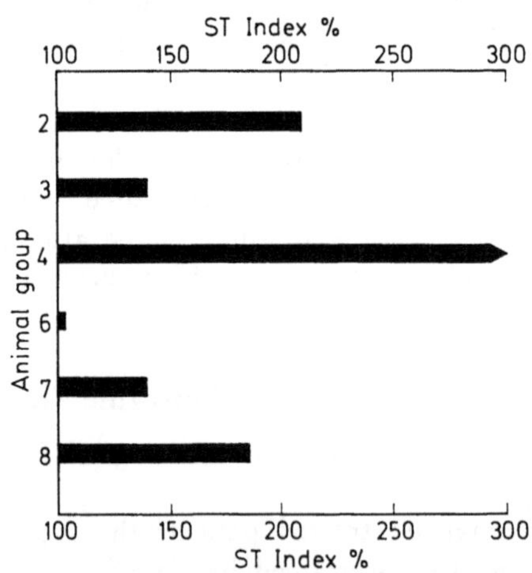

Fig. 10. Effect of antibodies against asparaginase on the inhibition of leukemia by Crasnitin treatment (6) and prevention of this effect by the combined treatment with actinomycin C (8). (Bars are numbered according to the schedule in Table 3.)

Table 3. *Immunological factors in crasnitin treatment*

1. Scheme of treatment

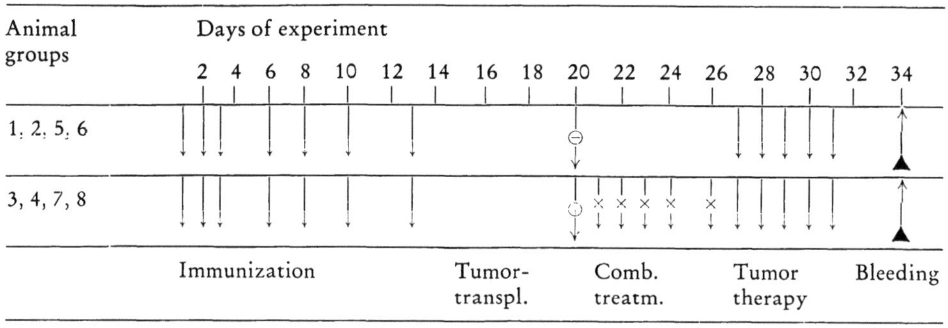

2. Animal groups

Group	Immunization	Combined treatment	Tumor therapy
1	Contr. NaCl 7×0.3 ml	Contr. NaCl 6×0.3 ml	Contr. NaCl 5×0.3 ml
2	Contr. NaCl 7×0.3 ml	Contr. NaCl 6×0.3 ml	Crasnitin 5×1000 U/kg
3	Contr. NaCl 7×0.3 ml	Actinomycin C 6×0.1 mg/kg	Contr. NaCl 5×0.3 ml
4	Contr. NaCl 7×0.3 ml	Actinomycin C 6×0.1 mg/kg	Crasnitin 5×1000 U/kg
5	Crasnitin 7×1000 U/kg	Contr. NaCl 6×0.3 ml	Contr. NaCl 5×0.3 ml
6	Crasnitin 7×1000 U/kg	Contr. NaCl 6×0.3 ml	Crasnitin 5×1000 U/kg
7	Crasnitin 7×1000 U/kg	Actinomycin C 6×0.1 mg/kg	Contr. NaCl 5×0.3 ml
8	Crasnitin 7×1000 U/kg	Actinomycin C 6×0.1 mg/kg	Crasnitin 5×1000 U/kg

Bar 2: NaCl pretreatment. Inhibition of EARAD 1-leukemia after Crasnitin therapy.

Bar 3: NaCl pretreatment. Leukemia inhibition after therapy with actinomycin C.

Bar 4: NaCl pretreatment. Inhibition of leukemia after combined therapy with Crasnitin plus actinomycin C.

Bar 6: Pre-immunization with Crasnitin. Prevention of the usual leukemia inhibition after Crasnitin therapy.

Bar 7: Pre-immunization with Crasnitin. Leukemia inhibition by therapy with actinomycin C.

Bar 8: Pre-immunization with Crasnitin. By the combined therapy with actinomycin C plus Crasnitin the prevention of leukemia inhibition in group 6 is reversed.

In addition to these animal experiments Truscheit demonstrated by immunoelectrophoresis that in group 6 the serum of mice showed a significant amount of antibodies against Crasnitin while in group 8 this amount was only small.

These results correspond with the prevention of Crasnitin induced tumor inhibition in group 6 and with the reversal of this result by the combined treatment with actinomycin C in group 8. With regard to the eventual formation of antibodies against the enzyme this finding suggests the use of cytostatic agents with immunosuppressive properties in combination with Crasnitin.

Summary

Under the experimental conditions used we demonstrated that within a certain range tumor inhibition increases with the dose of Crasnitin. However, beyond this range, higher doses do not further increase the rate of cures.

The therapeutic index may reach extraordinary high values, an indication for the leukemia specific mechanism of the action of Crasnitin.

Another investigation demonstrated the significance of an adaequate duration of enzyme treatment.

The effect on tumor inhibition of various treatment schemes demonstrated the relative influence of dose, interval and duration of therapy with Crasnitin.

The correlation of tumor inhibition in blood and subcutaneous tissues with dose and timing of Crasnitin pretreatment was studied. The results demonstrated a clear dependence of both factors and additionally striking differences of tumor inhibition in blood and subcutaneous tissues.

Another series of assays dealt with limiting factors of therapy. Crasnitin resistant tumors could be inhibited using actinomycin C (Sanamycin), cytosine-arabinoside, Melphalan and Natulan.

The same agents as well as Vincristine, and Proresid in combination with Crasnitin enhanced the effects of the enzyme. For this effect a certain sequence of the agents used appears to be essential.

The formation of antibodies to Crasnitin may further limit therapy. In our investigation of immunological factors, the inactivation of Crasnitin by such antibodies could be reversed by treatment with actinomycin C prior to enzyme therapy.

The names of agents used in this paper are registered trade marks of the following firms:

Crasnitin	Farbenfabriken Bayer AG., Leverkusen/Germany
Endoxan	Asta-Werke AG.
Melphalan	Burroughs Wellcome & Co.
Methotrexat	Lederle, Arzneimittel, Abt. der Cyanamid GmbH.
Myleran	Burroughs Wellcome & Co.
Natulan	Hoffmann-LaRoche AG.
Proresid	Sandoz AG.
Trenimon	Farbenfabriken Bayer AG., Leverkusen/Germany
Vincristin	Eli Lilly & Co.

Studies on the Glutaminase Activity of E. coli Asparaginase in Tissue Culture*

H. OERKERMANN, W. D. HIRSCHMANN, and R. GROSS

Medizinische Universitätsklinik Köln, Germany

With 6 Figures

The use of E. coli asparaginase in the treatment of neoplastic diseases is based on the assumption that asparaginase sensitive tumors or leukemias have lost the ability to synthesize L-asparagine and thus depend on the exogenous supply of this amino acid. Yet it is not always sufficiently considered that E. coli asparaginase also possesses a small amount of L-glutaminase activity [1] and in high dosage may become effective by depriving the cells of L-glutamine.

First we studied the effect of E. coli asparaginase on HeLa cells which we found to be highly sensitive. The cells became spindle-shaped and their growth was inhibited corresponding to the administered dosage of E. coli asparaginase. Large doses rapidly destroyed the whole culture (Figs. 1 and 2).

A decrease in the uptake of ^{14}C-leucine noted as early as one hour after the addition of E. coli asparaginase indicated a diminished protein synthesis. A reduced incorporation of ^{14}C-thymidine demonstrated the inhibition of the DNA turnover. The uptake of ^{14}C-uridine was normal or, in some of the experiments, even increased. Nevertheless, the incorporation of ^{14}C-uridine into the acid insoluble cell fraction was reduced (Fig. 3).

EAGLE and co-workers [2] have shown that HeLa cells are L-glutamine-dependent. Cultivating HeLa cells in EAGLE's Minimum Essential Medium (MEM) which contained neither asparagine nor glutamine we observed that the addition of L-glutamine improved the growth of the cells whereas the addition of L-asparagine did not. The combined addition of L-asparagine and L-glutamine gave no better results than that of L-glutamine alone (Fig. 4). These results suggest that the effects on HeLa cells mentioned above were due to the L-glutaminase component of E. coli asparaginase. We found further proof for this assumption in the observation that guinea pig serum which contains L-asparaginase but no glutaminase activity did not inhibit the growth of the HeLa cell cultures. Similar results were obtained by KIM and coworkers [3].

Subsequent experiments with HeLa cells in MEM revealed that the addition of L-glutamic acid improved the conditions for cell growth only to a slight extent. On

---

* This study was supported by the Deutsche Forschungsgemeinschaft.

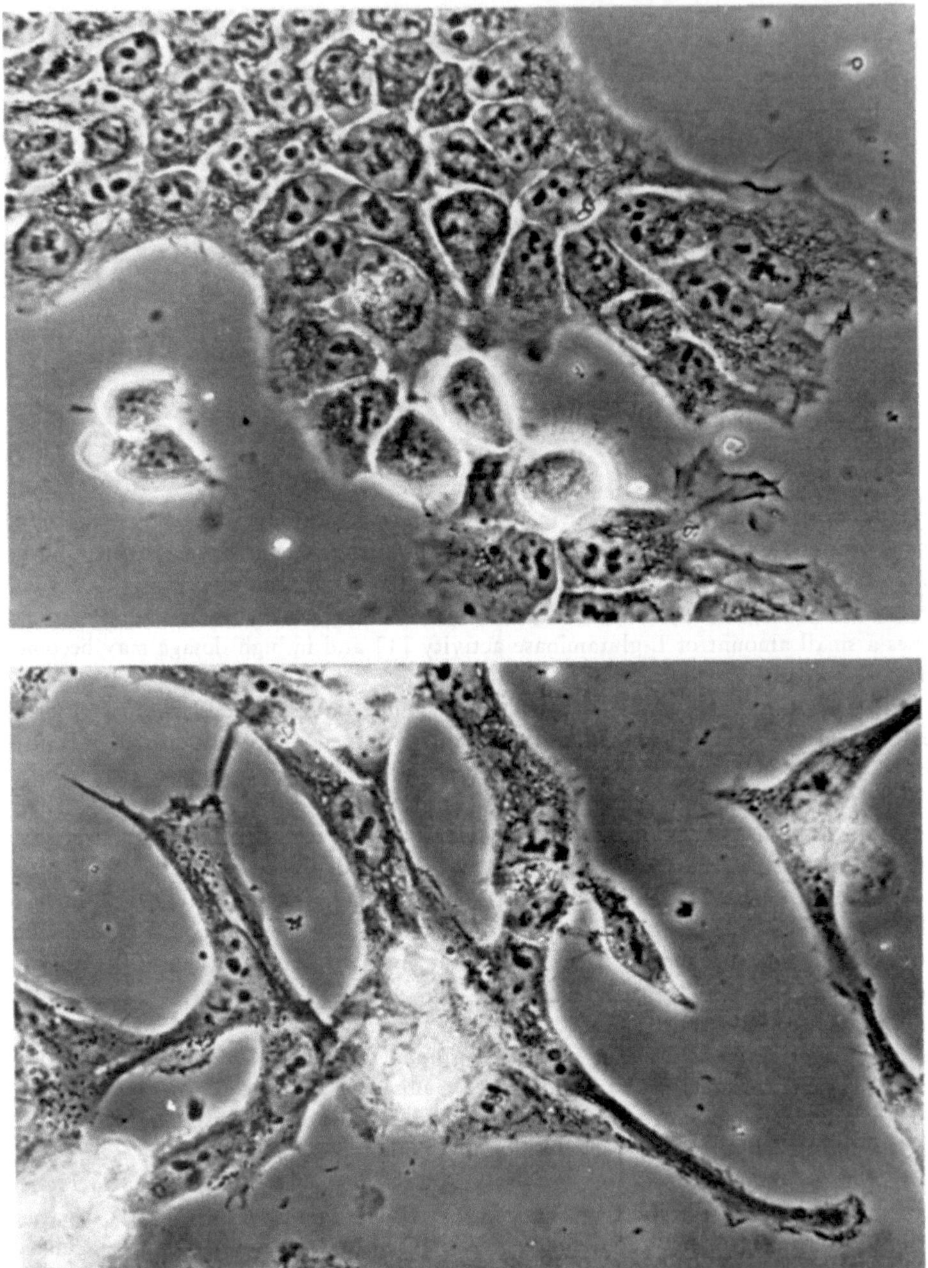

Fig. 1. Morphological changes of HeLa cells. Above: before treatment with EC-2 asparaginase; below: fourty-eight hours after the addition of EC-2 asparaginase

the other hand, in HeLa cells which had been cultivated for about six months with increasing doses of E. coli asparaginase and which had become more and more resistant the addition of L-glutamic acid stimulated the cell growth considerably (Fig. 5). We suppose that HeLa cells contain a small amount of L-glutamine synthetase and that their resistance to E. coli asparaginase is a result of an increase in their L-glutamine synthetase activity.

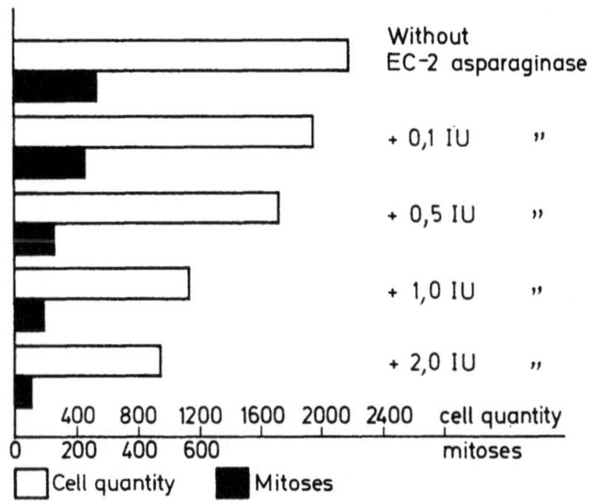

Fig. 2. Dose-responsive reduction of cell quantity and mitoses in HeLa cell cultures under the influence of EC-2 asparaginase

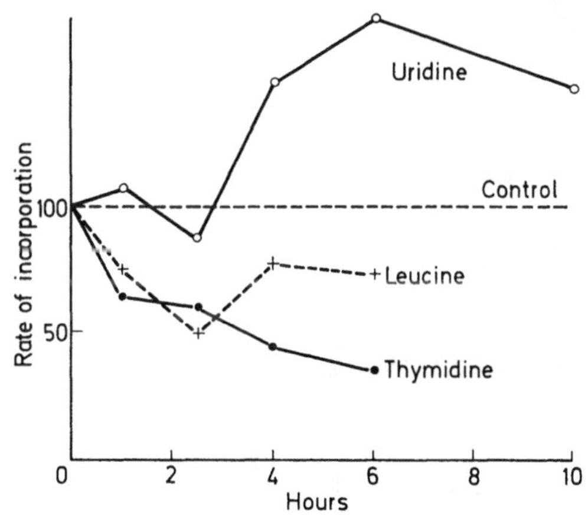

Fig. 3. The reduced incorporation of ^{14}C-leucine and ^{14}C-thymidine into HeLa cells as an effect of EC-2 asparaginase. The uptake of ^{14}C-uridine into the cells is augmented

Although the resistant HeLa cells showed continuous growth even with large doses of E. coli asparaginase a complete inhibition reappeared when the dosage exceeded a certain limit. We think this indicates that E. coli asparaginase, at least partially, passes the cell membrane and thus exerts an intracellular activity. In large doses of E. coli asparaginase the L-glutaminase activity would then exceed that of the elevated cellular L-glutamine synthetase of the resistant HeLa cells and cause a complete turnover of the newly synthesized L-glutamine.

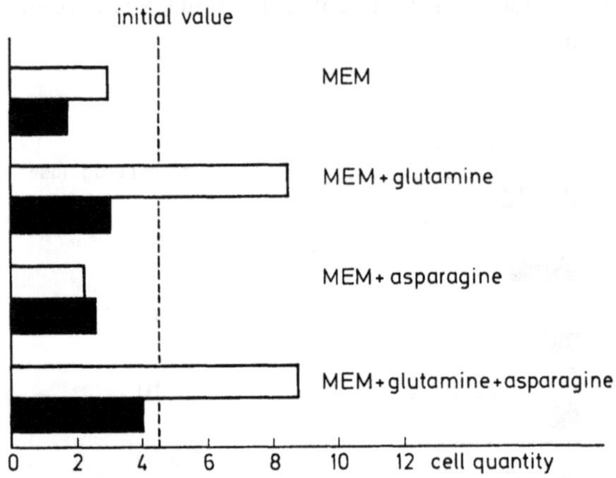

Fig. 4. The effect of the addition of L-glutamine, L-asparagine and L-glutamine+L-asparagine in HeLa cells cultivated in Eagle's Minimum Essential Medium (MEM). The black columns show the effect of the respective addition of EC-2 asparaginase

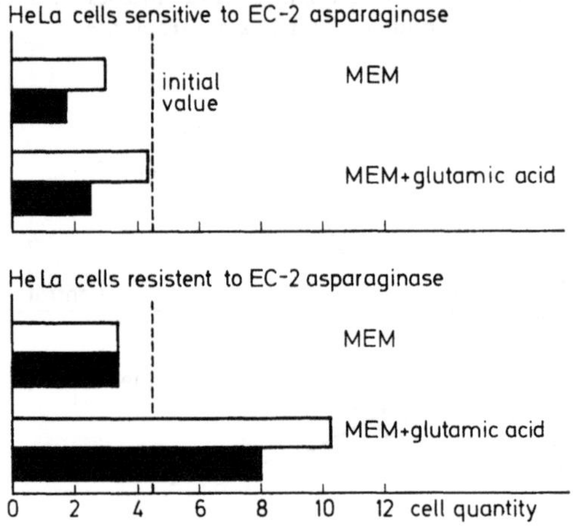

Fig. 5. Different utilization of L-glutamic acid by HeLa cells sensitive, and those resistant, to EC-2 asparaginase. The black columns show the effect of the respective addition of EC-2 asparaginase

HeLa cells are not dependent on L-asparagine but they may utilize it under certain conditions. HeLa cells cultivated in MEM containing L-glutamic acid and L-asparagine showed the same increase of growth as those cultivated in MEM with the addition of L-glutamine (Fig. 6). It is likely that L-asparagine favours the synthesis of L-glutamine from L-glutamic acid by the transfer of the amide group.

L-aspartic acid did not produce any stimulatory effect on HeLa cells cultivated in MEM. In combination with L-glutamine or L-glutamic acid L-aspartic acid had no additional effect.

Testing the effect of E. coli asparaginase on cultures of normal human leukocytes we observed that the neutrophil granulocytes died rapidly. This finding may

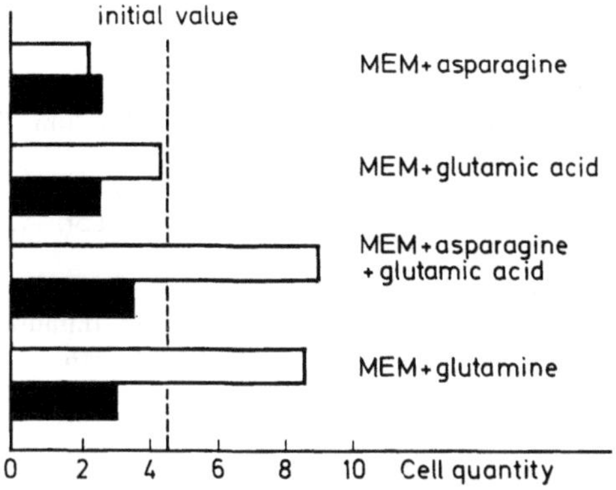

Fig. 6. Improvement of HeLa cell growth in the Minimum Essential Medium (MEM) by combined addition of L-asparagine and L-glutamic acid. The effect corresponds with that of L-glutamine. The black columns show the effect of the respective addition of EC-2 asparaginase

explain our clinical experience that in some cases of acute leukemia treated with E. coli asparaginase the initial decrease in peripheral blood leukocytes was not only caused by the fall of the blast cells but also by a diminution of the residual mature neutrophils.

In contrast to the neutrophils the eosinophils in culture proved to be resistant to E. coli asparaginase.

Blood monocytes were nearly as sensitive as the neutrophils. Macrophages and giant cells of the Langhans' type which were cultivated from human blood monocytes [4] died within a few days after the addition of E. coli asparaginase.

Non-stimulated human lymphocytes were not injured by E. coli asparaginase, whereas their blast-like transformation induced by phytohemagglutinin (PHA) was completely suppressed. This finding confirms similar results obtained by Astaldi and co-workers [5] and of Pappas [6].

We cultivated the lymphocytes in MEM and found that the PHA-induced transformation was L-glutamine dependent: The rate of transformation was increased by the addition of L-glutamine whereas with L-asparagine no rise of the transformation rate could be seen. L-asparagine even reduced the effect of L-glutamine when it was added to the MEM with L-glutamine simultaneously. These findings seem to show that E. coli asparaginase also suppresses the blast-like transformation of lymphocytes by its glutaminase activity.

In conclusion we want to state that the inhibitory effect of E. coli asparaginase on neoplastic diseases in some cases may be due to its L-glutaminase activity [7]. The lesion of normal leukocytes and their derivatives in vitro leads to the assumption that a therapy with E. coli asparaginase similarly may have side-effects on these cells in vivo. Some of the side-effects and perhaps even the immune suppressive effect also may be due to the glutaminase activity of E. coli asparaginase.

References

1. MEISTER, A., LEVINTOW, L., GREENFIELD, R. E., ABENDSCHEIN, P. A.: J. biol. Chem. **215,** 441 (1955).
2. EAGLE, H., WASHINGTON, C. L., LEVI, M., COHEN, L.: J. biol. Chem. **241,** 4994 (1966).
3. KIM, J. H., BOYSE, E. A., OLD, L. J., CAMPBELL, H. A.: Biochim. Biophys. Acta **158,** 476 (1968).
4. OERKERMANN, H: XII. Congr. Internat. Soc. Hematol. New York (N. Y.) 1968.
5. ASTALDI, G., BURGIO, G. R., KRC, J., GENOVA, R., ASTALDI, A. A., JR.: Lancet **1969,** 7591, 423.
6. PAPPAS, A. (Medizinische Universitätsklinik Köln, Germany): Personal communication.
7. OERKERMANN, H., HIRSCHMANN, W. D.: In: Chemo- und Immunotherapie der Leukosen und malignen Lymphome. Wien: Bohlmann-Verlag 1969, S. 316.

L-Asparaginase in the Treatment of Neoplastic Diseases of the Dog, Cat and Cow *

W. D. Hardy, Jr., and L. J. Old

Sloan-Kettering Institute for Cancer Research, New York, New York 10021, U.S.A.

With 7 Figures

Introduction

Asparagine-dependent neoplasms responsive to asparaginase therapy occur in the mouse [2, 3, 5, 9, 10], rat [9], dog [13, 14], and in man [6, 7, 11, 12] and are predominantly of lymphatic or hematopoeitic origin. Rarely, other tumor types, including a rat fibrosarcoma [8], a mouse mammary carcinoma [15], and two cases of human malignant melanoma [6, 12] may be suppressed by treatment with asparaginase.

In this study we have determined the incidence of asparaginase sensitive neoplasms in a series of 61 dogs, 9 cats and 3 cows.

Methods

Source of Asparaginase

Asparaginase was obtained from the following sources: *Escherichia coli* asparaginase (EC-2) from Bayer-Leverkusen, Wuppertal-Elberfeld, Germany; Merck, Sharp and Dohme Company, West Point, Penna., and Hakko Kyowa Co., Japan. Mammalian asparaginase, in the form of concentrated whole agouti serum, was supplied by Dr. Oswaldo de Lima, University of Recife, Recife, Brazil.

Source of Animal Tumors

Animals with naturally occurring tumors were obtained from the Henry Bergh Memorial Hospital of the A.S.P.C.A. and the Animal Medical Center, New York City and from veterinary practitioners in New York, New Jersey, and California.

* This work was supported in part by NCI grant CA 08748, a grant from the John A. Hartford Foundation, Inc., and The Henry Bergh Memorial Hospital of the American Society for the Prevention of Cruelty to Animals, New York.

Three cows were treated at the University of Pennsylvania, School of Veterinary Medicine, Philadelphia, Pennsylvania [1].

Diagnosis was made by biopsy in 58 animals, by cytological examination in 6 animals, by hematological examination in 7 animals and by clinical judgement in 2 animals.

Clinical Trials

The dose of asparaginase ranged from 100 to 3500 international units (IU) per kilogram daily given intraperitoneally for 10 consecutive days. Sixty-two of the 73 animals received doses between 100—400 IU/kg/daily.

One dog with lymphosarcoma received mammalian asparaginase in the form of concentrated whole agouti serum. The dog was given 100 IU/kg (20 IU/ml of concentrated agouti serum) daily for 4 consecutive days.

Three dogs with lymphosarcoma served as controls on standard therapy. They were treated with cyclophosphamide, 4 mg/kg/day per os for the first 3 days and 2 mg/kg/day per os thereafter combined with prednisolone, 1 mg/kg/day.

One dog with lymphosarcoma, at the owner's request, was not treated but was observed from the time of diagnosis until death.

Dogs with lymphosarcoma that responded after the initial 10 days of asparaginase therapy were divided into 4 groups and given different modes of maintenance therapy. Eight dogs received no maintenance therapy, 9 dogs received asparaginase once weekly in doses ranging from 650 to 1600 IU/kg, 5 dogs received 1 mg cyclophosphamide/kg/daily and 5 dogs were sacrificed immediately after the initial 10 days of asparaginase therapy.

The results were evaluated by determination of tumor size, blood counts, histological changes, lymphangiography and clinical observations. Measurement of selected peripheral lymph nodes in dogs with generalized lymphosarcoma and measurement of nonlymphomatous solid tumors were made before, during and after therapy. Lymphangiography was performed in 5 dogs with lymphosarcoma, hematological evaluation was utilized to monitor therapy in 50 animals and post-treatment histological examination was performed in 24 animals.

Results

Canine Lymphosarcoma

A high percentage of dogs with lymphosarcoma responded to chemotherapy with asparaginase. Dramatic therapeutic alterations were seen in 27 of 33 (82%) dogs with lymphosarcoma (Table 1). Reduction of peripheral lymphadenopathy, reduction in the number of abnormal circulating lymphocytes, increase in appetite and return of normal vigor were noted within 4—5 days after the start of asparaginase therapy. In one dog the right mandibular lymph node volume was 158 cubic centimeters (6.4 cm×5.6 cm×4.4 cm) before therapy and decreased to 14 cubic centimeters (2.8 cm×2.5 cm×2.0 cm) by the 5th day of therapy.

Fig. 1 and 2 show the response of a dog with generalized lymphosarcoma while Fig. 3 and 4 show the effect on lymphomatous tonsils. Sight returned within 10 days

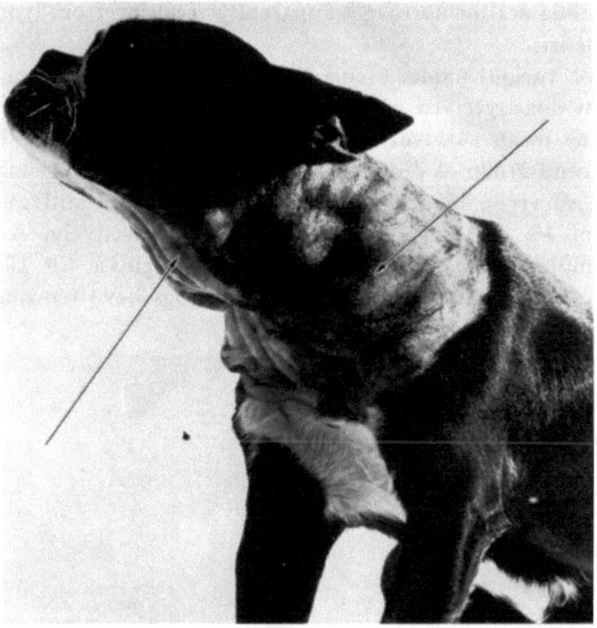

Fig. 1. Boston Terrier with generalized lymphosarcoma before L-asparaginase therapy. Note the enlarged mandibular and prescapular lymph nodes (arrows)

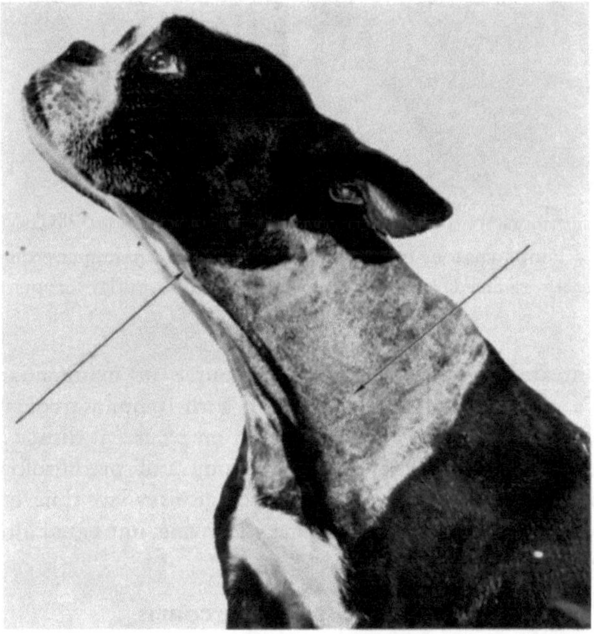

Fig. 2. After 10 days of L-asparaginase therapy the reduction in size of peripheral lymph nodes is evident (arrows)

to one dog with bilateral hemorrhages apparently resulting from lymphosarcomatous infiltration of the iris.

The results of various modes of maintenance therapy are summarized in Fig. 5. A group of eight dogs received no maintenance therapy after the initial 10 days of asparaginase. The mean survival time was 1.9 months (3, 3, 2, 2, 1.5, 1.5, 1.5, 1 months). A second group of 7 dogs which received large weekly maintenance doses of asparaginase survived longer. Six of these 7 dogs are still in remission with survival times of 15, 13, 3.5, 3, 1 and 1 months respectively. A third group of 5 dogs with lymphosarcoma was treated with asparaginase for 10 days and then maintained on cyclophosphamide. Three of these dogs have remained in remission, surviving for 2.25, 2 and 2 months.

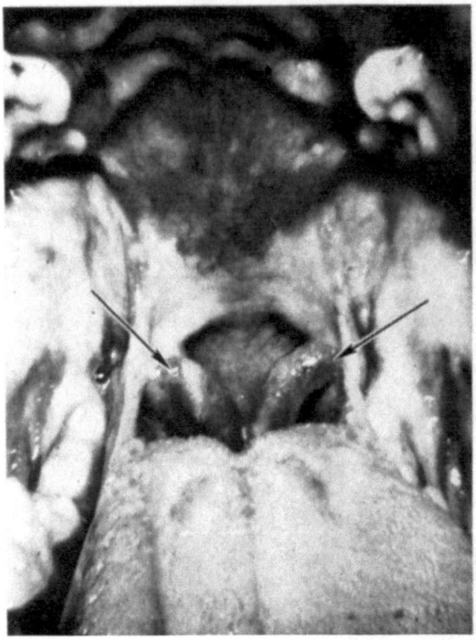

Fig. 3

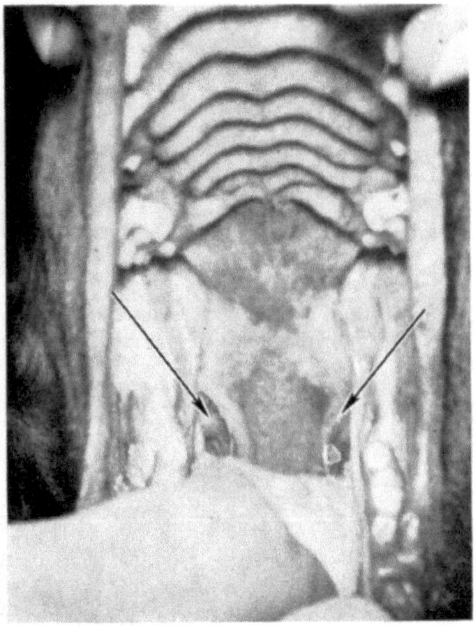

Fig. 4

Fig. 3. Enlarged lymphomatous tonsils of a dog before L-asparaginase therapy (arrows)
Fig. 4. Tonsils greatly reduced (arrows) and within the tonsillar crypts after 5 days of L-asparaginase therapy

Whole concentrated agouti serum (a rich source of mammalian asparaginase) rapidly induced a clinical remission in one dog with lymphosarcoma. This dog died one month later, without maintenance therapy, from recurrent disease.

The three dogs treated with cyclophosphamide and prednisolone survived for 1.25 months. Brick et al. [4] reported an average survival time of 2.5 weeks for 6 cases of untreated canine lymphosarcoma. The one untreated dog in our series survived for one month.

Canine Mast Cell Sarcomas

Mast cell sarcomas of the skin of the dog with recurrence at the site of surgical removal are common. Three of 6 dogs with mast cell sarcomas responded favorably

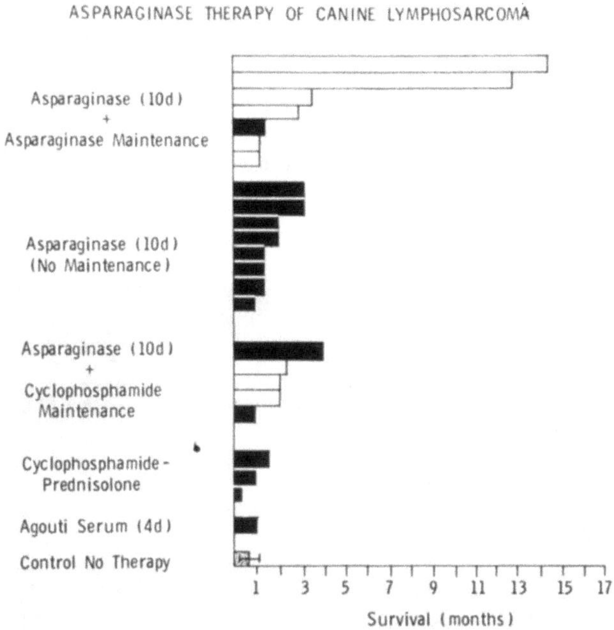

Fig. 5. Duration of remissions in 24 dogs with lymphosarcoma treated with L-asparaginase or other chemotherapeutic agents. Each bar represents an individual dog. White bars: no recurrence of disease. Black bars: recurrence of disease. The initial course of asparaginase therapy is given in days (d)

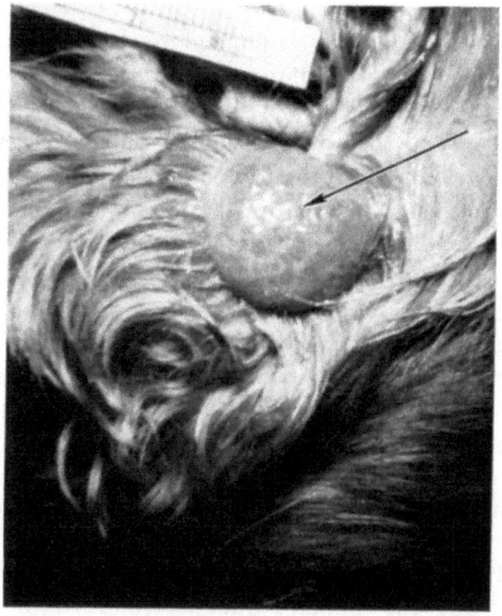

Fig. 6. Mast cell sarcoma before therapy (arrow) involving the ear skin of a Cocker Spaniel

to asparaginase. However, no maintenance therapy was given and tumor regrowth occurred in 2 of the 3 dogs within 2 months. Fig. 6 and 7 show the effect of asparaginase on a cutaneous mast cell sarcoma.

In the other instance, a young dog with a solitary mast cell sarcoma that recurred twice after surgical removal showed a good response to asparaginase. After asparaginase mediated tumor reduction was complete the surrounding skin was excised. Maintenance therapy was not attempted and the dog is free of recurrence 19 months later.

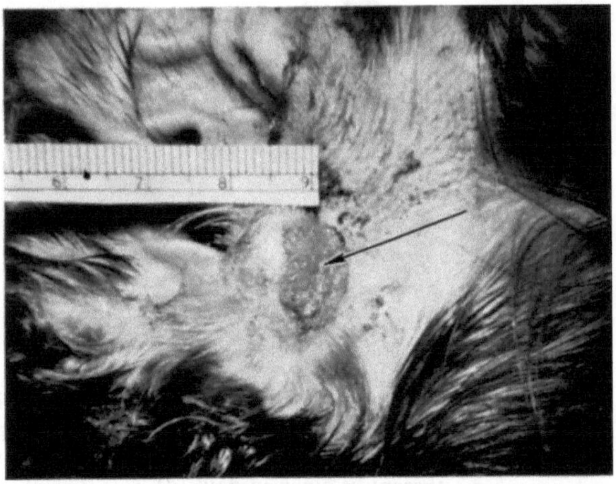

Fig. 7. After 6 days of therapy the tumor has regressed leaving an ulcerated area (arrow)

Canine Melanoma

One of 2 dogs with melanoma responded to asparaginase therapy. A German Shepherd dog was presented for examination because he was drooling and unable to eat, swallow or bark. Examination and biopsy revealed a large melanoma of the hard palate. After 5 days of therapy the tumor began to regress, drooling ceased and the dog was able to bark and swallow normally. No maintenance therapy was given and tumor regrowth occurred one month later, at which time, asparaginase therapy was reinstituted and tumor regression noted again after 5 days. Five weeks later the tumor recurred for the second time and the dog was sacrificed.

Seventeen other canine solid tumors including 4 squamous cell carcinomas, 2 mammary adenocarcinomas, 2 thyroid adenocarcinomas, 1 osteosarcoma and 1 fibrosarcoma did not respond to therapy with asparaginase (see Table 1).

Feline Tumors

Only 1 of 9 feline tumors was sensitive to asparaginase chemotherapy (Table 2). A cat with recurrent lymphosarcoma of the small intestine was anorectic, vomiting continually and had severe diarrhea. After a 10 day course of therapy the vomiting and diarrhea ceased and the animal's appetite returned to normal. However, no maintenance therapy was attempted and recurrence developed 2 months later.

Table 1. *Asparaginase sensitivity of various canine malignancies*

Tumor type	Number treated	Response
Lymphosarcoma	33	27 (82%)
Mast cell sarcoma	6	3 (50%)
Melanoma	2	1
Squamous cell carcinoma	4	0
Mammary adenocarcinoma	2	0
Thyroid carcinoma	2	0
Ovarian cystadenocarcinoma	1	0
Nasal adencarcinoma	1	0
Transitional cell carcinoma	1	0
Bile duct adenocarcinoma	1	0
Osteosarcoma	1	0
Multiple myeloma	1	0
Hemangiosarcoma	1	0
Mixed salivary gland tumor	1	0
Fibrosarcoma	1	0
Total	58	31

Table 2. *Asparaginase sensitivity of various feline malignancies*

Tumor type	Response
Mammary adenocarcinoma	—
Neurofibrosarcoma	—
Fibrosarcoma	—
Fibrosarcoma	—
Osteosarcoma	—
Lymphosarcoma	—
Lymphosarcoma	—
Lymphosarcoma	+
Lymphosarcoma	—

Bovine Lymphosarcoma

Three cows with generalized lymphosarcoma were given asparaginase at doses from 100 to 400 IU/kg/daily for 7 days. Marked reduction of lymph node size, increased food consumption and increased milk production was observed in one cow. Minimal clinical response and lymph node reduction was seen in the other 2 cows.

Toxicity

No significant toxic effects were observed in animals during the initial 10 day course of asparaginase therapy. However, 3 dogs developed hypersensitivity to the drug when long term maintenance therapy was attempted. In contrast the 3 long term surviving dogs tolerated well the large once weekly maintenance dose of asparaginase, with only occasional transient depression, incoordination and vomiting. Precipitating antibodies to the enzyme preparations are detectable in some animals, however, these appear to have little clinical significance.

In our study 3 types of tumors were sensitive to asparaginase: lymphosarcoma, mast cell sarcoma and melanoma. Asparaginase therapy has produced long term survivals in dogs with lymphosarcoma which are quite significant when one considers that the dog has only 1/6th the life expectancy of man.

One cat and 1 cow with lymphosarcoma also responded to asparaginase therapy. In conclusion, asparaginase is tolerated well by domestic animals and has striking antilymphoma properties in the dog which make it desirable for use in veterinary medicine.

Summary

Seventy-three animals (61 dogs, 9 cats, 3 cows) with spontaneous tumors were treated with L-asparaginase. Of these, 27 of 33 (82%) dogs with lymphosarcoma, 2 of 4 dogs with mast cell sarcoma and 1 of 2 dogs with melanoma responded with marked reduction in tumor size and clinical improvement. Three dogs with lymphosarcoma have survived 15, 13 and 3.5 months respectively, receiving large weekly maintenance doses of asparaginase. One dog with oral melanoma responded on two occasions.

Only 1 of 9 cat tumors was suppressed by asparaginase, the sensitive tumor being a recurrent lymphosarcoma of the small intestine. One of three cows with lymphosarcoma responded well to asparaginase with reduction of lymph node size while the other 2 showed only minimal clinical improvement. No significant toxic effects were observed in animals during the initial course of therapy. Three dogs receiving maintenance therapy developed hypersensitivity reactions. Precipitating antibodies against the enzyme preparations were detectable in the sera of several animals but they were not necessarily of clinical significance.

L-asparaginase is clearly applicable to clinical veterinary medicine, especially in the therapy and management of canine lymphosarcoma.

References

1. BLUM, J., JOHNSTONE, C., MARTIN, J.: In preparation.
2. BOYSE, E. A., OLD, L. J., STOCKERT, E.: Inhibitory effect of guinea pig serum on a number of new leukemias in mice. Nature (Lond.) **198,** 800—801 (1963).
3. — — CAMPBELL, H. A., MASHBURN, L. T.: Suppression of murine leukemias by L-asparaginase. J. exp. Med. **125,** 17—31 (1967).
4. BRICK, J. O., ROENIGK, W. J., WILSON, G. P.: Chemotherapy of malignant lymphoma in dogs and cats. J. Amer. vet. med. Ass. **153,** 47—52 (1968).
5. BROOME, J. D.: Evidence that the L-asparaginase activity of guinea pig serum is responsible for its antilymphoma effects. Nature (Lond.) **191,** 1114—1115 (1961).
6. HASKELL, C. M., CANELLOS, G. P., LEVENTHAL, B. G., CARBONE, P. P., BLOCK, J. B., SERPICK, A. A., SELAWRY, O. S.: L-asparaginase: Therapeutic and toxic effects in patients with neoplastic disease. New Engl. J. Med. **281,** 1028—1034 (1969).
7. HILL, J. M., ROBERTS, J., LOEB, E., KHAN, A., MACLELLAN, A., HILL, R. W.: L-asparaginase therapy for leukemia and other malignant neoplasms. J. Amer. med. Ass. **202,** 882—888 (1967).
8. JAMESON, E., AINIS, H., RYAN, R. M.: Action of guinea pig serum and human gamma globulin on the growth of a rat tumor. Science **124,** 980—981 (1956).
9. KIDD, J. G.: Regression of transplanted lymphomas induced *in vivo* by means of normal guinea pig serum. I. Course of transplanted cancers of various kinds in mice and rats given guinea pig serum, horse serum, or rabbit serum. J. exp. Med. **98,** 565—581 (1953).

10. Mashburn, L. T., Wriston, J. C., Jr.: Tumor inhibitory effect of L-asparaginase from *Escherichia coli*. Arch. Biochem. Biophys. **105**, 450—452 (1964).
11. Oettgen, H. F., Old, L. J., Boyse, E. A., Campbell, H. A., Philips, F. S., Clarkson, B. D., Tallal, L., Leeper, R. D., Schwartz, M. K., Kim, J. H.: Inhibition of leukemias in man by L-asparaginase. Cancer Res. **27**, 2619—2631 (1967).
12. — Schulten, H. K.: Hemmung maligner Neoplasien des Menschen durch L-asparaginase. Klin. Wschr. **47**, 65—71 (1969).
13. Old, L. J., Boyse, E. A., Campbell, H. A., Brodey, R. S., Fidler, J., Teller, J. D.: Treatment of lymphosarcoma in the dog with L-asparaginase. Cancer **20**, 1066—1070 (1967).
14. — — — L-asparagine and leukemia. Sci. Amer. **219**, 34—40 (1968).
15. Sugiura, K.: Effect of L-asparaginase (NSC-109,229) on transplantable and spontaneous tumors from mice and rats. Cancer Chemother. Rep. **53**, 189—194 (1969).

The Cytomorphological Effects of L-Asparaginase in Sensitive Cells

W.-H. Voigt, E. Grundmann, and R. Bierling

Institute of Experimental Pathology of Farbenfabriken Bayer AG., Wuppertal-Elberfeld, Germany

With 8 Figures

This report is concerned with light microscopic and, especially, electron microscopic changes taking place under the influence of Crasnitin [1] in laboratory animals and in vitro. The only morphological findings so far available are those of Borella et al. (1966) on ascitic cells in a case of lymphosarcoma. The guinea-pig-L-asparaginase which they used failed to produce significant effects on the lymphosarcoma cells examined. Our studies of the morphological pattern were intended to provide insight into the possible mechanism by which L-asparaginase acts on cells and tissues.

Material and Methods

50 mice were inoculated subcutaneously with 5 million leukemia EARAD 1 cells. Within a week, solid tumors 6 to 8 mm in diameter grew at the sites of inoculation.

Each of 36 animals received 1000 units Crasnitin per kg bodyweight (that means about 20 units/mouse) intraperitoneally. (The animal experiments were carried out in Dr. Bierling's laboratory.)

At 1, 2, 3, 4, 5, 6, 8, 12, 16, 24, and 48 hours after the injection of Crasnitin, 3 animals each were killed, and their tissues examined.

In an equally large group of mice, each animal was given 10 million cells of the Gardner mouse lymphosarcoma intraperitoneally. Seven to eight days after inoculation of the cells the animals were treated with Crasnitin like the EARAD 1 leukemia group. At that point the mice had developed many solid tumors of the intestinal loops and several millilitres of ascitic fluid.

Cells obtained from this ascitic fluid were isolated and embedded.

For in vitro testing of Crasnitin a KB strain was used in a 200,000 cells/ml culture. After 24 hours the cell cultures were treated with 10 units/ml Crasnitin in fresh culture medium. 4, 6, 8, and 24 hours after adding the preparation, the tissues were examined.

Results

1. Light Microscopic Findings

The solid tumors of EARAD 1 leukemia present the following picture in semithin sections: (Fig. 1) The leukemic cells are closely packed, show variably sized

[1] Registered trade mark: Bayer-Leverkusen, Germany.

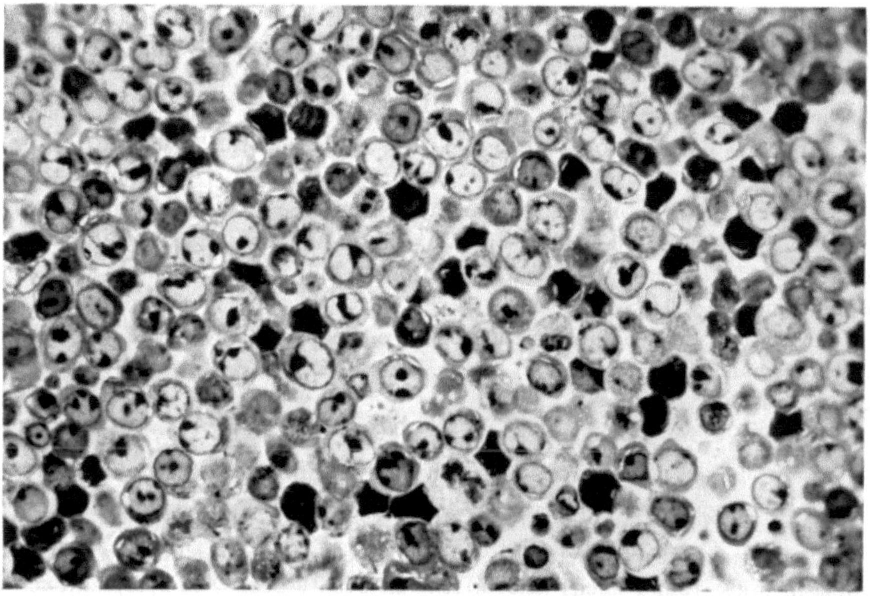

Fig. 1. Light micrograph of an untreated EARAD 1 tumor. ×540

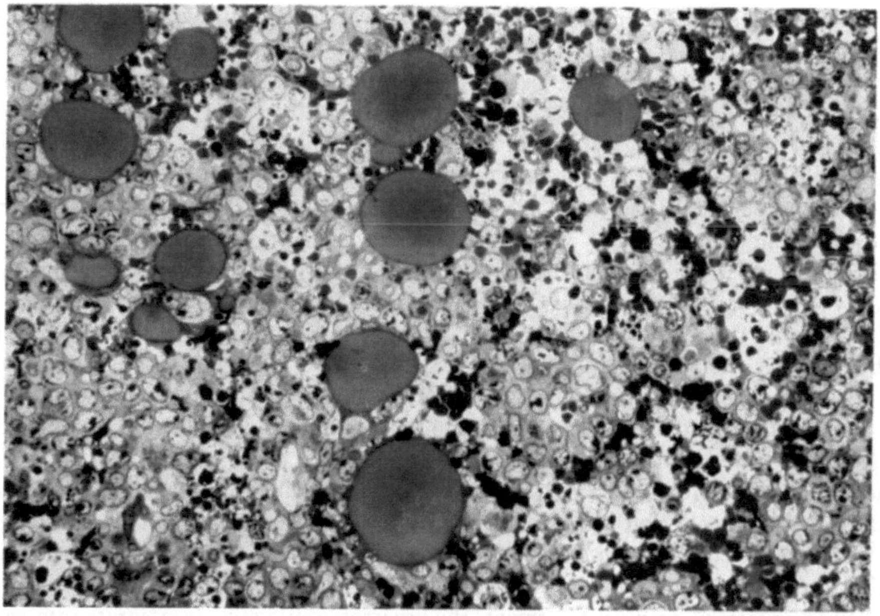

Fig. 2. The light micrograph shows EARAD 1 tumor complexes 6 hours after treatment with Crasnitin. ×350

commonly indented or round to oval nuclei with light karyoplasm and they are frequently in mitosis. 3 hours after Crasnitin treatment the leukemic cells look normal.

6 hours after treatment (Fig. 2) complexes are seen with cell remnants containing nuclear remains but also some intact leukemic cells. Some nuclei show early disintegration.

After 24 hours the following changes are prominent: coarser marginal chromatin, hyper- and hypochromatic nuclei, some of them in a state of rhexis. Also many cells are grossly swollen, have a large light cytoplasm and contain a pale nucleus. There are still some intact leukemic cells.

Even 48 hours after administration of the enzyme, single leukemic cell complexes are still unchanged. In most areas, however, intact tumor cells are no longer found; the tumors are very small.

2. Electron Microscopic Findings

The EARAD 1 tumor consists of cells, which have their external membrane directly adjacent to each other. They hardly differ in density and contrast from the cytoplasm. Most round nuclei also present an even aspect. The cytoplasm contains scattered mitochondria showing predominantly disc-shaped cristae in their light matrix. In the basic cytoplasm, free ribosomes appear, mostly single, but also in groups (Fig. 3). The endoplasmatic reticulum is only very poorly developed.

The first significant, though still slight changes are found in a few cells 4 hours after Crasnitin treatment: The karyoplasm appears somewhat coarser. In the cytoplasm, small vesicular membranous structures are found relatively frequently.

8 hours after the administration of Crasnitin, the changes become more marked. Near blood vessels, the cells still remain essentially unchanged. However, zones of different density are frequently seen in the nuclei. Further away from the immediate blood supply, optically lighter cells stand out distinctly from the other tissue with its uniform contrast. The cytoplasm of the light cells is loosened. Ribosomes are less densely distributed.

After prolonged action of Crasnitin, the mitochondria in several cells undergo the following changes: Their matrix becomes denser and while the membranes of the cristae run parallel in the untreated cells, they now begin to diverge, and optically empty spaces appear between them. With continuing action of the enzyme, the ribosomes in the cytoplasm rearrange themselves so that the previously separate ribosomes become polysomes.

The aspect of a relatively uniform tissue structure gradually vanishes. Different degrees of density of the organelles become marked in more and more cells distinguishing them from the cells in their immediate vicinity (Fig. 4). Thus, 24 hours after the start of Crasnitin treatment, most of the tumor cells show an increase of cytoplasmic membranes with attached ribosomes. Definite loosening of the tumor tissue is visualised. Generally, the cell contact is decreasing: The cells separate from each other and tend to round off.

48 hours after Crasnitin treatment, the ergastoplasmic sacs disintegrate into small vesicles and gradually dissolve. Polysomes revert to separate ribosomes. Many cells are still in mitosis.

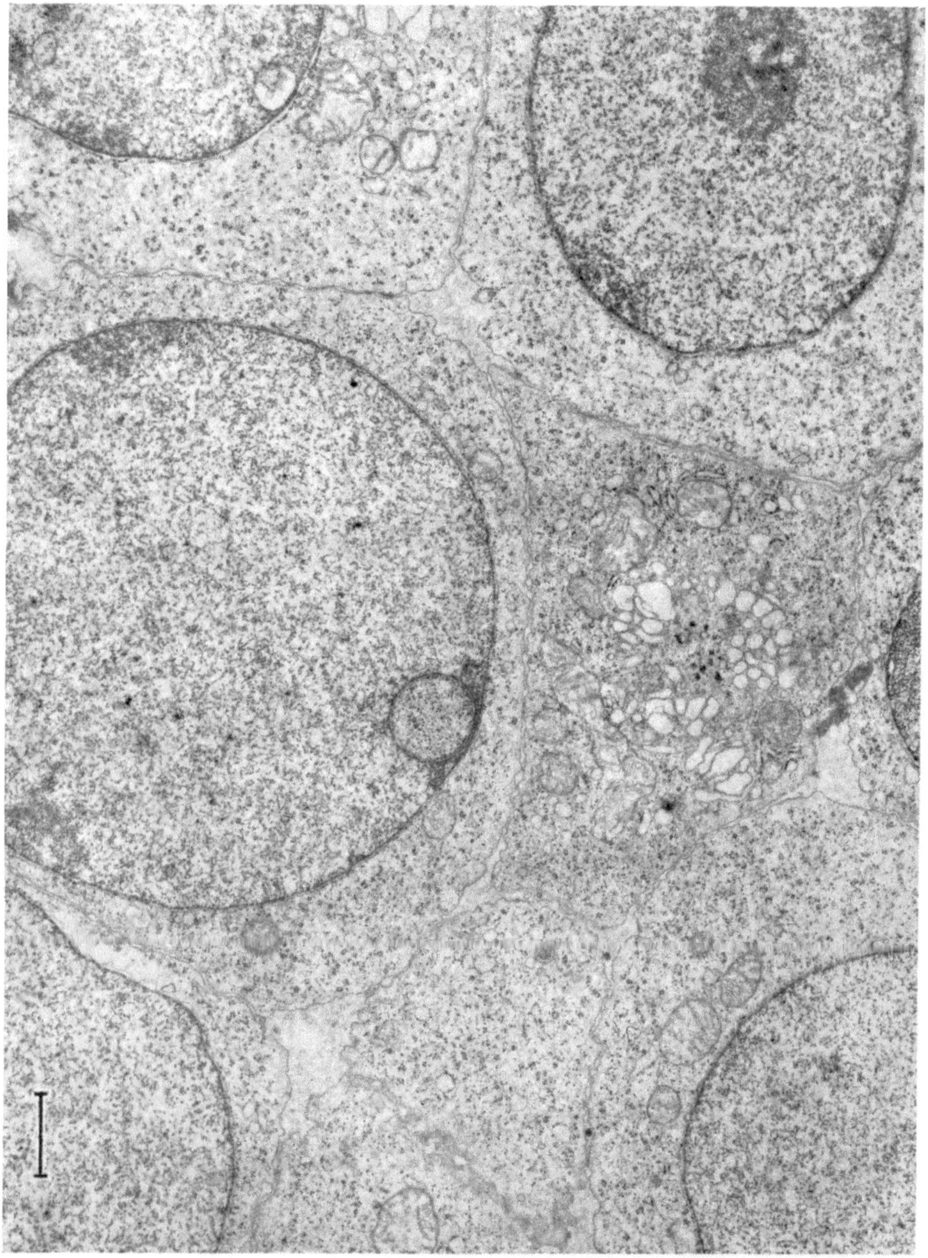

Fig. 3. Electron micrograph of an untreated EARAD 1 tumor. The cells hardly differ in density and contrast from the cytoplasm. ×11,200

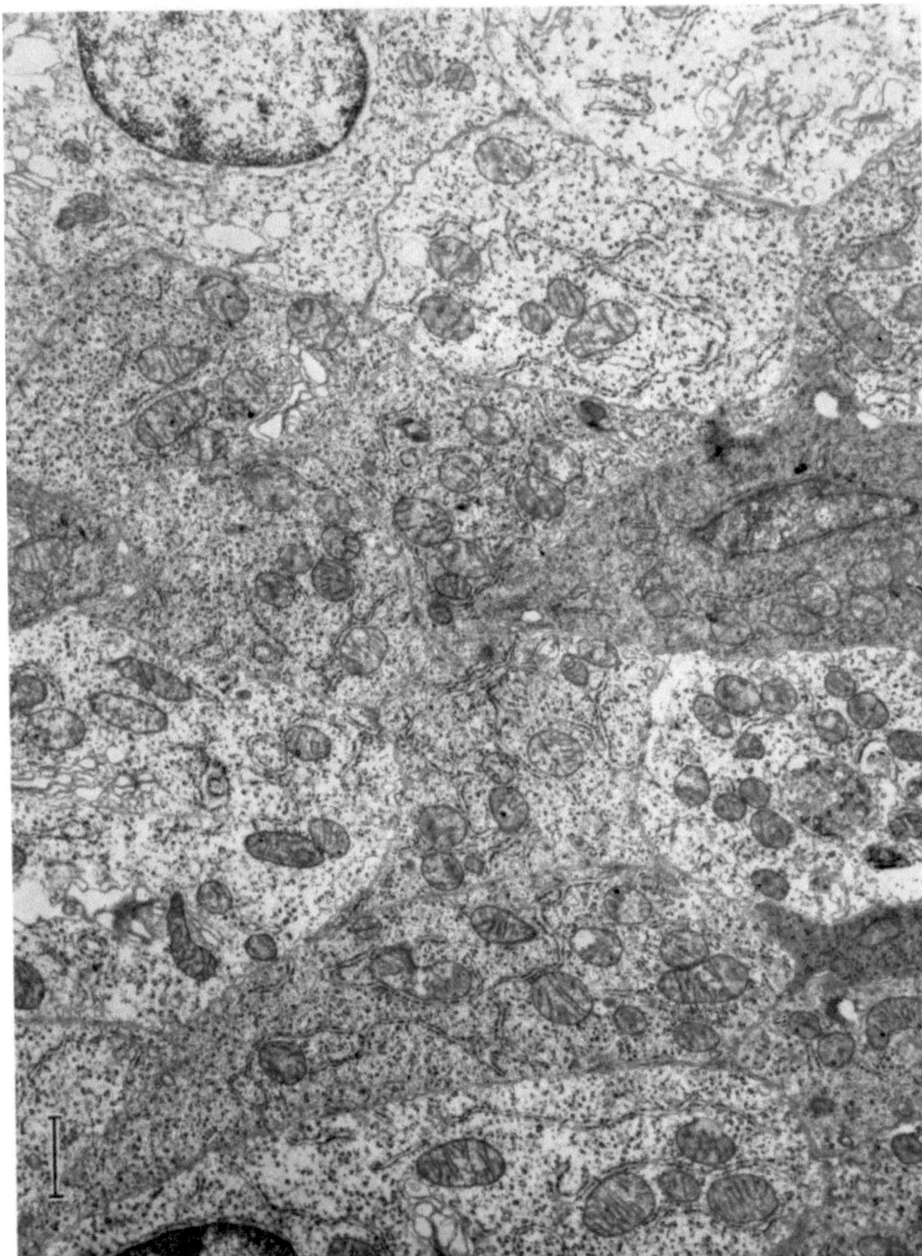

Fig. 4. After prolonged action of Crasnitin the aspect of a relatively uniform tissue structure gradually vanishes. Different degrees of density of the organells become marked in more and more cells by which they are distinguished from the cells in their immediate vicinity. ×10,300

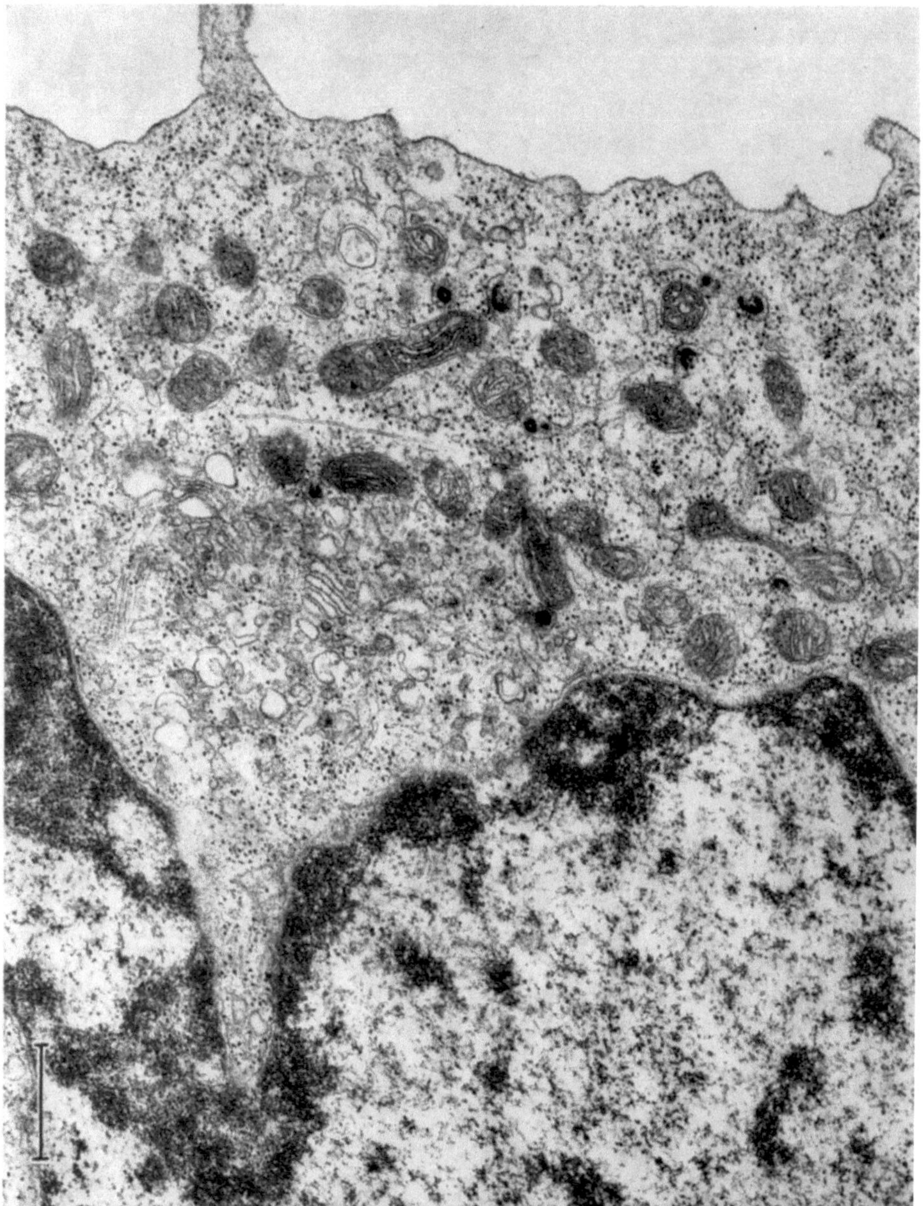

Fig. 5. Part of ascites cell of the untreated Gardner lymphoma with many separate ribosomes. ×15,200

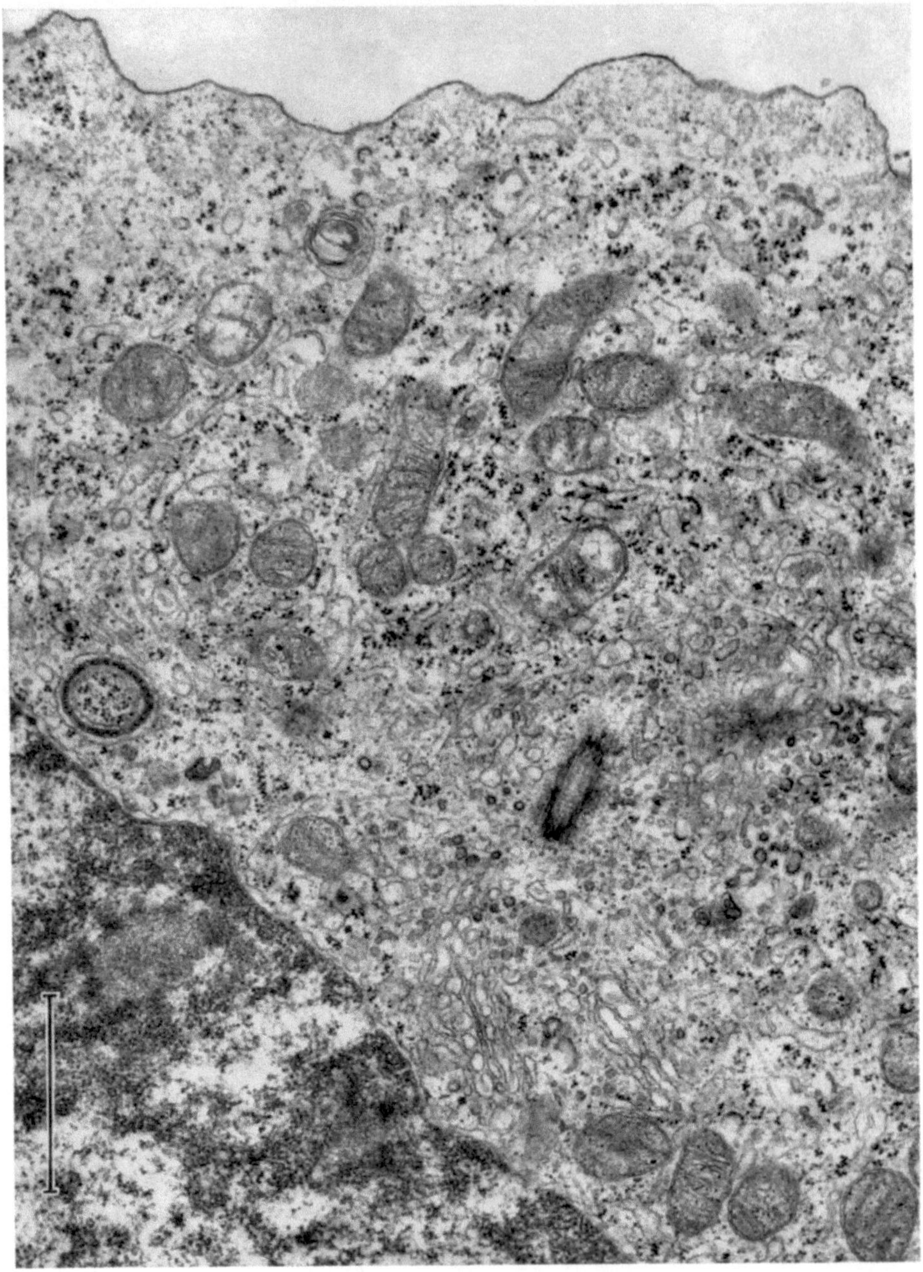

Fig. 6. Part of ascites cell of Gardner lymphoma with aggregation of ribosomes to polysomes 16 hours after Crasnitin action. ×26,600

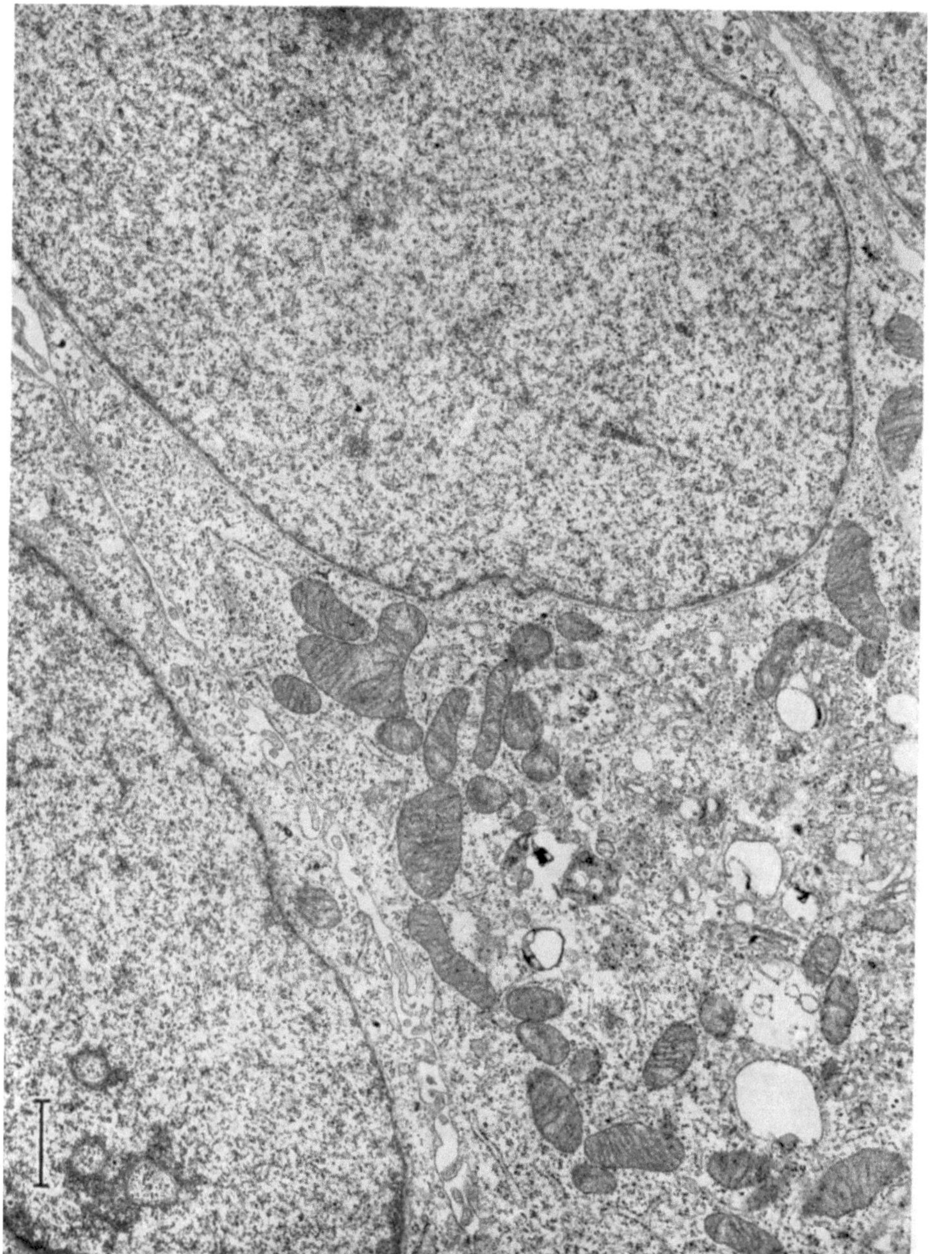

Fig. 7. Untreated cells of the KB strain in tissue culture. The cytoplasm contains many mitochondria, in the matrix of which narrow cristae are embedded side by side. ×12,100

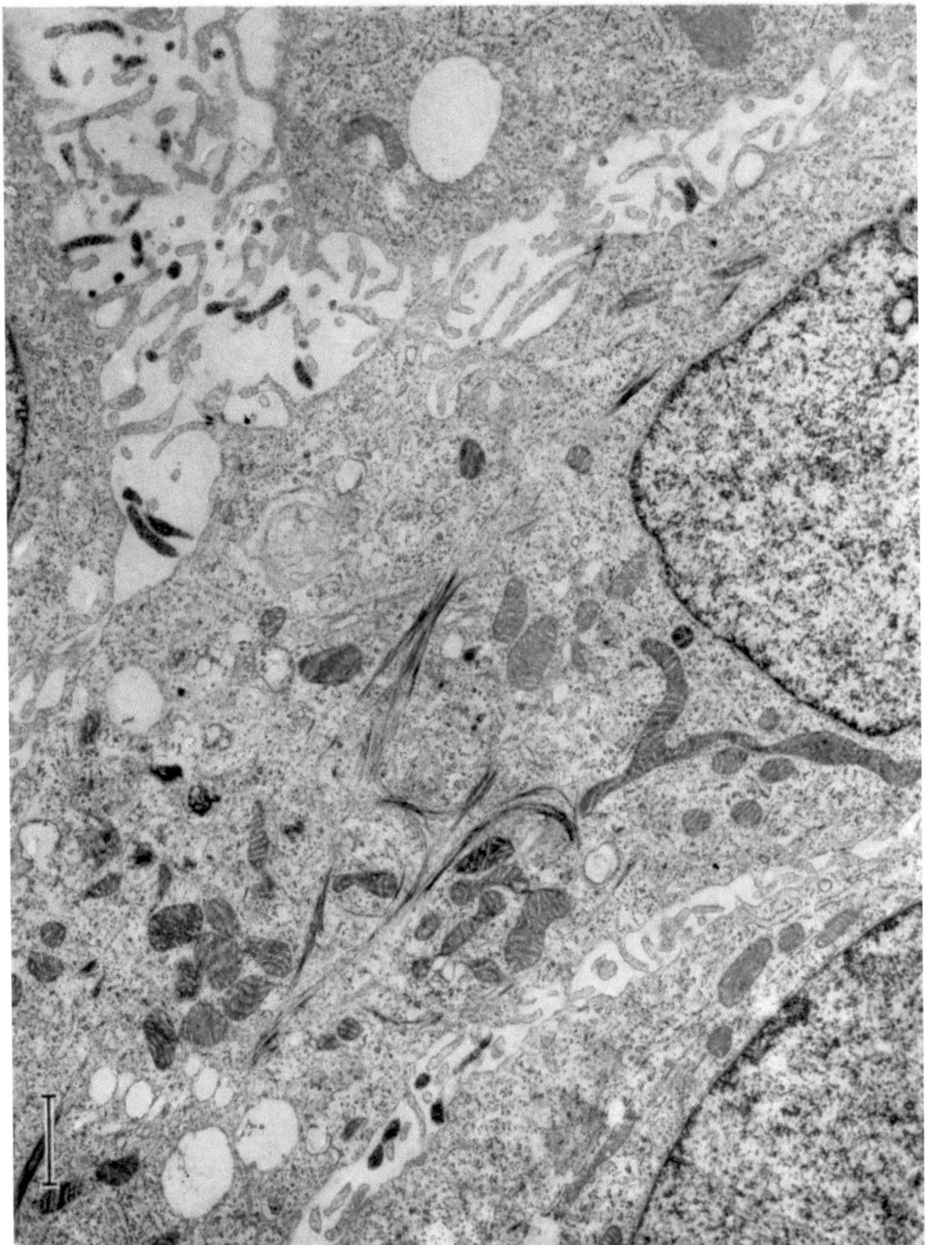

Fig. 8. 24 hours after enzym action KB cells in tissue culture contain prominent mitochondria. They are marked by a very dense matrix, in which the light clefts between the separated cristae membranes stand out clearly. ×12,100

In the Gardner lymphoma, principally the same changes are found in the examined ascites cells. Gardner lymphoma cells, too, do not normally possess an endoplasmatic reticulum but they have many separate ribosomes (Fig. 5). After 16 hours of Crasnitin action, the aggregation of ribosomes to polysomes is particularly marked, as already described for EARAD 1 (Fig. 6). The mitochondria remain essentially unchanged in this phase, though this is not true for all cells.

The density of the mitochondrial matrix, observed in EARAD 1 cells, is also present in several cells of the Gardner lymphoma.

After a more prolonged action of Crasnitin the ascites cells round off. The polysomes revert to individual ribosomes, the karyoplasm become increasingly coarse, while the mitochondria swell and thereby become optically emptier.

The untreated cells of the KB strain which often have delicate digitate protrusions on their surface, usually form a dense lawn of cells. The cytoplasm contains many mitochondria, in the matrix of which narrow cristae are embedded side by side (Fig. 7). In addition to a more or less strongly developed ergastoplasm, there are always free ribosomes, usually single.

After 24 hours of enzyme action the following features become prominent: the delicate protrusions of the cell surface are often replaced by plump lobular cell extensions. More ribosomes have aggregated to polysomes. The total number of ribosomes has decreased. In many cells, the mitochondria are now prominent in the cytoplasm. They are characterized by a very dense matrix, in which the light clefts between the separated cristae membranes stand out clearly (Fig. 8). The cytoplasmic filamentous bundles also show more contrast.

Summary

Our light microscopic and electron microscopic findings show that after the administration of Crasnitin changes of the histological structure occur in solid tumor tissue as well as in single cells of the ascites of mouse leukemias and, in a similar form, in cell cultures of the KB-strain which are sensitive to the enzyme. These changes do not begin immediately after Crasnitin treatment but they become visible only after several hours. Even 48 hours after administration of the enzyme, we often found cells or tissue areas which did not show any morphological differences from the untreated controls. Mitoses were also still observed at that time. This seems to be one of the reasons why Borella et al. (1966) in their investigation using guinea-pig asparaginase did not find any morphological changes of lymphoma cells.

The most marked changes are those of the ribosomes and mitochondria and also the formation of a coarse ergastoplasm. After Crasnitin treatment, ribosomes first appear more often as polysomes, and with continuing action again become single and decrease in number.

It is generally accepted that the formation of polysomes represents an increase in protein synthesis and that the coarse endoplasmic reticulum, representing increased protein synthesis for "export", is found in all protein secreting cells.

An explanation for this apparent discrepancy could lie in a temporary compensation for the amino acid depletion.

Findings similar to ours, namely a marked condensation of the mitochondrial matrix and simultaneous widening of the intra-cisternal clefts, were described by Jagendorf-Elfvin and Eliasson (1969) as a sign of glutamine deficiency of liver cells. Whether these changes are a sign of aminoacid-deficiency generally, or whether they present a specific reaction of the cell, we cannot yet answer.

Crasnitin also possesses glutaminase activity, although to a minor degree. Thus, the possibility cannot be dismissed that at least part of the changes which we have found are related to its glutaminase activity. Studies on this score are being continued.

References

Borella, L., Journey, J., Hiramoto, R.: In vivo and in vitro effects of the L-asparaginase fraction of guinea pig serum on the 6C3HED ascites lymphosarcoma. Cancer Res. **26/1**, 2451—2460 (1966).

Jagendorf-Elfvin, M., Eliason, E.: Reversible changes in the ultrastructure of Chang liver cell mitochondria following incubation of the cells in a glutamine-deficient medium. J. Cell. Biol. **41**, 905—909 (1969).

Inhibitation by L-Asparaginase from E. coli of Human Malignant Melanoma Cells Growing in vitro

P. Alexander, G. Hamilton Fairley, I. D. Hunter-Craig, R. L. Ilonopisov, and M. G. Lewis

Chester Beatty Research Institute, Belmont, Sutton, Surrey, England

Introduction

Techniques for the short-term culture of human malignant melanoma have been developed in this laboratory so as to investigate immunologically mediated host reactions to this disease (Lewis et al., 1969). In these studies the patient's own serum was added to the tumour cells *in vitro* and the existence of complement-dependent autoantibodies to some melanomas was demonstrated. To test if melanoma cells were sensitive to L-asparaginase, the cells were treated in exactly the same way except that instead of autologous serum *E. coli* L-asparaginase from Bayer was added to the cultures.

Experimental Procedure

Immediately after removal the tumour was placed in tissue culture medium 199 and within 24 hours of receipt cells were separated mechanically by scraping with a scalpel. The resulting suspension contained also cells other than melanoma but there was seldom difficulty in distinguishing the tumour cells microscopically. The cell suspension was adjusted so as to contain 10^6 tumour cells in 2 ml of a medium consisting of 80% TC. 199 and 20% heat inactivated foetal bovine serum and the L-asparaginase at different concentration expressed as units/ml (u/ml). Wherever possible the tests were run with

a) No L-asparaginase:
b) 5 u/ml L-asparaginase:
c) 20 u/ml L-asparaginase:
d) 40 u/ml L-asparaginase.

In a few cases where there was insufficient tumour material L-asparaginase was only tested at the highest (i. e. 40 u/ml) concentration. Each was run in duplicate.

The culture method was based on that described by Pulvertaft (1965). The culture chamber is formed by a ring of Teflon which sits on a microscope slide and is closed on the top by a coverslip. The chamber was then inverted so that coverslip was on top and in this way dead cells and debris dropped off and made it possible to examine the melanoma cells that adhered to the glass directly by phase-contrast microscopy. Interference with growth was recognized by failure of the cells to adhere to the coverslip and the reading was carried out between five to seven days after setting up. While ability to adhere to glass is an arbitrary criterion for damage, in a few cases the cells that had dropped off the coverslip were examined and found to be non-viable on the basis of a dye-exclusion test with trypan blue. In the absence of L-asparaginase, virtually every melanoma provided cells that adhered to the cover glass, which could be identified as tumour cells and could be maintained for at least ten days. Some melanomas grew as round cells, while others were dendritic. A positive effect of L-asparaginase was obvious on inspection in that the coverslip was virtually devoid of tumour cells. No case was encountered where toxicity was in doubt; either the cultures with L-asparaginase were undistinguishable from those without or the number of cells adhering to the glass was reduced to less than 20% of the control.

Results

Table 1 shows that of the sixty malignant melanoma tested, 30% were inhibited *in vitro* by L-asparaginase. Of the 18 sensitive tumours, 15 were tested at all three concentrations of L-asparaginase. 11 of the 15 were inhibited already at 5 u/ml, while 4 required higher concentrations (see Table 2).

All of these melanomas were also tested with the patient's own serum in the culture medium to determine if complement-dependent cytotoxic auto-antibodies were present. Table 3 shows that there is no correlation between sensitivity to

Table 1. *In vitro sensitivity of malignant melanoma to L-asparaginase*

Total number of Melanoma studied	60
Positive (i. e. sensitive)	18 (30%)
Negative	42 (70%)

Table 2. *Sensitivity of malignant melanoma to varying concentrations of L-asparaginase*

Of the 18 asparaginase sensitive tumors		
inhibited by	5 units/ml	—11 cases
inhibited only by	20 units/ml	— 2 cases
inhibited only by	40 units/ml	— 2 cases

(three of the positive tumours were tested only at 40 units/ml).

Table 3. *Sensitivity of melanoma cells to L-asparaginase in vitro in relationship to the presence of cytotoxic autoantibodies*

	Number tested	% with auto-antibodies
Asparaginase sensitive	18	30
Asparaginase resistant	42	38

L-asparaginase and the immune reactivity against the melanoma cells; *in vitro* sensitivity to L-asparaginase was found in the same proportion amongst patients with and without autoantibodies. Since autoantibodies were confined almost entirely to patients in whom the disease was still localized (LEWIS et al., 1969), it is obvious that sensitivity to L-asparaginase, as revealed by this *in vitro* test, is not related to the stage of the disease.

Discussion

In vitro sensitivity provides no indication of clinical usefulness. Six patients in this series — all of whom gave a positive *in-vitro* test — were treated with L-asparaginase but none appeared to benefit (HAMILTON FAIRLEY et al., 1969). In one case the serum from a patient undergoing treatment with L-asparaginase contained sufficient of the enzyme to stop tumour cells, which had been removed by biopsy, from growing *in vitro*, yet there was no effect on the tumour *in vivo*. One reason for this failure could be that *in vivo* tumour cells are exposed to a concentration of the enzyme which is very much lower than that found in the serum (cf. HALL, 1969); another factor could be that normal cells may supply the tumour cells with nutritional factors and that this "feeding" is more difficult to prevent *in vivo* than *in vitro*.

Unfortunately, the experiments described here do not make it possible to determine the mode of action of L-asparaginase in this system. While the tissue culture medium 199 does not contain asparagine, the foetal serum used in the test had not been dialysed and it is, therefore, probable that some asparagine was available. Furthermore, the preparations did not consist only of melanoma cells and there was a variable but significant number of normal cells in every one of the cultures. The possibility that these contaminating cells "feed" the melanoma cells with essential nutrients including, in some cases, asparagine cannot be excluded. The fact that four of the tumours were only inhibited at very high concentrations of L-asparaginase could be explained if the asparagine had to be "intercepted" as it passes from one cell to another. The lowest concentration of the enzyme used was more than adequate to deplete the medium of free asparagine and the need for the high concentrations indicates that this reaction alone is insufficient to explain the results. Indeed, already at 5 u/ml the level of glutamine in the medium would also be significantly reduced and it is somewhat surprising that 70% (i. e. those insensitive to L-asparaginase) of the melanoma tested grew apparently normally in the presence of 40 u/ml of L-asparaginase.

Many obvious experiments to distinguish between the various possibilities suggest themselves and we are very conscious of the obvious shortcomings of this investigation. The reason for this is the shortage of the amount of tumour available for experiment. In many cases, the number of cells that can be obtained from the tumour handed to us is only of the order of 20 million and this is just sufficient for one series of experiments. When large numbers of cells have been obtained, then these were in general used for immunological procedures such as autoimmunization.

We have attempted to resolve the possible role of the glutaminase activity by using the enzyme found in Agouti serum which is devoid of all glutaminase activity. By salt precipitation a material having an asparaginase activity of about 2 u/mg of protein was obtained but this proved to be toxic to several of the melanoma cells tested, including those that were uneffected by the *E. coli* L-asparaginase. Obviously, further purification is necessary before the mammalian L-asparaginase can be used in this type of test. Preliminary experiments have been performed using dialysed serum and synthetic media containing 1) neither asparagine nor glutamine; 2) asparagine only; 3) glutamine only; 4) both glutamine and asparagine. The results so far obtained are difficult to interpret because all of the 11 tumours tested (2 of which were sensitive to L-asparaginase and 9 were not) showed the same general pattern; no growth in medium (1); poor growth in (2) and (3) and good growth in (4).

Summary

Cells separated from malignant melanoma were set up in short-term tissue culture using the Pulvertaft technique. *E. coli* L-asparaginase was added to the cultures at three concentrations, 5, 20 and 40 units/ml. An effect of asparaginase was recognised by the failure of the tumour cells to adhere to the coverslip. Of sixty melanomas examined 18 (30%) were sensitive to the presence of asparaginase, whereas 70% were uneffected even by the presence of 40 u/ml in the medium. Most of the tumors that were sensitive showed this effect fully at 5 u/ml but there were 4 tumours in which inhibition of growth was only seen at 20 u/ml and above. Neither the asparagine-sensitive nor the asparagine-resistant cells required the presence of asparagine in the medium for growth. But there is the possibility that the need of some melanoma cells for asparagine is being met by "feeding" from contaminating fibroblasts. Since the *E. coli* enzyme also deaminates glutamine it is possible that the effects seen may be due wholly or in part to glutamine deprivation.

Acknowledgment

This investigation has been supported by grants to the Chester Beatty Research Institute (Institute of Cancer Research; Royal Cancer Hospital), from the Medical Research Council and the British Empire Cancer Campaign for Research.

References

HALL, J. G.: This Symposium (1969).
HAMILTON FAIRLEEY, G., MALPAS, J. S., GALTON, D. A. G.: This Symposium (1969).
LEWIS, M. G., IKONOPISOV, R. L., NAIRN, R. C., PHILLIPS, T. M., HAMILTON FAIRLEY, G., BODENHAM, D. C., ALEXANDER, P.: Brit. med. J. **3**, 547 (1969).
PULVERTAFT, R. J. V.: J. clin. Path. **18**, 261 (1965).

Influence of L-Asparaginase Preparations of E. coli and Agouti Serum on the Homograft Reactivity in the Mouse

Hans Karl Schulten [1] and Gaetano Giraldo [2]

Sloan Kettering Institute for Cancer Research New York 10021, U.S.A.

With 2 Figures

Immunosuppression by E. coli L-asparaginase was first reported by Bertelli and his coworkers [3] who observed prolonged survival of skin allo- and xenografts in mice treated with high doses of the enzymepreparation. Hobik described inhibition of the graft-versus-host reaction in mice and rats receiving E. coli L-asparaginase [8]. Suppression of phytohemagglutinin-induced transformation of human lymphocytes was reported by Astaldi et al. [1] and by Ohno [12].

We have studied the effect of L-asparaginase on the resistance of mice to grafts of allogeneic and syngeneic tumors. Two types of enzymes were used: E. coli L-asparaginase, which also has L-glutaminase activity, and agouti serum L-asparaginase, which lacks L-glutaminase activity [5, 13].

In the allogeneic system the grafted tumor was an L-asparaginase-resistant subline of the radiation-induced leukemia EARAD 1 [4]. This leukemia originated in a $(C57BL/6 \times A)F_1$ mouse; its H-2 type is $H\text{-}2^b/H\text{-}2^a$. The recipents were $BALB/c \times C57BL/6)F_1$ mice, their H-2 type being $H\text{-}2^d/H\text{-}2^b$. The minimal number of EARAD 1 cells required for successful grafts in these incompatible recipients was 10^7. A subcutaneous inoculum of this size was used in all experiments.

Fig. 1 shows average growth curves of the subcutaneous grafts in three groups of mice. The control group received injections of saline. The subcutaneous grafts in this group reached an average diameter of 16 mm after 16 days. The second group received E. coli L-asparaginase 1000 IU/kg/day for a period of 11 days, beginning on the day of inoculation of the leukemia cells, by intraperitoneal injection. The average diameter of the grafts in this group after 16 days was 23 mm. The third group was treated with a ten-fold larger dose of E. coli L-asparaginase for the same period of time. In this group the average graft size was 26 mm. The initial delay in leukemia growth in the L-asparaginase-treated animals may be due to the L-glutaminase activity of the E. coli L-asparaginase preparation since leukemia EARAD 1 like many other cell lines requires L-glutamine in culture [9]. Or it may

---

[1] present address: Medizinische Klinik der Universität, 5 Köln-Lindenthal, Germany.

[2] Public Health Service Fellow (Fellowship No. FO 5 TW 1412—01).

be that the greater size of the early tumors in the untreated group is accounted for by oedema and cellular infiltration whiich accompanies the rejection of leukemia allografts [7]. The survival time was shortest for the group receiving 10,000 IU/kg/day of L-asparaginase, longer for the group treated with 1000 IU/kg/day and longest for the control group which was sacrificed 10 days after the last mouse that was treated with L-asparaginase had died from generalized leukemia. At autopsy (Table 1) the control mice showed only local tumors at the site of the graft. In other experiments, where control mice were not sacrificed, these tumors regressed completely later on. 3 of 4 mice treated with 1000 IU/kg/day of L-asparaginase showed circumscribed metastases in liver, spleen and kidney but no diffuse leukemic process. By contrast, 3 of 4 mice treated with 10,000 IU/kg/day had diffuse generalized leukemia of the type seen when this leukemia is passed in syngeneic recipients.

The question arose as to whether the immunosuppressive effect of E. coli L-asparaginase observed in this type of experiment was associated with its L-glutaminase activity. Experiments with agouti serum, which contains L-asparaginase but has no

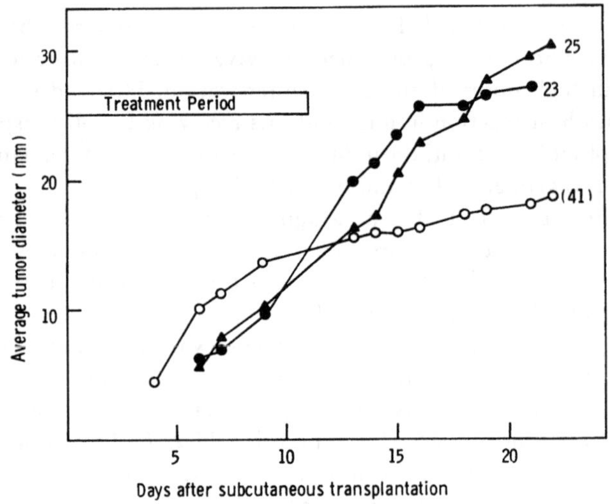

Fig. 1. Effect of E. coli L-asparaginase on the growth of leukemia EARAD 1 in (BALB/c ×C57BL/6)F_1 hosts (groups of 4 mice). ○——○ Saline i. p.; ▲——▲ L-asparaginase 1000 IU/kg/day i. p.; ●——● L-asparaginase 10,000 IU/kg/day i. p.

Table 1. *Times of death and patterns of growth in the three groups of mice shown in Fig. 1*

Dose (IU/kg/day)	Localized tumor	Circumscribed metastases	Generalized leukemia	Survival time (days)
—	4/4	—	—	41 [a]; 41 [a]; 41 [a]; 41 [a];
1,000	—	3/4	1/4	23; 23; 24; 31
10,000	—	1/4	3/4	21; 21; 22; 28

[a] Sacrificed.

L-glutaminase activity showed, however, that this was not the case. Agouti serum was partially purified four-fold by the method of MEISTER et al. [11]. Whole serum was precipitated with half saturated Na_2SO_4, the precipitate dissolved in cold water and after adsorption with calcium phosphate gel the supernatant was dialysed against phosphate buffered saline. The final product contained 20 IU of L-asparaginase per ml per 80 mg protein. Table 2 shows the effect of the agouti serum frac-

Table 2. *Effect of agouti serum L-asparaginase and of rabbit serum on the growth of leukemia EARAD 1 in (BALB/c×C57BL/6)F$_1$ hosts*

Treatment	Total graft regression	Localized tumor	Circum-scribed metastases	Gener-alized leukemia	Survival time (days)
Saline	4/4	—	—	—	91 [a]; 91 [a]; 91 [a]; 91 [a];
Agouti serum (1000 IU L-asparaginase/kg/day) [b]	—	1/4	2/4	1/4	23; 25; 28; 31
Rabbit serum	2/4	2/4	—	—	39; 45; 91 [a]; 91 [a]

[a] Sacrificed.
[b] Concentrated by the method of MEISTER et al. [11] to 20 IU L-asparaginase per ml.

tion on the rejection response of incompatible recipients to subcutaneous EARAD 1. The agouti serum fraction was administered subcutaneously for a period of 13 days, beginning on the day of inoculation of the leukemia cells at a dose of 20 IU L-asparaginase or 80 mg protein per mouse in 1 ml. There were two control groups: one injected with saline, the other injected with rabbit serum at a dose equivalent to the dose of the agouti serum fraction in terms of protein, according to the same schedule. It is evident that the mice receiving agouti serum died earlier than the control mice. At autopsy 1 was found to have generalized leukemia, and 2 had circumscribed metastases in liver and spleen. Two of the mice injected with rabbit serum died with large local tumors but showed no metastases at autopsy. The other two mice and those of the saline control group rejected the grafts completely. They were sacrificed and autopsied after three months and were free of tumor. Although we have not ruled out the alternative possibilities of immunosuppression by natural heteroantibody or by antigenic competition [6] this experiment indicates that L-glutaminase activity is not essential for the immunosuppressive effect of L-asparaginase preparations. This is also suggested by OHNO's observation that L-asparagine was more potent than L-glutamine in counteracting the inhibitory effect of E. coli L-asparaginase on the P.H.A. induced lymphocyte transformation *in vitro* [12], and by a recent report of OSOBA [14], which refers to enhanced antibody induction *in vitro* in the presence of added L-asparagine.

Having established that L-asparaginase inhibits the rejection response to allografted tumors we turned to the question of the potency of the enzyme in comparison to other immunosuppressive agents. In initial experiments of this sort the effect of L-asparaginase on the growth of grafts of a strongly antigenic methylcholanthrene-induced sarcoma in syngeneic mice was compared with that of the most potent immunosuppressive agent known, antilymphocyte serum. The antilymphocyte serum was raised in rabbits by injecting 10^9 mouse thymocytes on three occasions, with two week intervals. Its cytotoxic titer against mouse lymphocytes was 1 : 2000. Fig. 2 shows the growth curves of subcutaneous grafts of sarcoma Meth-A in three groups of BALB/c mice in one of these experiments. The control group received no treatment. One group was treated with 10,000 IU of E. coli L-asparaginase per kg per day for 15 days beginning two days before the tumor was grafted. A third group received 0.5 ml of antilymphocyte serum two days before the tumor graft, 0.2 ml on the day of inoculation and 0.1 ml every other day for a period of 15 days. After 20 days the average graft diameter was 12 mm in the control group, 15 mm in the group receiving L-asparaginase and 18 mm in the group treated with antilymphocyte serum. The corresponding survival times were 48, 37 and 35 days. It is evident that, although L-asparaginase inhibited the rejection response the antilymphocyte serum was more potent in this respect.

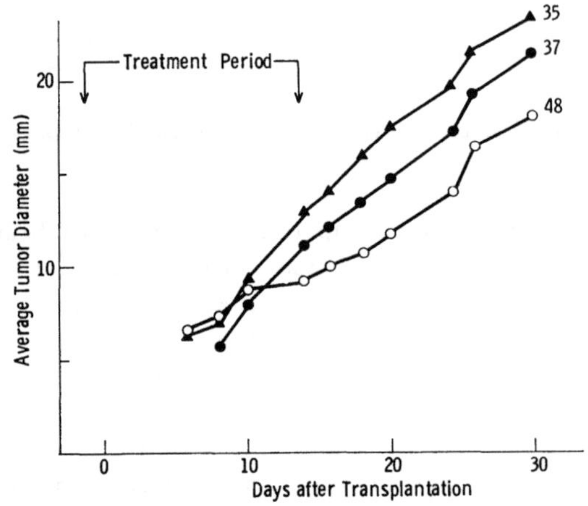

Fig. 2. Effect of E. coli L-asparaginase and antilymphocyte serum on the growth of transplants of sarcoma Meth-A in BALB/c mice. ○——○ No treatment; ▲——▲ Antilymphocyte serum; ●——● E. coli L-asparaginase

If one considers the available evidence there can be no doubt that L-asparaginase inhibits immune responses, particularly those of the cell-associated type. Since both E. coli L-asparaginase and agouti serum are effective, it seems more likely than not that this inhibition is the consequence of L-asparagine deprivation. It is not clear, at this point, whether this effect is sustained through long periods of therapy or whether immunological competent cells can adapt to the presence in the blood of L-asparaginase, a phenomenon that was first described by BECKER and BROOME in the regenerating liver of the rat [2]. In our experiments, an initial immunosuppressive effect of short duration could have sufficed to make possible the proliferation of the tumor grafts to a point where fully recovered immunologic competence would have been ineffective.

References

1. Astaldi, G., Burgio, G. R., Krč, J., Genova, R., Astaldi, A. A., Jr.: Lancet **1969 I,** 423.
2. Becker, F. F., Broome, J. D.: Science **156,** 1602 (1967).
3. Bertelli, A., Donati, L., Trabucchi, E.: Arch. ital. Pat. **11,** 3 (1968).
4. Boyse, E. A., Old, L. J., Campbell, H. A., Mashburn, L. T.: J. exp. Med. **125,** 17 (1967).
5 Campbell, H. A., Mashburn, L. T., Boyse, E. A., Old, L. J.: Biochemistry **6,** 721 (1967).
6. Despont, J. P., Cruchaud, A.: Nature **223,** 838 (1969).
7. Gorer, P. A.: Ann. N. Y. Acad. Sci. **73,** 707 (1958).
8. Hobik, H. P.: Naturwissenschaften **4,** 217 (1969).
9. Kim, J. H., Boyse, E. A., Old, L. J., Campbell, H. A.: Biochim. biophys. Acta (Amst.) **158,** 476 (1968).
10. McElwain, T. J., Hayward, S. K.: Lancet **1969 I,** 527.
11. Meister, A., Levintow, L., Greenfield, R. E., Abendschein, P. A.: J. biol. Chem. **215,** 441 (1955).
12. Ohno, R.: Proc. Amer. Ass. Cancer Res. **10,** 66 (1969).
13. Old, L. J., Boyse, E. A., Campbell, H. A., Daria, G. M.: Nature **198,** 801 (1963).
14. Osoba, D.: J. exp. Med. **129,** 141 (1969).

Studies on the Immunosuppressive Activity of L-Asparaginase

R. MARAL, J. C. GUYONNET, L. JULOU, Y. DE RATULD, and G. H. WERNER
Research Laboratories, Société des Usines Chimiques Rhône-Poulenc 94-Vitry-sur-Seine, France

With 4 Figures

I. Introduction

The immunological study of L-asparaginase is of interest for two main reasons:

first, this enzyme is immunogenic; this effect may explain the appearance of resistance in mice bearing a leukemia which is sensitive to the drug (WARAVDEKAR and GOLDIN, 1969) (personal unpublished findings);

secondly, L-asparaginase shows immunosuppressive activities in a number of tests.

Here we shall only consider the immunosuppressive activity of L-asparaginase, which we studied by various techniques:

a) effect of L-asparaginase on the production of antisheep red blood cell agglutinins in mice;

b) effect of L-asparaginase on the number of hemolysin-producing spleen cells in the mouse;

c) effect of L-asparaginase on the phenomenon of immuno-cyto-adherence of spleen cells (I.C.A.) in the mouse;

d) effect of L-asparaginase in the mouse on the tolerance of homologous skin grafts and effect of L-asparaginase on the proliferation of adult hen's lymphocytes on the chorioallantoic membrane of the chick embryo (graft versus host reaction);

e) effect of L-asparaginase on the blastic transformation of dog lymphocytes induced by phytohemagglutinin or by mixed culture of lymphocytes from two donors;

f) effect of L-asparaginase on the adjuvant-induced polyarthritis in the rat.

For this study, we have used L-asparaginase (or: L-asparagine-amidohydrolase, EC 3.5.1.1.) type EC_2, isolated from *Escherichia coli* which we received from Farbenfabriken Bayer (titer of this preparation: 150 I.U./mg).

II. Effect on the Production of Anti-Sheep-Hemagglutinins

1. Method

Animals: R III/Rho male inbred mice, about 6 weeks old.

Antigen: Sheep red blood cells; intravenous injection of 10^8 cells in 0.2 ml saline on day 0.

L-asparaginase: daily dose: 100 or 200 I.U./kg i. p.; treatment at various intervals (from day −8 up to day +7).

Hemagglutination reaction: performed on day +10; two-fold serial dilutions of serum were made in saline (0.50 ml/tube), a 1% suspension of sheep red blood cells in saline was added (0.50 ml/tube); the results were read after 24 hours.

2. Results

The results are summarized in Table 1.

$$\text{The ratio: } \frac{\text{hemagglutinating titer in serum of control mice}}{\text{hemagglutinating titer in serum of treated mice}}$$

was considered significant when higher than 4. Under these conditions, L-asparaginase was active when administered before the injection of the antigen and during a prolonged period (from 5 to 8 treatments). A prolonged treatment after injection of antigen did not affect the immune response.

Table 1. *Production of anti-sheep hemagglutinins in the mouse*

Asparaginase daily dose (I.U./kg i. p.)	Treatment on days	Result A/B [a]
100	−2 0 +2	1.3
	−2 0 +2	1.8
200	−2	0.8
100	0	1.0
200	+2	1.2
100	0 +1 +5 +6 +7	0.6
100	−6 −5 −2 −1 0	34
200	−8 −7 −6 −5 −4 −2 −1 0 +1 +2	23

[a] $A/B = \frac{\text{Hemagglutinin titer in control mice}}{\text{Hemagglutinin titer in treated mice}}$.

III. Number of Hemolysin-Producing Spleen Cells

1. Method

We used a modification of the technique described by JERNE (JERNE and NORDIN, 1963).

Female 1 month old (C.O.B.S.) mice (Charles River-France) were injected intravenously with 10^8 sheep red blood cells per mouse on day 0. L-asparaginase (100 I.U./kg i. p.) was given on days 0, +1 and +2. On day +3, the spleens were removed and a suspension of spleen cells was prepared, containing $0.25 \cdot 10^7$ spleen cells in 3 ml of Eagle medium with 10% guinea pig serum. These 3 ml of suspension were poured in Petri dishes (95 mm diameter) onto a layer of 3 ml of agar (Difco

Noble Agar) at 1% in saline, containing $0.66 \cdot 10^8$ sheep red blood cells/ml. The dishes were incubated for 20 hours at 37° in a humid atmosphere. The number of hemolytic plaques was then determined for each dish.

2. Results

The results are given in Table 2. The inhibitory effect of L-asparaginase on the average number of hemolysin-producing cells was considerable, in spite of the fact that the enzyme was administered *after* the antigen.

Table 2. *Hemolysin-producing mouse spleen cells*

Experiment	Asparaginase dose (I.U./kg i. p.)	Average number of hemolysis plaques for 0.25×10^7 spleen cells	Ratio $\frac{\text{control}}{\text{treated}}$
1	0	268	
	100	64	4.1
	200	38	6.9
2	0	163	
	100	60	2.7
	200	21	7.8

IV. Immuno-Cyto-Adherence (I.C.A.)

1. Method

We studied the effect of L-asparaginase on the phenomenon of immuno-cyto-adherence (NOTA et al., 1964; BIOZZI et al., 1966; BACH et al., 1968, 1969). Several types of I.C.A. tests were performed:

a) *in vitro:* spontaneous I.C.A. (12 000 splenic cells/µl)
induced I.C.A. (6 000 splenic cells/µl)

b) *in vivo:* spontaneous I.C.A. (12 000 splenic cells/µl)
induced I.C.A. (6 000 splenic cells/µl)

c) we also studied the effect of serum from asparaginase-treated animals on spontaneous I.C.A. (12 000 splenic cells/µl).

These techniques are illustrated in figures 1 and 2.

2. Results

a) The *in vitro* results are summarized in Table 3. In these tests L-asparaginase, like azathioprine, inhibited the formation of spontaneous "rosettes"; it did not effect induced "rosettes", however.

b) Results obtained *in vivo* are summarized in Table 4. L-asparaginase inhibited the *in vivo* production of "rosettes". Again, this effect was more marked on spontaneous "rosettes" than on induced "rosettes"; on the latter, L-asparaginase was less active than azathioprine.

c) *Effect of serum of asparaginase-treated mice on spontaneous I.C.A.*

We used female 1 month old C.O.B.S. mice (Charles River-France). The mice were treated with 100 I.U./kg of L-asparaginase i. p.; their serum was collected at various intervals after the injection of the enzyme; the effect of the serum on spontaneous I.C.A. was studied, by determination of the serum dilution which reduced by 50% the number of spontaneous "rosettes" (ID_{50}). The results are shown in figure 3: The peak of activity in the serum was reached after 2 hours,

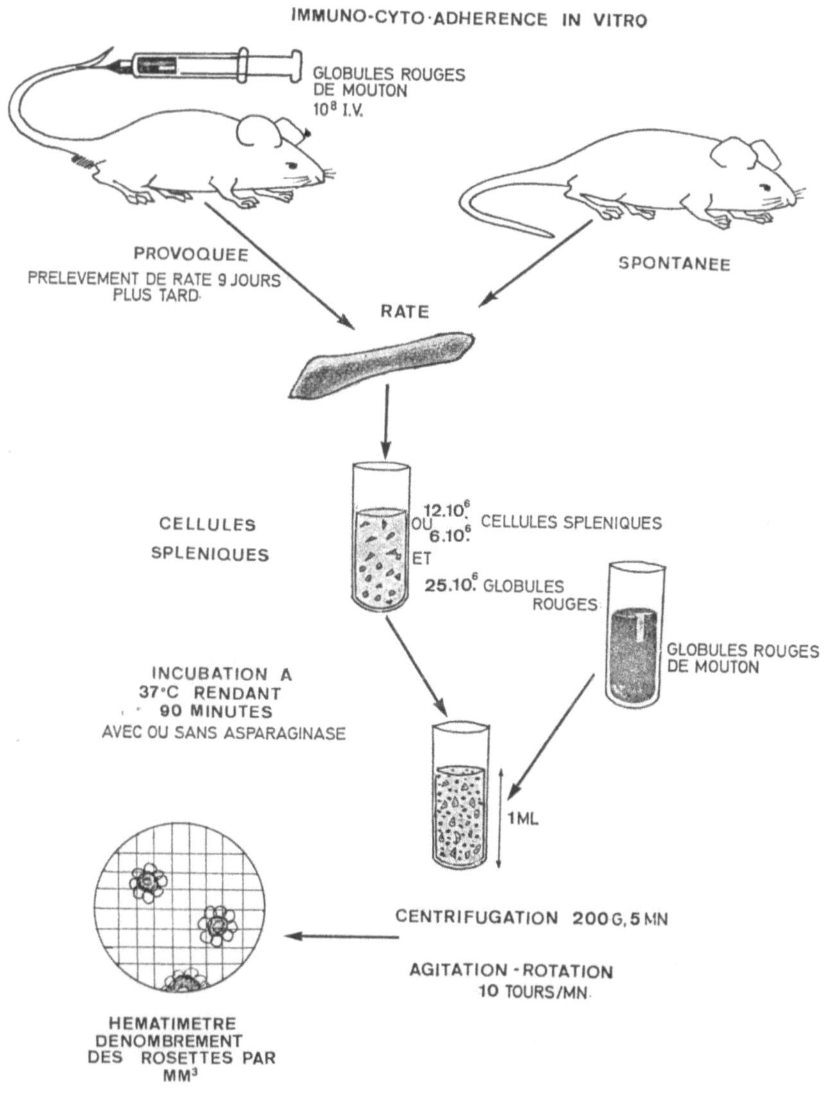

Fig. 1. Immune-Cyto-Adherence in vitro

corresponding to an average serum dilution of 1 : 96. We know that a 50 per cent inhibition of spontaneous "rosettes" formation is produced by 0.24 I.U./ml (IC_{50}). Therefore, the theoretical concentration of the enzyme in the blood is $0.24 \times 96 = 23$ I.U./ml. As we treated the mice with 100 · I.U./kg of L-asparaginase i. e. 2 I.U. for 20 g mouse, we found in the blood a theoretical amount of asparaginase which was markedly higher than the amount actually given. This discrepancy might be explained by assuming that the circulating blood contains a factor which activates the enzyme.

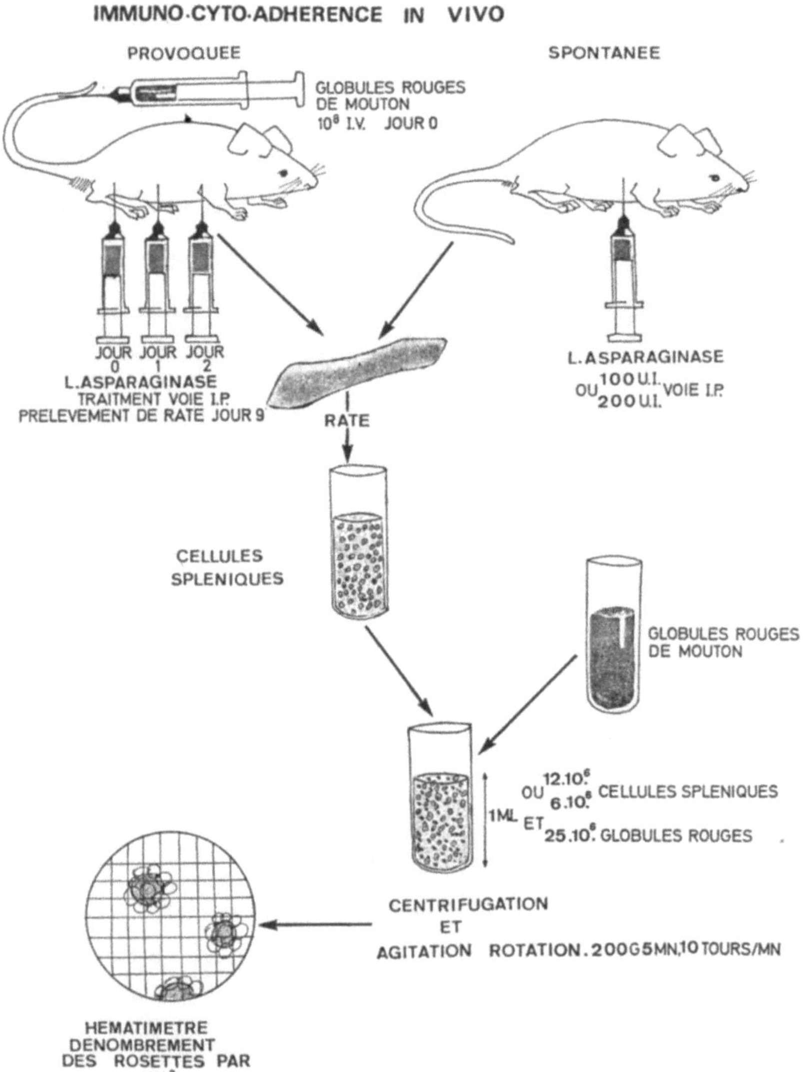

Fig. 2. Immune-Cyto-Adherence in vivo

Table 3. *Effect of asparaginase on Immune-Cyto-Adherence (I.C.A.) in vitro*

I.C.A.	L-asparaginase			Azathioprine		
	50% inhibitory concentration (IC_{50})	50% cytotoxic concentration (CC_{50})	Ratio $\frac{CC_{50}}{IC_{50}}$	50% inhibitory concentration (IC_{50})	50% cytotoxic concentration (CC_{50})	Ratio $\frac{CC_{50}}{IC_{50}}$
Spontaneous	0.24 I.U./ml [a]	10 I.U./ml [b]	41	6 μg/ml	100 μg/ml	16,6
Induced	> 20 I.U./ml		< 1	200 μg/ml		< 1

[a] 0.24 I.U./ml = 1.6 μg/ml.
[b] 10 I.U./ml = 6.6 μg/ml.

Table 4. *Effect of asparaginase on Immune-Cyto-Adherence (I.C.A.) in vivo. Number of "rosettes" for 1000 spleen cells*

I.C.A.	L-Asparaginase			Azathioprine		
	Dose I.U./kg i. p.	"Rosettes" ‰	Ratio $\frac{\text{control}}{\text{treated}}$	Dose mg/kg i. p.	"Rosettes" ‰	Ratio $\frac{\text{control}}{\text{treated}}$
Spontaneous	0	0.5	—	0	0.7	—
	200	0.1	5	75	0.1	7
	100	0.3	1.6	50	0.2	3.5
Induced	0	12.3	—	0	10.9	—
	200	6.2	1.9	100	2.8	3.9
	100	10.8	1.1	50	4.9	2.2

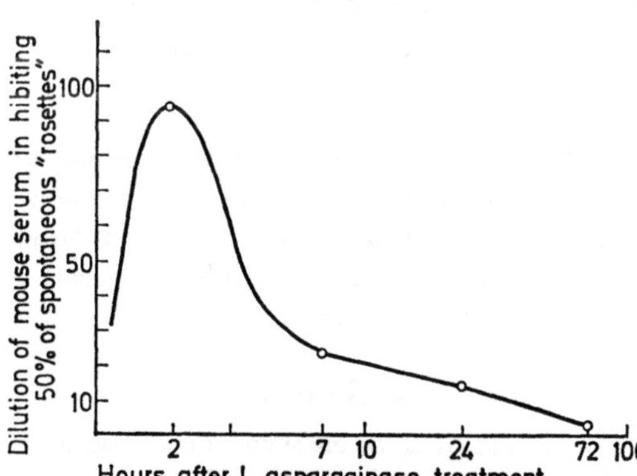

Fig. 3. Effect of the serum of asparaginase-treated mice on spontaneous rosette formation in vitro

V. Homologous Grafts

A. Homologous Skin Grafts in the Mouse

1. Method

The mice were 2 months old. The skin grafts were performed using female inbred AKR/Rho mice as donors and female inbred RP XXI/Rho mice as recipients. The animals were treated for one or two weeks before grafting and thereafter until the grafts had been rejected.

2. Results

The results are summarized in Table 5. Under our experimental conditions (the dose of L-asparaginase was fairly low), treatment with asparaginase did not prolong the survival of the skin grafts. It is noteworthy that HOBIK (1969) described an immunosuppressive activity of asparaginase in the mouse on the graft reaction against the host. (GvHR: splenic index.) SCHULTEN et al. reported in a recent paper (SCHULTEN et al., 1969) that L-asparaginase treatment (1000 and 10,000 I.U./kg i. p.) allowed the growth in the mouse of a non-histocompatible tumor.

Table 5. *Homologous skin grafts in mice. AKR/Rho ♀ → RP XXI ♀*

Experiment	Asparaginase daily dose I.U./kg i. p.	Average time (in days) until graft rejection	
		Control mice	Treated mice
1 [a]	100	11.0±0.1	11.3±0.2
2 [b]	200	11.0±0.1	11.0±0.3

[a] Treatment begun one week before grafting.
[b] Treatment begun two weeks before grafting.

B. Inoculation of Adult Fowl Lymphocytes Onto the Chick Embryo Choriollantoic Membrane

1. Method

The inoculation of adult fowl lymphocytes (5×10^6 lymphocytes per membrane) onto the chorioallantoic membrane of chick embryos of 10 days incubation leads to the formation of characteristic nodular lesions, which represent the reaction of immunologically competent cells to histocompatibility antigens present in the membrane (BOYER, 1960; BURNET and BOYER, 1960).

2. Results

When injected in the air sac of chick embryos, at a dose of 500 µg/egg (75 I.U.), asparaginase did not decrease the number of nodular lesions caused by the inoculation of adult fowl lymphocytes onto the chorioallantoic membrane. It should be noted that, among a number of compounds studied by this technique, only cyclophosphamide has shown some activity.

VI. Transformation of Lymphocytes Into Lymphoblasts

A. Stimulating Effect of Phytohemagglutinin on the Blastic Transformation of Lymphocytes (NOWELL, 1960; ROBBINS, 1964)

At the highest concentration studied (50 µg/ml or 7 I.U./ml in the culture medium), asparaginase caused a 40% inhibition of the blast formation of dog lymphocytes induced by phytohemagglutinin (present at a 2.5% concentration in the medium). This observation confirms the results of MCELWAIN et al. (1969), OHNO (1969) and ASTALDI (1969).

B. Lymphoblast Formation in Mixed Lymphocytes Cultures

It is known that the mixed culture of lymphocytes from 2 donors of the same species causes the transformation into lymphoblasts of a certain percentage of the cells (BACH and HIRSCHHORN, 1964; BAIN and LOWENSTEIN, 1964).

Using mixed dog lymphocyte cultures, we have found that, at concentrations varying between 7 and 100 µg/ml (1 to 15 I.U./ml), L-asparaginase caused a practically total inhibition (80 to 100%) of the lymphoblastic transformation of the cells. In the control mixed cultures, without L-asparaginase, 20 to 30% of the cells were transformed. It should be noted that the minimum essential medium of Eagle, used in our cultures, does not contain any asparagine.

The fact that L-asparaginase exerted a stronger inhibitory effect on the lymphoblastic transformation in mixed cultures than on that induced by phytohemagglutinin, is in favor of the assumption that the compound has a specific activity on the immunological reactivity of the lymphocytes.

VII. Adjuvant-Induced Polyarthritis in the Rat

1. Method

Polyarthritis was provoked in the rat following a technique similar to that of DELBARRE, et al. (1968), by injecting 0.1 ml of a 0.6% suspension of *Mycobacterium butyricum* in an emulsion in vaseline oil into the foot-pad of a hind leg. Unter these conditions, one can observe the appearance of a polyarthritis, together with secondary lesions on the tail and on the ears, 10 to 12 days after injection of the mycobacteria.

The animals were observed daily for 12 days, beginning 10 days after the injection of the mycobacteria, and an arthritis index (0, 1, 2, 3 or 4), proportional to the severity of the lesions, was given to the uninjected hind leg, to the fore legs, to the tail and to the ears.

2. Results

A preliminary study showed that, when given to the rat at a daily dose of 200 I.U./kg i. p. for 21 days beginning on the day of the inoculation of the mycobacteria, L-asparaginase exerted a marked inhibitory effect on the development of the polyarthritis. These results are illustrated by Fig. 4: between the 16th and 21st day of treatment, the average arthritis index of treated animals was about 50% lower than the average arthritis index of the untreated control animals.

This interesting aspect of the pharmacological activity of L-asparaginase is now being studied in greater detail.

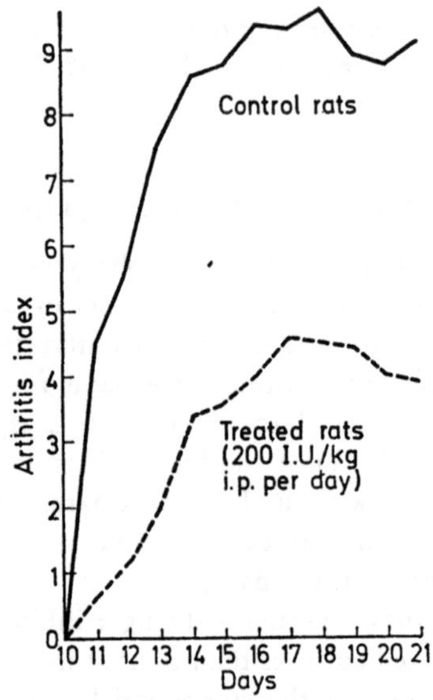

Fig. 4. Adjuvant-induced polyarthritis in the rat. Preventive activity of L-asparaginase

VIII. Conclusions

The immunosuppressive activity of L-asparaginase varies according to the immunological tests used in this study. These tests belong essentially to two groups: those based on humoral immunity (anti-sheep hemagglutinin) and those bringing into play cell-bound immunity phenomena (transformation of lymphocytes into lymphoblasts). The other tests (such as hemolysin-producing spleen cells, immuno-cytoadherence) are more difficult to classify, because they probably involve both types of immunity. Finally, the adjuvant-induced polyarthritis is reminiscent of autoimmune diseases.

It is therefore established that L-asparaginase is capable, on the one hand, of inhibiting the production of circulating antibodies and, on the other hand, of interfering with some phenomena of cell-bound immunity, such as the lymphoblastic transformation of lymphocytes. In addition, this enzyme can also exert an inhibitory effect on an auto-immune disease, examplified by the adjuvant-induced arthritis in the rat.

For these reasons, a precise localization of the site of action of L-asparaginase in the complex scheme of immunological phenomena is not possible; our results, together with those of other authors, show, however, that the enzyme can act not only on some sensitive malignant cell lines (asparagine-dependent) but also on normal cells of the thymus, the spleen and the bone marrow, which play a role in immunological phenomena.

Among the various mechanisms which have been considered by HUMPHREY (1969) to explain the immunosuppressive activity of drugs, it is logical to assume that the enzyme interferes with some processes of cellular protein synthesis, particularly that of immunoglobulins.

Summary

The immunosuppressive activity of L-asparaginase was studied by means of several *in vivo* and *in vitro* tests.

The enzyme was found to exert a significant inhibitory effect on the production of anti-sheep hemagglutinins in the mouse, on the number of hemolysin-producing mouse spleen cells (even when it was administered after the antigen), on the number of spontaneously occurring "rosettes" in the phenomenon of immuno-cyto-adherence and also on the blastic transformation *in vitro* of dog lymphocytes induced by phyto-hemagglutinin or in mixed cultures. On the other hand, L-asparaginase treatment (at a low dose) did not increase the survival time of homologous skin grafts in the mouse and did not affect the production of nodular lesions in the chorioallantoic membrane of chick embryos inoculated with adult fowl lymphocytes. Finally, L-asparaginase exerted a significant preventive effect on the adjuvant-induced polyarthritis in the rat.

It may be concluded that L-asparaginase is capable of inhibiting the production of circulating antibodies and also of interfering with some phenomena associated with cell-bound immunity.

References

ASTALDI, G., BURGIO, G. R., GENOVA, R., ASTALDI, A. A.: Lancet **1969 I**, 423.
BACH, F. H., HIRSCHHORN, R.: Science **143**, 815 (1964).
BACH, J. F., ANTOINE, B.: Nature **217**, 658 (1968).
— DARDENNE, M., FOURNIER, C.: Nature **222**, 998 (1969).
BAIN, B., LOWENSTEIN, L.: Science **145**, 1315 (1964).
BIOZZI, G., STIFFEL, C., MOUTON, D., LIACOPOULOS-BRIOT, M., DUCREUSEFOND, C., BOUTHILLIER, Y.: Ann. Inst. Pasteur **110**, 7 (1966).
BOYER, G.: Nature **185**, 327 (1960).
BURNET, F. M., BOYER, G.: Nature **186**, 175 (1960).
DELBARRE, F., BROUILHET, H., KAHAN, A.: C. R. Soc. Biol. (Paris) **162**, 58 (1968).
HOBIK, H. P.: Naturwissenschaften **56**, (4), 217 (1969).
HUMPHREY, J. H.: Antibiot. et Chemother. (Basel) **15**, 1 (1969).
JERNE, N. K., NORDIN, A. A.: Science **140**, 405 (1963).
MCELWAIN, T. J., HAYWARD, S. K.: Lancet **1969 I**, 527.
NOTA, N. R., LIACOPOULOS-BRIOT, M., STIFFEL, C., BIOZZI, G.: C. R. Acad. Sci. (Paris) **259**. 1277 (1964).
NOWELL, P. C.: Cancer Res. **20**, 462 (1960).
OHNO, R.: Proc. Amer. Ass. Cancer Res. **10**, 66 (1969).
ROBBINS, J. H.: Science **146**, 1, 648 (1964).
SCHULTEN, H. K., GIRALDO, G., BOYSE, E. A., OETTGEN, H. F.: Lancet **1969 I**, 644.
WARAVDEKAR, V. S., GOLDIN, A.: Proc. Amer. Ass. Cancer Res. **10**, 95 (1969).

Experimental Immunosuppression with L-Asparaginase

K. Lauenstein, E. Grundmann, H. P. Hobik, and W.-P. Madaus

Institute of Experimental Pathology, Farbenfabriken Bayer AG.,
Wuppertal-Elberfeld, Germany

During the last year several papers were published dealing with an immunosuppressive action of Escherichia coli L-asparaginase. Hobik described the inhibition of the graft-versus-host reaction in rats and mice. Bertelli, Donati and Trabucchi, using very high doses of L-asparaginase, found a prolongation of the rejection time of allogeneic and xenogeneic skin grafts in mice. Schulten, Giraldo, Boyse and Oettgen showed an effect of L-asparaginase on the homograft response. These experiments were presented by Dr. Schulten during this symposium. Several other reports deal with the inhibition of phythaemagglutinin-induced blastic transformation of human lymphocytes in vitro by L-asparaginase.

All these experimental models are concerned with the inhibition of cell-bound immunity. In his preceding paper Dr. Maral and his group presented evidence that the formation of humoral antibodies is also influenced by L-asparaginase.

Our paper is concerned with the inhibition of both humoral and delayed type immune responses.

In Table 1 we have summarized our results regarding the heterohaemagglutinin titres in mice. Using a variety of therapeutic schemes we were not able to demon-

Table 1. *The effect of Crasnitin*[1] *on the heterohemagglutinin titre of the mouse. CFW-mice. 0.2 ml 5% sheep red cells suspension i.v. on day 0. Titres estimated in the pooled sera of each group*

Dosis IU/kg i. p.	No. of animals	Therapy on the days	Titre on day	Mean $\log_2$ titre of the therapy group	Mean $\log_2$ titre of the control group
150	10	+1	7	5	5
300	10	+1	7	4	5
600	10	+1	4	6	6
600	10	0	4	5	6
600	10	+1	4	6	6
600	10	+2	4	6	6
600	10	−1 until +2 daily	4	6	6
1000	10	−8 until +4 daily	7	5	6
1200	10	+1	7	6	6
2000	10	−20 until +4 daily	7	5	6
3000	10	−20 until +4 daily	7	5	6

[1] Registered trade mark: Bayer-Leverkusen, Germany.

strate any effect of Crasnitin on the synthesis of agglutinins against sheep red cells. On the other hand Dr. MADAUS in our group found an inhibition of plaque forming cells using the Jerne technique. This fits in well with Dr. MARAL's results, this technique being much more sensitive than the estimation of agglutinins.

Since the sheep red cell model presents more of a secondary than a primary immune response, we immunized mice with bovine transferrin as a model of a primary humoral immune response.

In Table 2 it is noted that there is a significant inhibition of the antibody titre by Crasnitin.

Table 2. *Effect of Crasnitin on the antitransferrin formation of mice. NMRI-mice. Bovine transferrin (Mann Res. Lab.). Gradient plate technique. Therapy daily for 6 weeks starting 1 week before antigen. P calculated by the t-test*

No. of animals	Crasnitin IU/kg i. p.	Mean body weight after 6 weeks therapy	Mean $\log_2$ titre ± SD	Significance P
9	Controls	37.0	8.7 ± 1.3	
10	1500	32.2	6.4 ± 1.9	0.03
10	3000	30.4	2.6 ± 3.6	<0.001

Table 3. *Inhibition of the graft-versus-host-reaction of the mouse by Crasnitin. Three months old (C57/Bl/6×CPB/N)-F1-mice. Therapy starting on the second day after spleen cell injection for 5 resp. 10 days. Estimations of the spleen weights on day 15. P calculated by the t-test*

	No. of animals	Mean values of spleen weights mg ± SD	Significance P
Controls 0.9% NaCl 10×i. p.	10	78 ± 10	—
21.8×10⁶ spleen cells i. p. 0.9% NaCl 10×i. p.	7	310 ± 90	—
21.8×10⁶ spleen cells i. p. 1000 IU/kg Crasnitin 5×i. p.	9	107 ± 10	<0.001
21.8×10⁶ spleen cells i. p. 500 IU/kg Crasnitin 10×i. p.	10	149 ± 60	<0.001

In Tables 3, 4, and 5 we have demonstrated an inhibition of cell-bound immunity in three different in vivo systems. Table 3 shows the influence of Crasnitin on the graft-versus-host reaction of mice. These results have already been published. Doses of below 500 IU/kg were not effective. On 3 months old F1-hybrids of Wistar I and BD III rats the same reaction was influenced by 1000 IU/kg Crasnitin in a similar manner.

It must be stressed that in these and the following experiments the effective dose of Crasnitin was always higher than 500 to 1000 IU/kg. Secondly we only get an effect by treatment before or immediately after exposure to antigen. This means that Crasnitin acts on a very early stage of the immune response. Finally all rodents treated over a longer period developed anti-asparaginase antibodies.

Table 4 demonstrates the influence of Crasnitin on the allogeneic skin transplantation of two inbred mice strains. There is a significant prolongation of graft survival when doses higher than 2000 IU/kg daily are used. Even with these doses the effect is moderate.

Using colony rats (Table 5) we obtained the same results.

Table 4. *Allogeneic skin transplantation between C3H and B6D2F1 mice*

Crasnitin daily i. p. until graft rejection Start of therapy	IU/kg	No. of animals	Mean reaction time Days ± SD	Mean body weight after graft rejection	Significance P
1 day after transplantation	Controls	9	19.5 ± 1.2	23.2	
	150	9	20.3 ± 1.4	23.4	—
	300	9	20.8 ± 1.1	23.0	—
10 days before transplantation	Controls	14	20.4 ± 1.0	20.9	
	1000	14	21.0 ± 1.5	20.1	0.1
21 days before transplantation	Controls	9	19.6 ± 2.3	25.2	
	2000	8	22.8 ± 2.3	22.7	<0.001
21 days before transplantation	Controls	9	21.0 ± 2.1	27.4	
	3000	9	30.6 ± 10.7	23.7	<0.001
7 days before transplantation	Controls	10	20.9 ± 1.7	24.7	
	3000	9	26.9 ± 3.8	22.7	<0.001
	4000	8	31.1 ± 3.1	21.1	<0.001

Table 5. *Effect of Crasnitin on the allogeneic skin transplantation of rats. Male Wistar I rats. Therapy from 3 weeks before transplantation until graft rejection*

Crasnitin IU/kg i. p.	animals No. of	Mean body weight after rejection	Mean rejection time Days ± SD
Controls	4	346	15.6 ± 2.0
2000	4	299	32.2 ± 10.3
3000	3	330	46.1 ± 12.8

How does Crasnitin act on immunocompetent cells? We assumed that the mechanism involved would be the same as in leukemic cells. It would be reasonable to expect this mechanism to operate also in in vitro immune models, for example in the PHA-induced blastic transformation. But recently doubts arose as to wheter this holds true also for in vivo experiments.

Some other possibilities are glutamine depletion, antigenic competition or other unknown or unspecific effects. To exclude antigenic competition we have started experiments in our laboratory and are attempting to induce low dose immunotolerance against L-asparaginase and then we will repeat some of our tests using these animals.

In summary Crasnitin has an immunosuppressive effect in rodents. This effect can be obtained in vivo only with doses higher than 500 to 1000 IU/kg. Both immune systems, the humoral and the cell-bound immune response can be inhibited. It has not been proved yet, that Crasnitin acts on the immune systems by asparagin depletion.

References

ASTALDI, G., BURGIO, G. R., BISCATTI, G., ASTALDI, A., JR., FERFOGLIA, L.: Lancet **1969 I**, 643.
— — KRČ, J., GENOVA, R., ASTALDI, A. A.: Lancet **1969 I**, 423.
BERTELLI, A., DONATI, L., TRAUBUCHI, E., JR.: Arch ital. Pat. **11**, 475 (1969).
HOBIK, H. P.: Naturwissenschaften **56**, 217 (1969).
MADAUS, W.-P.: Klin. Wschr. **48**, 240 (1970).
MCELWAIN, T. J., HAYWARD, S. K.: Lancet **1969 I**, 527.
OHNO, R.: Proc. Amer. Ass. Cancer Res. **10**, 66 (1969).
SCHULTEN, H. K., GIRALDO, G., BOYSE, E. A., OETTGEN, H. F.: Lancet **1969 I**, 644.
SCHWARTZ, R. S.: Nature (Lond.) **224**, 275 (1969).

Part V
Animal Toxicity

Experimental Studies on the Toxicity of Crasnitin in Animals

D. Lorke and D. Tettenborn

Institute of Toxicology, Farbenfabriken Bayer AG., Wuppertal-Elberfeld, Germany

With 4 Figures

Crasnitin [1] (L-asparaginase) is a new therapeutic agent in the treatment of acute lymphoblastic leukemia. In the development of new drugs thorough toxicological investigations are always carried out and this applied also to Crasnitin.

We tested Crasnitin for

1. Acute toxicity
2. Subchronic toxicity (3 months)
   a) rats
   b) dogs
3. Antigenicity
4. Pyrogenicity
5. Embryotoxicity and teratogenicity.

The investigations were generally carried out by intravenous application. If it was not possible after repeated treatment to inject Crasnitin intraveneously, the injections were given intraperitoneally.

1. Acute Toxicity

The acute toxic effect is shown in the first table.

We used five species: Mouse, rat, cat, dog and rabbit.

The LD_{50} for mouse and rat lies above 200,000 U/kg. It was not possible to inject higher doses because of the limited solubility of Crasnitin.

Cats and dogs were more sensitive. The LD_{50} was about 50,000 U/kg.

The rabbit is an exception. Some animals already died after receiving doses of 500 or 1000 U/kg, while others survived 10,000 U/kg. We have no explanation for this unusual behaviour.

In all five species we found: decreased motility, anorexia, weakness and weight loss. In addition vomiting was observed in cats and dogs.

---

[1] Registered trade mark: Bayer-Leverkusen, Germany.

The weight loss after a single dose is shown in Fig. 1.

This figure gives the weight curve of mice which have been injected with varying doses of Crasnitin. One can clearly observe that the treated animals lost weight immediately after injection.

During the following days the treated animals gained weight though not to the same extent as the controls.

In rats the loss of weight is dose-related and the recovery is more rapid (see Fig. 2).

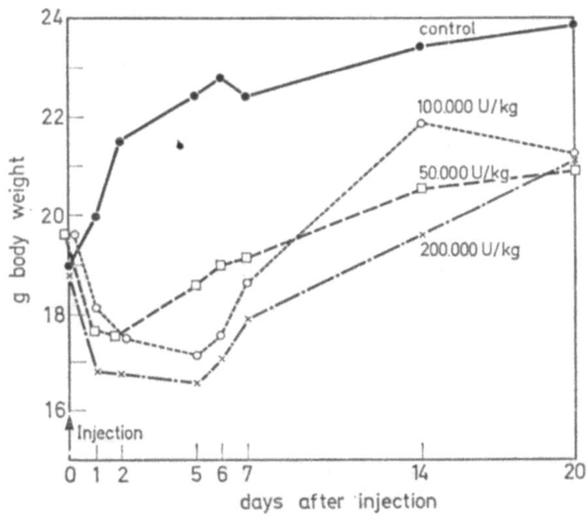

Fig. 1. Weight changes after single injections of varying doses of Crasnitin in mice

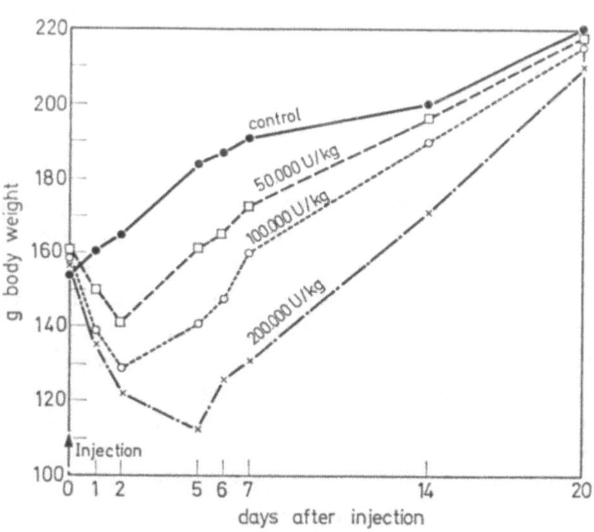

Fig. 2. Weight changes after single injections of varying doses of Crasnitin in rats

Table 1. *Results of the acute toxicity tests in animals*

Species	LD_{50}—U/kg	Symptoms
Mice	> 200,000	Decreased motility, ataxia, weakness, ventral position, heavy breathing, cyanosis; weight loss
Rats	> 200,000	Symptoms as in mice
Cats	ca. 50,000	Vomiting, decreased motility, anorexia, weight loss
Dogs	ca. 50,000	Vomiting, decreased motility, weakness, anorexia, weight loss, exsiccosis, haemoconcentration
Rabbits	varying results: death from 500—10,000 U/kg	Decreased motility, weakness, anorexia, weight loss, lateral position, salivation, tremor P.M.: in rare cases enterocolitis or edema of lungs

2. Subchronic Toxicity

a) Rat

Groups of ten male and ten female rats were treated daily with Crasnitin intraperitoneally (5 times a week) receiving the following doses: 200, 800 and 3000 U/kg.

The amount of solution at all dose levels was 10 ml/kg. The animals were treated for a period of three months.

The animals tolerated the treatment without any effects on their behaviour. A slightly slower weight gain, however, was observed in the male rats treated with 800 or 3000 U/kg, whereas female rats, receiving the same doses, tolerated them without any change in their weight curve (Fig. 3).

No biochemical or haematological differences were apparent between the test and control animals.

Gross pathology showed no damage and all organ weights were within the normal range.

Histological investigations by LUCKHAUS, SAWADA and HOBIK revealed a mild swelling of the liver cells with a slight periportal fatty infiltration. The thymus showed broadening of its cortex.

b) Dog

The method of our subchronic toxicity test in dogs was as follows. Three female and three male pure bred beagle dogs were used in each group. They were housed individually during the treatment period of 3 months and received the same dose levels as the rats: 200, 800 or 3000 U/kg. The following investigations were carried out: General behaviour, weight, haematology, clinical chemistry, liver function test, urine analysis, gross pathology, histopathology; special investigations: ECG, ophthalmic investigations. All dogs survived, although they had shown clear signs of toxicity.

Doses of 3000 U/kg caused vomiting in the dog one to two hours after injection. Vomiting became less frequent and, after a treatment period of four weeks, vomiting ceased altogether.

Considerable loss in weight occurred especially in the animals of the highest dose group during the first period of treatment. This was not the case in the control group (Fig. 4).

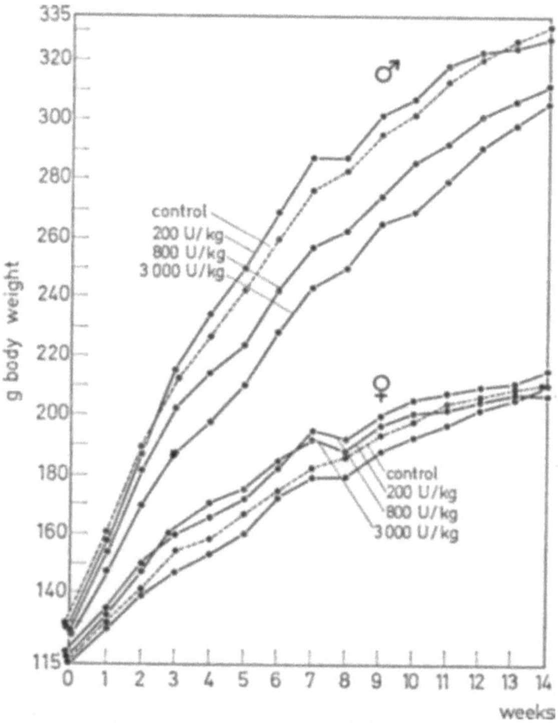

Fig. 3. Growth curve of rats in the subchronic toxicity test

The results of the biochemical and haematological investigations were not impressive, in contrast to the marked weight loss and symptoms. A slight increase in BSP-retention in one dog and a temporary rise in activity of GOT and GPT in another dog point to a slight damage of the liver. Interim autopsy of some dogs after four weeks showed that the thymi were completely atrophied. Dogs killed at the end of the 3 month test period did not show complete thymic atrophy. The thymi were, however, reduced in size.

Only one dog of the highest dose group showed slight fatty infiltration of the liver cells in the form of very fine droplets.

3. Antigenicity

The antigenicity tests were carried out in guinea pigs in standard fashion.

The animals were sensitized by two individual doses of Crasnitin. The immune reaction was evoked 14 days later by giving the same dose. Table 2 shows the results.

We tested two different batches of Crasnitin, using Ov-Albumin as a positive control.

Our test demonstrated that Crasnitin has a marked antigenic effect.

4. Pyrogenicity

According to the DAB-7th edition, we injected Crasnitin intraveneously in rabbits and the temperatures were measured by the use of an automatic temperature recorder.

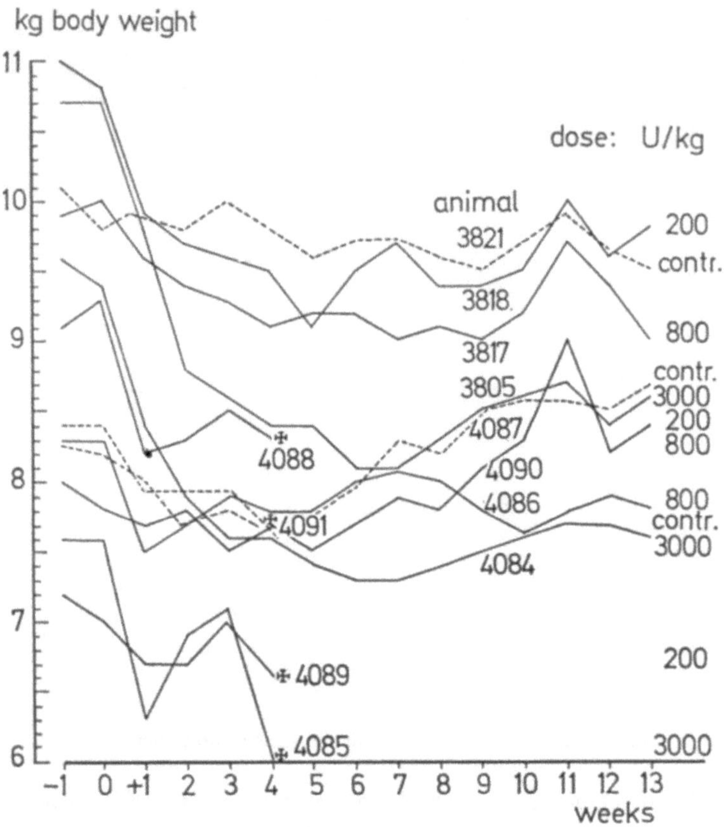

Fig. 4. Weight changes in female dogs during the subchronic toxicity study

Table 2. *Results of antigenicity tests in guinea pigs*

Preparation batch	Dose	Number of animals	Number of animals with symptoms: without symptoms	slight symptoms	severe symptoms	Exitus	Number of animals with lethal shock in %
L-asparaginase 9868 batch	500 U/kg	11	9	1	0	1	9
	1000 U/kg	12	6	0	0	6	50
	2000 U/kg	12	5	1	3	3	25
L-asparaginase 11269 batch	500 U/kg	12	10	1	0	1	8
	1000 U/kg	11	11	0	0	0	0
	2000 U/kg	10	6	1	1	2	20
Ovalbumin	0.3 mg/kg	12	6	4	1	1	8
	1.0 mg/kg	10	3	0	4	3	30

At the beginning of our tests, 200 U/kg were injected; at the moment 1000 U/kg are injected. Only if these doses are tolerated without producing a rise in temperature are the batches released.

5. Teratogenic Effect

ADAMSON and FABRO published in 1968 in Nature that it was possible to cause malformations with L-asparaginase in rabbits. We tested Crasnitin for its embryotoxic and teratogenic effect in rats.

These investigations were carried out in accordance with the recommendations of the FDA:

Treatment from the 6. to the 15. day of pregnancy
Dose levels: 300, 1000, 3000, 10,000 U/kg
Number of dams per group: 10
Caesarian section one day before birth
Careful investigations of the fetuses
The results of our studies are summarized in Table 3.

Table 3. *Results of investigations on teratogenicity and embryotoxicity in rats*

Dose	Weigt gain of the dams in gm: during the whole period of pregnancy	Weigt gain of the dams in gm: from the 6th to 15th day of pregnancy	Number of: Implantations	Number of: Fetuses	Number of: Resorptions	Weight of the fetuses gm	Number of malformations	Stunted fetuses < 3 gm
1 ml/animal saline solution	+134.8	+34.0	11.9	8.6	3.3	4.14	0	0.2
300 IU	+ 99.8	+13.7	11.9	6.3	5.6	3.60	0	0.4
1,000 IU	+100.0	+ 7.5	11.1	4.3	6.8	3.17	0.5	2.5
3,000 IU	+ 55.3	— 9.3	11.3	2.1	9.2	2.87	2.3	5.3
10,000 IU	+ 21.7	—23.8	11.6	0	11.6			

We found a dose related decrease of the weigth gain of the dams during the treatment period and during the whole period of pregnancy.

No significant differences were observed in the number of implantations. Crasnitin has no influence on the implantation.

The mean number of fetuses was diminished, and this abnormality was dose-related.

Then, Crasnitin had a marked influence on resorption. 10,000 U/kg destroyed all fetuses.

The weight of the fetuses was decreased and (see the last column) the number of the stunted fetuses was increased. These changes were also dose-related.

The malformations which we found are shown in Table 4.

300 U/kg caused no abnormalities. Higher doses produced a dose-related increase of malformations.

In our rat strain malformed babies are rarely observed. Therefore we can say that these malformations were caused by the treatment with Crasnitin, and we can confirm that Crasnitin produces malformations. In addition we found that the embryotoxic and teratogenic effects of Crasnitin are clearly dose-related.

Table 4. *Type of malformations in rat fetuses after treatment with Crasnitin*

Control	none	
300 U/kg	none	
1,000 U/kg	2 Fetuses	Microphthalmia
	1 Fetus	Malformation of the vertebral column
3,000 U/kg	1 Fetus	Exenteria
	4 Fetuses	Microphthalmia
	2 Fetuses	Sternal cleft
10,000 U/kg	all Fetuses	resorbed

Conclusions

We have compared the results of our animal studies with the side effects observed during treatment of human patients in Table 5.

Vomiting, loss of appetite and weight loss were seen both in humans and in animals. Batches which were pyrogenic produced fever in humans and in rabbits. Allergic reactions were also found by tests carried out in guinea pigs.

Table 5. *Comparison of toxic effects in animals with side effects in humans*

	Animal	Man
Nausea/Vomiting	+	+
Anorexia	+	+
Weight loss	+	+
Fever	+	+
Antigenicity	+	+
Liver damage	(+)	+
Coagulopathy	—	+
Disturbance of lipid metabolism	—	+
Atrophy of the thymus	+	?

By contrast we found only a slight indication as to liver damage in animals while severe liver damage has been reported in man.

Two other side effects have only been observed in man, namely changes in the coagulation system and in lipid metabolism. The atrophy of the thymus has only been seen in animals.

From our animal investigations it has been possible to anticipate some of the risks incurred when administering Crasnitin to human patients.

Part VI
Resistance Problems

The Effect of Asparaginase on Some Animal-Tumors

T. A. CONNORS and M. JONES

Chester Beatty Research Institute,
Institute of Cancer Research: Royal Cancer Hospital, Fulham Road, London, S.W. 3, England

With 1 Figure

Some time ago, when the clinical potential of asparaginase therapy was relatively unknown, the Chester Beatty Research Institute was asked by a number of organisations to provide facilities for the routine anti-tumor screening of asparaginases isolated on a large scale and from sources other than *E. coli*. During the course of these investigations a number of observations have been made on the properties of asparaginase enzymes tested against animal tumor systems.

An initial survey of the action of an *E. coli* asparaginase against a number of animal tumors revealed that the majority of available tumors were quite insensitive even to large dose levels of the enzyme (up to 20,000 i.u./kg daily for five days), but that two other mouse tumors besides the Gardner lymphosarcoma, the R1 and the TLX5 lymphoma showed some response to five daily injections of 320 i.u./kg daily. Table 1 shows that this dose level of the enzyme is sufficient to cure animals bearing the Gardner lymphosarcoma, all treated animals surviving at fifty days after treatment with no signs of tumor. Treatment of the TLX5 and R1 lymphomas leads to a considerable extension of survival time (about 20 days as compared with 8—9 days in control animals) but all animals eventually succumb to the continued growth of the tumor.

As a result of this preliminary survey the screening test proposed for these preparations was an initial test against the highly sensitive Gardner lymphosarcoma in order to detect compounds with even a minimal *in vivo* asparaginase activity,

Table 1. *Effect of asparaginase on three mouse tumors 320 i.u./kg daily×5 intraperitoneally*

Tumor	Range of survival times (days)	% increase in life span
Gardner	No deaths at 50 days	"Cures"
R1 lymphoma	17—22	118
TLX5 lymphoma	19—22	152

followed by the retesting of active compounds against the more resistant R1 and TLX5 lymphomas in order to distinguish between highly active and moderately active derivatives.

Materials and Methods

Tumors. The Gardner lymphosarcoma was obtained from Dr. J. D. BROOME in 1968. It is routinely passaged in both ascitic form, by the intraperitoneal injection of 2×10^6 cells in 0.1 ml saline containing penicillin and streptomycin, and in solid form by the subcutaneous implantation of tumor fragments. Solid tumors may also be obtained from ascites cells by subcutaneous injection. The tumor is carried in CBA/LAC mice not the C3H strain in which it was originally induced.

The R1 lymphoma was obtained in 1959 on transplantation of the thymus of a CBA mouse which had received a total dose of 1950 r (X-rays; cobalt source) over a period of 13 weeks. The tumor has, since 1967, been passaged in CBA/LAC mice by transplantation of 10^6 ascites cells. It is of interest that a subcutaneous injection of 10^6 ascites cells is followed by a rapid dissemination of the tumor, all animals dying 9 days after transplantation. Bioassay of organs at 8 days after subcutaneous injection showed that spleen, lung, liver and kidneys contained up to 10% of their weight in tumor cells with large numbers of tumor cells in circulating blood. The primary tumor at the site of injection is never more than 200 mg in weight at the time of death.

The TLX5 tumor was induced in a CBA mouse in 1967 in a similar manner to the R1 lymphoma, following a course of X-irradiation and transplantation of the subsequently enlarged thymus. Since induction it has been carried in CBA/LAC mice. Similarly to the R1 lymphoma, subcutaneously injected cells appear to disseminate rapidly killing animals about 9 days after subcutaneous injection of 2×10^6 ascites cells, although in this case, the primary tumor may weigh as much as 1 gm at the time of death.

Screening Tests

The routine screening tests are carried out in mice 3 days after subcutaneous injection of 10^6 ascites cells (or 7 days after transplantation of tumor fragments in the case of the Gardner lymphosarcoma, when the tumor becomes palpable). The preparation under test is administered intraperitoneally in 0.1 ml of saline at doses ranging from 10 to 1280 i.u./kg. Assay of chemotherapeutic effectiveness in the case of the R1 and TLX5 lymphomas is by measurement of survival time and estimation of cell kill by reference to a survival time/cell inoculum correlation previously obtained. For the Gardner lymphosarcoma, tumors are dissected out and weighed, and the weights of treated groups are compared with the weight of a control untreated group.

For a direct comparison of the effect of asparaginase on all three tumors, animals bearing the ascites tumors were injected three days after transplantation, with intraperitoneal doses of asparaginase (Bayer, Crasnitin) in 0.1 ml of saline at doses ranging from 1.2 to 20,000 i.u./kg daily for 5 days and in all cases effectiveness measured by extension of survival time compared with controls.

CBA/LAC female mice about 6 weeks old and 20—25 gm weight were used in all experiments.

Results

Screening tests using preparations of asparaginase from *E. coli* (E.C. 2) have given similar results, irrespective of their method of purification, having tumor effective doses (I.D. 90) against the Gardner lymphosarcoma of about 40—160 i.u./kg administered intraperitoneally as a single dose to animals bearing the 7 day old solid tumor. The least toxic preparations have an LD_{50} of about 320,000 i.u./kg giving a therapeutic index (LD_{50}/ID_{90}) of about 8000 by far the largest index so far observed in any test of an anti-tumor agent against a tumor bearing animal. Asparaginases derived from sources other than *E. coli* have generally been found to be less potent, with ID_{90}'s of greater than 160 i.u./kg but no less toxic—with a consequently smaller therapeutic index. No chemical modification of an asparaginase enzyme has been found to give more potent derivatives.

Table 2 shows the relationship between survival time and the number of cells injected for the Gardner lymphosarcoma. The tumor grows rather slowly, having a doubling time of approximately 24 hrs., although the numbers of animals used are

Table 2. *Gardner lymphosarcoma. Relationship between survival time and number or cells injected (i. p.)*

No. cells	Range of survival times (days)	Median survival time (days)
10^7	12—16	14.1
10^6	15—21	16.5
10^5	15—21	18.8
10^4	19—27	20.7
10^3	22—28	24.4

too small to enable the calculation of an exact doubling time or to calculate cell kill in a quantitative manner. Although this tumor is not growing in the strain in which it was induced it can be seen that one can still obtain 100% tumor takes at inocula as low as 1000 cells. Table 3 shows similarly for the R1 lymphoma, the relationship between number of tumor cells injected and survival time. This tumor grows quicker than the Gardner, having a doubling time of about 10 hrs., and is remarkably consistent, especially at the higher cell numbers, in the day at which it kills the animals. Tumors can arise following the injection of as few as 10 cells. The TLX5 tumor (Table 4) shows a pattern similar to that seen for the R1 lymphoma.

Fig. 1 shows the response of the Gardner lymphosarcoma and the R1 and TLX5 lymphomas to various dose levels of asparaginase (Bayer: Crasnitin). The enzyme is injected intraperitoneally into animals, three days after transplantation of 10^6 cells of either of the three tumors. At low dose levels (2.4—40 i.u./kg) all tumor lines

Table 3. *R1 lymphoma. Relationship between survival time and number of cells injected (i. p.)*

No. cells	Range of survival times (days)	Median survival time (days)
10^6	8	8.0
10^5	9	9.0
10^4	11	11.0
10^3	13—15	13.3
10^2	13—15	13.9
10^1	14—18 (5/10 takes)	15.4

Table 4. *TLX5 lymphoma. Relationship between survival time and number of cells injected (i. p.)*

No. cells	Range of survival times (days)	Median survival time (days)
10^7	9—10	9.4
10^6	10	10.0
10^5	11	11.0
10^4	12—13	12.2
10^3	13—15	14.0

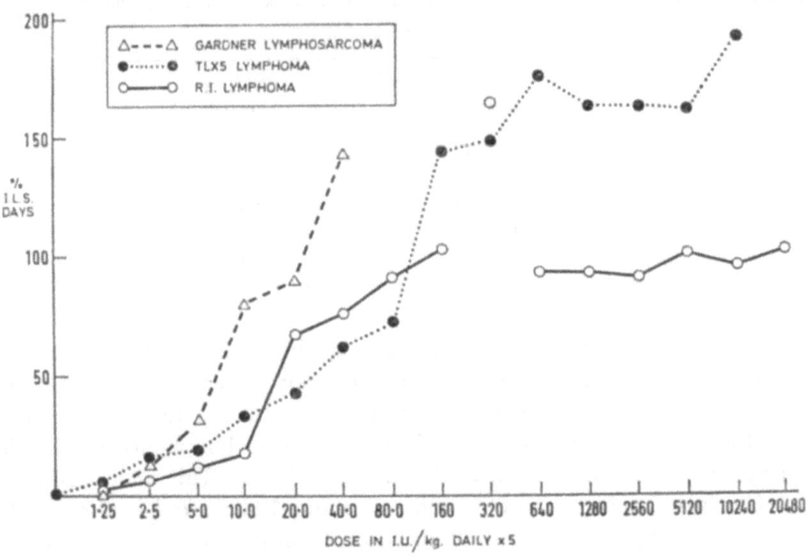

Fig. 1. The effect of asparaginase (Bayer: Crasnitin) on the survival time of mice bearing the Gardner lymphosarcoma or the R1 and TLX5 lymphomas. Only the survival time of animals dying within 50 days of transplantation are used in the calculation of the increase in life span (ILS) compared with controls. The atypically high value for animals with the R1 lymphoma receiving 320 i.u./kg of asparaginase was due to an unusually high number of cures (4/10) together with two animals showing a survival time of 40 days

respond to the treatment, the maximum effective dose which results in complete "cures" of the Gardner lymphosarcoma, and maximum extension of survival time for the R1 lymphoma, being in both cases about 40 i.u./kg daily for five days. At dose levels higher than 40 i.u./kg animals with the Gardner tumor show no signs of the tumor 50 days after treatment and are considered cured, while animals bearing the R1 lymphoma still die from the tumor with an extended survival time similar to that obtained at 40 i.u./kg. Cures of animals bearing the R1 lymphoma and survival times of 36—40 days do occur in a small proportion of cases with a tendency to increasing numbers of cures at very high dose levels. The dose response for the TLX5 tumor is similar to that seen for the R1 lymphoma. There is a response at low doses increasing to a maximum effect at about 80 i.u./kg. There then follows a plateau with no greater effect at increasing dose levels. Cures are extremely rare at all doses below 1280 i.u./kg but above this dose level they occur in an inconsistent fashion but again more frequently at dose levels above 5120 i.u./kg.

Table 5. *Development of a resistant line of the R1 lymphoma*

Passage	Range of survival times (days)	Median survival time (days)
1	Control 8—9	8.6
(4,000 i.u./kg daily×5)	Treated 18—19	18.4
2	Control 8—9	8.4
(4,000 i.u./kg daily×5)	Treated 11—13	12.2
3	Control 7—8	7.6
(4,000 i.u./kg daily×5)	Treated 9—10	9.6
4	Control 7—8	7.8
(4,000 i.u./kg daily×5)	Treated 9—10	9.8
5	Control 7—8	7.6
(4,000 i.u./kg daily×5)	Treated 9—10	9.4
8	Control 7—9	8.0
(16,000 i.u./kg daily×5)	Treated 9—11	9.4
11	Control 8—9	8.2
(16,000 i.u./kg daily×5)	Treated 9—10	9.2

Table 5 shows the development of resistance of the R1 lymphoma to asparaginase. Ten animals in passage one are transplanted with approximately 10^6 tumor cells intraperitoneally. Five of these mice are then given from day 3, five daily doses of 4000 i.u./kg of asparaginase. The effect on the survival time of the treated animals is considerable, but not curative in any case. One animal from this treated group serves as the donor for the second passage and half the animals in the group again receive asparaginase while the remainder serve as controls. In the treated group there is, again an extension of survival time, but not as large as that seen with the first treatment indicating a rapid development of resistance. For the third passage, again using a treated animal from the preceeding passage as donor, there is an extension of survival time in the treated animals but smaller than that observed in the first two treatments. Thereafter by continuing the same process for up to eleven passages there is always a difference between treated and control groups of about 1—2 days. It has proved impossible to obtain this increase in survival time by non-specific procedures such as the daily injection of large volumes (1 ml) of saline or water.

Discussion

The numbers of animals used to obtain the data for the correlation between cell survival and number of cells injected have been too small (10 per group) to make precise calculations, but there are some features of interest arising from the study of the response of these animal tumours to asparaginase. Although the TLX5 and R1 lymphomas were considered from the data in Table 1 to be more resistant to asparaginase than the Gardner lymphosarcoma, this appears to be due to a small proportion of resistant cells rather than to a lowered sensitivity of all the tumor cell population. Both the TLX5 and the R1 respond to low dose levels of asparaginase (2.4 to 80 i.u./kg). At dose levels higher than these there is no increased effect on the tumors and, if this proves to be a general phenomenon, one must question the validity of employing large doses (up to 5000 i.u./kg) in clinical chemotherapy. The clinical toxicity observed with asparaginase may be due mainly to the complete removal of asparagine from circulating blood and, if so, would not increase with doses above the low levels required to keep the blood free from asparagine. However, there is also the possibility that some of the side effects may be due to contaminants of the preparation and these could be avoided by the use of minimum effective dose levels.

There is also an indication that, at extremely high dose levels, asparaginase is having another action against the TLX5 tumor. Although not consistent, there were more cures at extremely high dose levels of asparaginase (2560 i.u./kg + above). This effect at very high dose levels could be due to the enzyme acting on another substrate or possibly due to traces of a contaminant.

At effective dose levels of asparaginase the survival time of animals transplanted with 10^6 TLX5 or R1 lymphoma cells increases from the control value of 8—9 days to a value of about 18—20 days. This is greater than the theoretical survival time for animals transplanted with a single cell and would mean that, of the original 10^6 cells transplanted, there was only a single cell that was not sensitive to treatment. It is difficult to see, however, if this is the case, why more cures are not obtained at effective dose levels of asparaginase. If the resistant colony of cells is such a small proportion of the total tumor cell colony one would expect that, on transplantation, a fairly large number of transplants would contain no resistant tumor cells at all and would, therefore, be curable on asparaginase treatment. A more likely explanation is that the proportion of resistant cells in the colony is larger than that predicted from the cell inoculum/survival curve. Asparaginase does not kill these cells but either increases their generation time, or holds them up at some stage of the cell cycle, so that the extension of survival time observed is not a true measure of cell kill.

The studies on the development of a line of the R1 lymphoma, resistant to asparaginase, are also indicative that asparaginase can effect the growth of tumor cells without necessarily killing them. As shown in Table 5 resistance develops rapidly in a predictable manner until the fourth passage. Further passaging of the tumor in the presence of asparaginase then always produces a constant extension of survival time which by reference to Table 3, would indicate a cell kill between 90 and 99%. Since resistance has obviously developed rapidly over the first three passages, it is difficult to see how, afterwards, there could remain a sensitive fraction of cells affected at each passage by asparaginase but capable of regrowth in the next passage where they are again susceptible to asparaginase treatment. A more probable explanation is that, after the fourth passage, all cells are resistant to the cytotoxic action of the agent but they are, nevertheless, affected in a non-lethal manner. The extension in survival time observed in each passage could be a result of an extension of cell generation time, or perhaps, a hold up of growth when the enzyme is present in high concentration, until the cells can induce sufficient amounts of asparagine synthetase.

This phenomenon obviously requires further investigation since if asparaginase has this action on resistant cells it is important to recognise it when the enzyme is being used in combination with drugs such as cytosine arabinoside which are uniquely effective against cells in DNA synthesis. Any treatment that may affect the S period or temporarily inhibit DNA synthesis might exert a protective action against the cytotoxicity of drugs such as cytosine arabinoside.

Summary

Experience with three animal tumours has shown that one (the Gardner lymphosarcoma) is highly sensitive to asparaginase while two others (the R1 and TLX5 lymphomas) are less sensitive to the extent that cures are not obtainable at dose levels sufficient to deplete the circulating blood of asparagine. The lack of sensitivity of these two tumors is apparently due to the presence of a small fraction of resistant cells, since all three tumors respond to low doses of asparaginase and the maximum effective dose is of the same order in all cases. No evidence has been found that high dose levels of asparaginase such as those used clinically (about 2000 i.u./kg), are any more effective than lower dose levels (about 40 i.u./kg) although, at extremely high dose levels, asparaginase may be having another effect. There is also some evidence that cells resistant to asparaginase *may* be held up for a short period by high dose levels of asparaginase.

Acknowledgment

This work was supported by grants to the Chester Beatty Research Institute, Institute of Cancer Research from the Medical Research Council and the British Empire Campaign for Cancer Research.

Studies of Resistance to L-Asparaginase in Human Leukemia

GEORGE P. CANELLOS and CHARLES M. HASKELL

Solid Tumor Service, Medicine Branch, National Cancer Institute Bethesda, Maryland, U.S.A.

With 4 Figures

The biochemical basis for the treatment of neoplastic disease with L-asparaginase is the demonstration that exogenously derived asparagine is an amino acid essential for growth in some tumors [1, 2]. It was further shown that the L-asparaginase sensitive murine tumor cells were deficient in an asparagine biosynthetic mechanism which was present in resistant cells [3]. In mammalian tissues, an *in vitro* enzymatic synthesis of asparagine from aspartate in the presence of glutamine, ATP, and magnesium has been described [4, 5].

A survey of asparagine synthetase activity in a large number of murine tumors showed a close correlation between absence of the enzyme and *in vivo* sensitivity to L-asparaginase [6]. Furthermore, a marked elevation of enzyme activity was noted to occur in resistant 6C3HED lymphoma cells following administration of L-asparaginase [7]. At the inception of clinical trials, cell cultures with human leukemic cells revealed some correlation between *in vitro* asparagine dependency and clinical effectiveness of the drug [8]. This suggested that an alteration in asparagine biosynthesis in human leukemic cells might be the basis of clinical resistance. Asparagine synthetase activity was examined in a group of leukemic patients prior to and following L-asparaginase treatment. In addition, serial enzymatic studies, as well as determination of intracellular asparagine levels, were performed in representatives of the sensitive and resistant groups.

Patients and Methods

Investigations were performed in patients with leukemia on the clinical research wards of the National Cancer Institute. A group of eighteen patients had determinations of leukocyte asparagine synthetase prior to treatment with L-asparaginase. The number of patients with each type of leukemia and whether they were sensitive (S) or resistant (R) to L-asparaginase are enumerated as follows: acute lymphoblastic leukemia (5 R, 4 S); acute granulocytic leukemia (3 R); chronic granulocytic leukemia (4 R, 1 S); and, chronic lymphocytic leukemia (1 R). The nine patients with repeat determinations during or after therapy included the following: acute lymphoblastic leukemia (2 R, 3 S); chronic granulocytic leukemia (2 R, 1 S); chronic lymphocytic leukemia (1 R).

All patients were treated with *E. coli* L-asparaginase at a dose of 200 International Units per kilogram. The usual duration of therapy was three weeks with the exception of one patient with granulocytic leukemia who was treated for only three days because of pronounced toxicity coincident with a marked anti-leukemic effect.

It was possible to perform serial studies of leukemic leukocyte asparagine synthetase and intracellular asparagine during treatment in two patients with granulocytic leukemia, one of whom was sensitive to L-asparaginase and the other resistant.

Cells were obtained from bone marrow aspirates or from peripheral blood specimens obtained by plasmapheresis. Leukemic cells were separated by Dextran sedimentation or by differential centrifugation, and washed an average of five times with three to four volumes of a balanced salt solution. Thorough washing of cells was particularly critical during L-asparaginase therapy, since even trace contamination with L-asparaginase could obliterate the asparagine formed in the subsequent assay. Acetone powder extracts were prepared and assayed for asparagine synthetase as previously described [9]. Incubations in duplicate or triplicate were performed for thirty minutes at 37° in a 1.0 ml incubation medium containing 100 μmoles Tris at pH 7.8, 8 μmoles $MgCl_2$, 20 μmoles L-glutamine, 8 μmoles disodium ATP, 2 μmoles L-aspartic acid, 0.4 μc ^{14}C-L-aspartic acid (u. l., New England Nuclear Corp.), and 1—4 mg of enzyme protein. The reaction was terminated by 1.0 ml 10% trichloracetic acid, the pH was readjusted to 5—7 with 5 *N* KOH, and 0.5 mg asparagine carrier was added. ^{14}C-asparagine formed was then separated from ^{14}C-aspartic acid by eluting the reaction mixture through an Alumina Column (Fisher Co.) with 0.5 *N* acetic acid. Radioactivity was determined in a liquid scintillation spectrometer, and results expressed as mμmoles asparagine formed per mg protein per hour of incubation. Asparagine synthesis in this system was confirmed by the complete removal of the elutable radioactivity following incubation of the reaction product with *E. coli* L-asparaginase. Intracellular asparagine was measured in aqueous extracts of washed leukocytes which were boiled for ten minutes in capped polycarbonate tubes. The enzymatic assay was similar to that outlined by HANDSCHUMACHER [10] and described in detail by COONEY et al. [11] for plasma and red cell asparagine.

Observations and Discussion

In all patients studied before treatment, asparagine synthetase was all but undectable in leukemic cells and thus could not be used to predict subsequent response to L-asparaginase therapy. As illustrated in Fig. 1, the activity of the enzyme did not change in those patients in whom an antileukemic effect occurred. However, a seven-fold rise in enzyme activity occurred in those patients unresponsive to treatment.

In order to define the effect of L-asparaginase administration on asparagine synthetase activity and intracellular L-asparagine levels, serial studies were performed on a patient with granulocytic leukemia who was markedly sensitive to L-asparaginase and compared with a patient with the same disease who was totally resistant. In the resistant patient asparagine synthetase levels were greatly increased and remained elevated throughout the eleven day period of study. During this period there was a steady decline of intracellular L-asparagine to indeterminate levels while on asparaginase (Fig. 2). In contrast, the patient with L-asparaginase sensitive cells showed no elevation of enzyme activity despite rapid diminution of L-asparagine

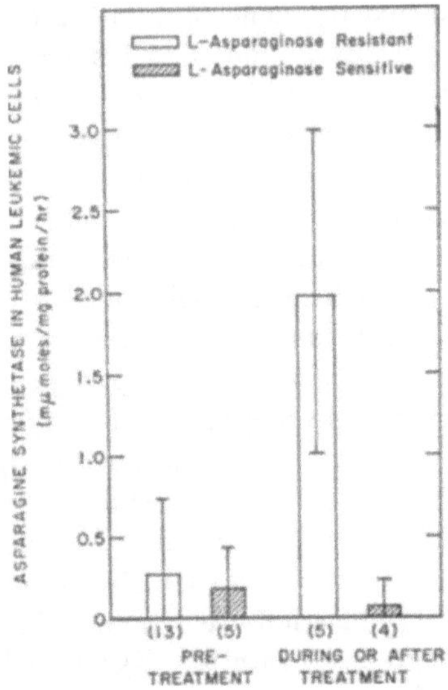

Fig. 1. Asparagine synthetase activity of leukemic cells from eighteen patients before and in nine cases during or after asparaginase treatment. The mean and one standard deviation of asparagine synthetase for each group are expressed as mμmoles asparagine formed per mg protein per hour. The number of patients in each response group are in parentheses. (Reprinted with permission from Pergamon Press)

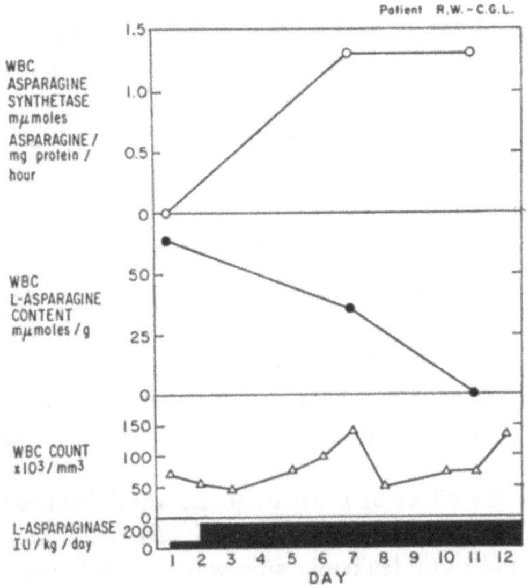

Fig. 2. Asparaginase resistance. Leukemic leukocyte asparagine synthetase and asparagine levels during asparaginase administration

levels (Fig. 3). There was also a marked decrease in the leukocyte count after only a relatively small dose of drug further illustrating the extreme sensitivity of his cells. These observations suggest that the mode of resistance by human leukemic cells involves, at least in part, the ability to respond to exogenous asparagine depletion by an increase in asparagine synthetase. Every patient refractory to L-asparaginase demonstrated a significant increase in endogenous asparagine synthesis apparently in quantities sufficient to maintain cellular metabolism. The absence of myelotoxicity with asparaginase treatment suggests that normal bone marrow cells might have adequate asparagine synthetase activity to adapt to the stress. Normal marrow studies from two patients with non-hemopoietic neoplasms treated with asparaginase indicate a rise in enzyme activity similar to resistant leukemic cells (unpublished observations). With respect to the cellular response to asparaginase, these clinical biochemical studies demonstrate a close correlation to the reported observations of asparaginase resistance in murine tumor systems [6, 7]. As opposed to the refractory murine tumor, asparagine synthetase in resistant human cells was undetectable prior to treatment and became measurable only during periods of exogenous asparagine deprivation.

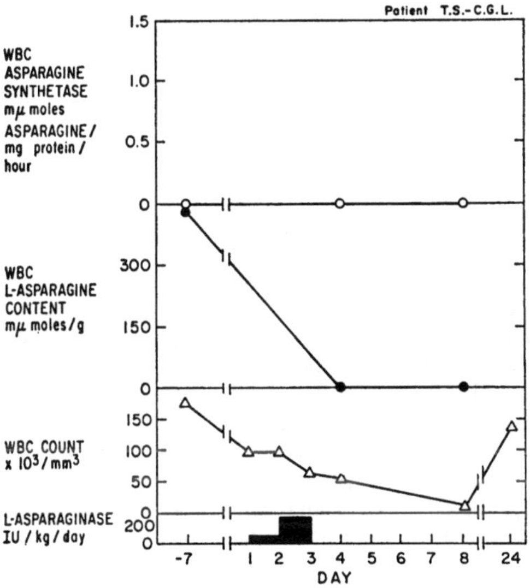

Fig. 3. Serial determination of asparagine and asparagine synthetase in leukemic leukocytes in a patient responsive to L-asparaginase

The control mechanism by which asparagine synthetase activity increases following asparaginase remains unexplained. There is evidence in mammalian systems that asparagine synthetase can be inhibited by its product [5, 7], as well as enzymes derived from *Lactobacillus arabinosus* and *Streptococcus bovis* [12, 13]. A comparable effect was seen in the human enzyme as shown in Fig. 4 which illustrates the inhibitory effect of increasing concentrations of L-asparagine on asparagine synthetase extracts derived from human myeloblastic leukemic cells. Leukocyte asparagine levels fall to unmeasurable levels following asparaginase and this decrease may thus reduce the level of inhibition of the enzyme already present.

Another mechanism which could account for the rise of asparagine synthetase is derepression of enzyme protein synthesis following depletion of the repressor amino acid, in this instance asparagine. This has already been shown to occur in asparagine synthetase from *Lactobacillus arabinosus* and *Escherichia coli* [12, 14]. An understanding of the metabolic pattern of resistance to asparaginase might permit pharmacologic means by which it can be overcome.

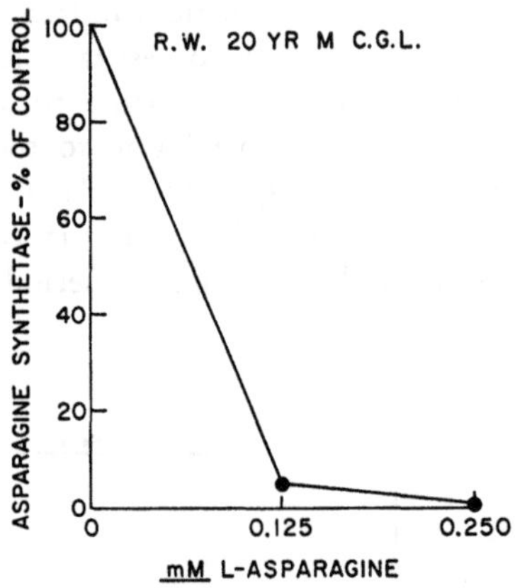

Fig. 4. Asparagine inhibition of asparagine synthetase derived from leukemic leukocytes

Summary

Asparagine synthetase was studied in leukocytes of eighteen leukemic patients prior to administration of L-asparaginase. Nine of this group had repeat assays during or immediately following treatment in order to determine whether sensitive and resistant patients differed in their response to asparagine deprivation. Prior to treatment, the enzyme was barely measurable in leukemic cells. In five patients refractory to asparaginase the mean level of asparagine synthetase rose seven fold higher over pretreatment levels. Four patients responding to asparaginase therapy did not increase the level of asparagine synthetase.

Determination of intracellular asparagine levels in a sensitive and resistant patient revealed a marked depression in both patients although the resistant patient showed a pronounced rise in asparagine synthetase activity.

Acknowledgements

The authors are indebted to Miss Marla Paul for her skilled technical assistance and Drs. Brigid Leventhal and Robert Graw for their assistance in these studies. The authors are also grateful to Drs. Max Tishler and R. Denkewalter of Merck, Sharpe and Dohme who supplied the E. coli L-asparaginase used in these studies.

References

1. Broome, J. D.: Evidence that the L-asparaginase of guinea pig serum is responsible for its antilymphoma effects. II. Lymphoma 6C3HED cells cultured in a medium devoid of L-asparagine lose their susceptibility to the effects of guinea pig serum *in vivo*. J. exp. Med. **118**, 121 (1963).

2. SOBIN, L. H., KIDD, J. G.: A metabolic difference between two lines of lymphoma 6C3HED cells in relation to asparagine. Proc. Soc. exp. Biol. (N. Y.) **119**, 325 (1965).
3. BROOME, J. D., SCHWARTZ, J. H.: Differences in the production of L-asparagine in asparaginase-sensitive and resistant lymphoma cells. Biochim. biophys. Acta (Amst.) **138**, 637 (1967).
4. PATTERSON, M. K., ORR, G.: L-asparagine biosynthesis by nutritional variants of the Jensen sarcoma. Biochem. biophys. Res. Commun. **26**, 228 (1967).
5. — — Asparagine biosynthesis by the Novikoff hepatoma. J. biol. Chem. **226**, 191 (1968).
6. HOROWITZ, B., MADRAS, B. K., MEISTER, A., OLD, L. J., BOYSE, E. A., STOCKERT, E.: Asparagine synthetase activity of mouse leukemias. Science **160**, 533 (1968).
7. PRAGER, M. D., BACHYNSKY, N.: Asparagine synthetase in asparaginase resistant and susceptible mouse lymphomas. Biochem. biophys. Res. Commun. **31**, 43 (1968).
8. OETTGEN, H. F., OLD, L. J., BOYSE, E. A., CAMPBELL, H. A., PHILIPS, F. S., CLARKSON, B. D., TALLAL, L., LEEPER, R. D., SCHWARTZ, M. K., KIM, J. H.: Inhibition of leukemias in man by L-asparaginase. Cancer Res. **27**, **2619** (1967).
9. HASKELL, C. M., CANELLOS, G. P.: L-asparaginase resistance in human leukemia: asparagine synthetase. Biochemical Pharmacology **18**, 2578 (1969).
10. HANDSCHUMACHER, R. E.: Mechanisms of control of tumor growth: asparaginase and asparagine analogs in Exploitable Molecular Mechanisms and neoplasia. Williams & Wilkins Co. 1969.
11. COONEY, D. A., CAPIZZI, R., HANDSCHUMACHER, R. E.: Cancer Res. (in press).
12. RAVEL, J. M., NORTON, S. J., HUMPHREYS, J. S., SHIVE, W.: Asparagine biosynthesis in *Lactobacillus arabinosus* and its control by asparagine through enzyme inhibition and repression. J. biol. Chem. **237**, 2845 (1962).
13. BURCHALL, J. J., REICHELT, E. C., WOLIN, M. J.: Purification and properties of the asparagine synthetase of *Streptococcus bovis*. J. biol. Chem. **239**, 1794 (1964).
14. CEDAR, H., SCHWARTZ, J. H.: The asparagine synthetase of *Escherichia coli*. J. biol. Chem. **244**, 4112 (1969).

The Antigenicity of E. coli-Asparaginase

H. E. Reis and C. G. Schmidt

Innere Klinik und Poliklinik (Tumorforschung) der Ruhr-Universität, Klinikum Essen, Germany

With 3 Figures

Allergic reactions are among the side effects of E. coli-asparaginase. In the blood of patients with and without allergic reactions during treatment with asparaginase Oettgen [1] could first demonstrate precipitating and complement-binding antibodies. In our own patients Gallmeier [2] also found precipitating antibodies. One of these patients, who was in the hospital during June 1968, produced the precipitating antibodies during treatment of an acute myelocytic leukemia. To study whether these antibodies were directed against the enzyme itself or against antigens without enzyme activity we fractionated the asparaginase preparation used in this patient by isoelectric focusing and tested the reactions of the fractions obtained with the patient's serum. (For these studies E. coli-asparaginase of the Farbenfabriken Bayer was used.)

The column for isoelectric analysis and the carrier ampholytes were manufactured by L.K.B.-Producter, Stockholm, Sweden. The preparation of the column was carried out according to the method of Vesterberg and Svensson [3]. The asparaginase sample for each experiment was 20 mg. The final voltage was 500 Volts and the run lasted 72 hours in the pH-range from 3 to 10 and 48 hours in the pH-range from 4 to 6. After that time 1 ml samples were collected and the absorbance at 280 mμ was determined. The pH-measurement was performed on every fifth sample and in the top-sample of each absorption peak. For the determination of the asparaginase activity a modification of the method described by Mashburn and Wriston [4] was used. The ammonia liberated from asparagine was determined using the reaction of Berthelot.

Antigenic determinants of the enzyme preparation and of the fractions were demonstrated by the technique of Ouchterlony [5], using the serum of the patient who developed precipitating antibodies against asparaginase during intravenous treatment for acute myelocytic leukemia.

The elution curve from the column containing asparaginase in carrier ampholytes of the pH-range pH 3 to 10 showed the asparaginase to be focused only in one band, with an isoelectric point at pH 5.1. The more accurate analysis in the pH-range pH 4 to 6 is seen in Fig. 1. In that pH-range the asparaginase elution curve shows three absorption peaks at 280 mμ with isoelectric points at pH 5.26, pH 5.07

and pH 4.89. Since the resolving power of the method in our hands was in the order of 0.03 pH units the duplicate results varied in that range.

To investigate, whether or not the three protein fractions possessed enzyme activity, the asparaginase activity of the samples was determined. As seen from the asparaginase activity curve only the first two peaks of the protein absorption curve had enzyme activity. In the third protein peak no comparable amount of enzyme activity could be demonstrated. From the shoulder of the asparaginase activity curve it can be assumed, that a third enzyme fraction may be situated between the second and the third protein peak. A further separation was not possible in that pH-range.

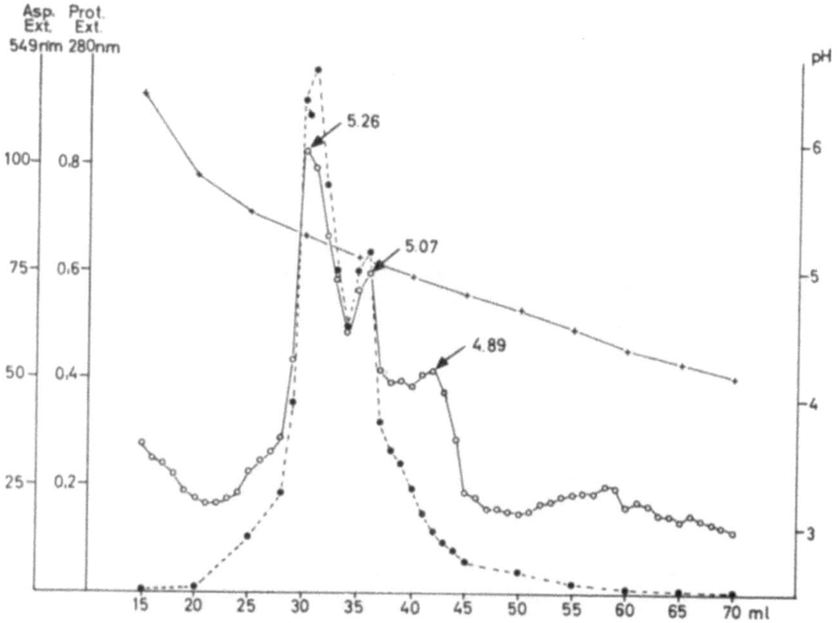

Fig. 1. Isoelectric focusing of asparaginase in carrier ampholytes of the pH-range 4 to 6. Eluate in ml on the left "Asp.": asparaginase activity curve at 549 nm; on the left "Prot.": Protein absorption at 280 nm; on the right: pH-values. o—o Protein absorption curve; ●—● asparaginase activity curve; +—+ pH-curve

The next step was to find out, whether one of the isoelectric fractions with asparaginase activity acted as antigen or whether perhaps only the third protein fraction was antigenic. To answer this question, we reacted the three protein fractions with the patient's serum containing precipitating antibodies in Ouchterlony tests. The samples of each peak with the greatest absorption intensity were used.

Fig. 2 shows the immunodiffusion plate. Central well: the antiserum; peripheral wells: Down two times the whole asparaginase-preparation and in the clockwise direction follows fraction 1, 2 and 3. As seen from the picture all three fractions and the whole asparaginase preparation gave identical precipitation lines.

Since the isoelectric focusing of asparaginase in the pH-range 4 to 6 gives only analytical values of different fractions and their isoelectric points but not a sufficient purification of the fractions, one can not conclude, however, that all fractions have the same antigen.

Fig. 3 shows that the top sample of the first peak may not have contamination from the third and the third not from the first. To be sure, that we got a sample in which no contamination of the first peak from the third occurs, we investigated a sample of the rising branch of the first (28) and a sample of the descending branch of the third peak (44). Both gave precipitin lines of identity when compared with the whole asparaginase preparation and the other fractions.

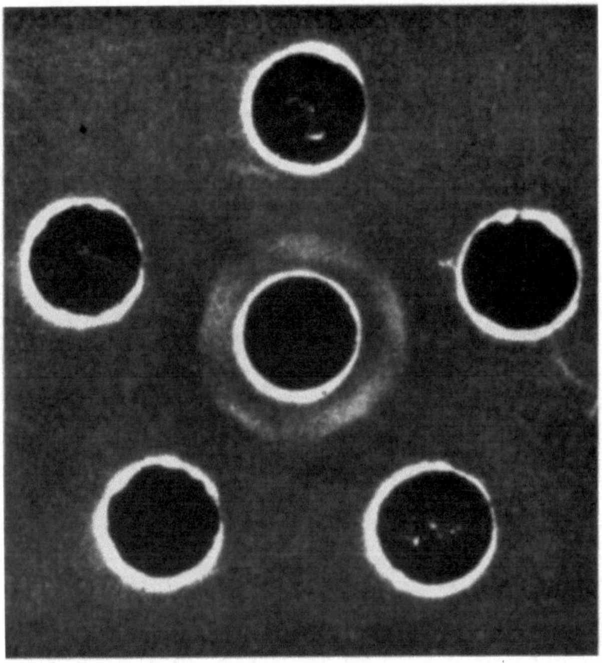

Fig. 2. Immunodiffusion. Demonstration of precipitating antibodies against asparaginase. Whole asparaginase preparation and the isoelectric fractions. Central: the antibody containing serum of the patient. Peripheral: down 2× whole asparaginase preparation; the clockwise direction follows Asp. F1, F2, F3

These results demonstrate, that the asparaginase preparation used was heterogenous by isoelectric focusing and that it consisted at least of two enzyme-active protein components. This corresponds with the results reported by Dr. Mashburn yesterday [6]. The third fraction did not seem to possess a comparable amount of asparaginase activity. The results demonstrate further, that the antigenicity at least of the first peak is due to an asparaginase active component. Wether all three fractions possess the same antigen or not can not be concluded from the experiment, because we could not purify the fractions in the used carrier ampholytes of two pH-steps. Other physico-chemical properties and the question of wether the third protein fraction may be a denaturated enzyme component that lost nearly all of the enzyme activity, have not yet be investigated because of insufficient purification. The carrier ampholytes of one or one half pH-step that are now becoming available may allow it to investigate these questions.

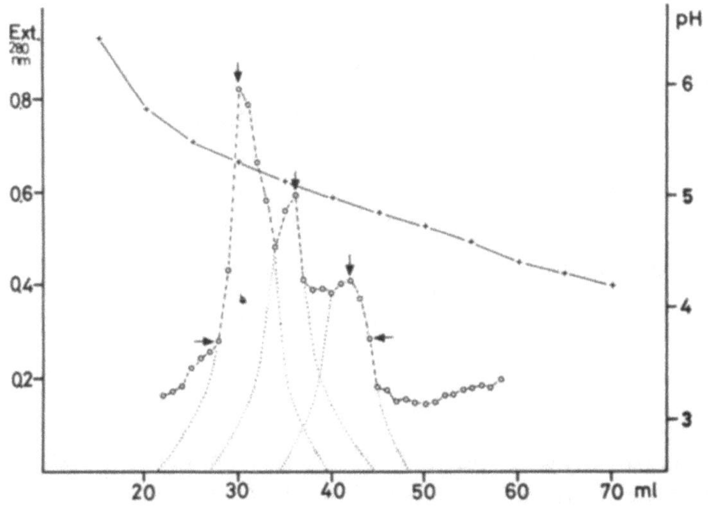

Fig. 3. The distribution of the three isoelectric protein fractions and the contamination possibilities. The samples tested in the immunodiffusion test are marked

References

1. OETTGEN, H. F., SCHULTEN, H. K.: Hemmung maligner Neoplasien der Menschen durch L-asparaginase. Klin. Wschr. **47**, 65 (1969).
2. SCHMIDT, C. G., GALLMEIER, W. M.: Zur Enzymtherapie der Leukämien. Dtsch. med. Wschr. **93**, 2299 (1968).
3. VESTERBERG, O., SVENSSON, H.: Isoelectric fractionation, analysis and characterization of ampholytes in natural pH-gradients. IV. Further studies on the resolving power in connection with separation of myoglobulin. Acta chem. scand. **20**, 820 (1966).
4. MASHBURN, L. T., WRISTON, J. C.: Tumor inhibitory effect of L-asparaginase. Biochem. biophys. Res. Commun. **12**, 50 (1968).
5. OUCHTERLONY, Ö.: Diffusion—in-gel methods for immunological analysis. II Progr. Allergy **6**, 30 (1962).
6. MASHBURN, C. T.: Some physicochemical aspects of L-asparaginase therapy. Intern. Symp. about experimental and clinical effects of L-asparaginase. October 1969, Wuppertal-Elberfeld, Germany.

Studies on Antibody Formation in Patients Treated with L-Asparaginase

A. DOHLWITZ, S. FRANZÉN, A. HOLMGREN, A. KILLANDER, D. KILLANDER, L. WIDE, and L. ÅHSTRÖM

Radiumhemmet and Dept. of Pediatrics, Karolinska Hospital;
Dept. of Chemistry II, Karolinska Institutet, Stockholm 60
and Dept. of Clinical Chemistry, University of Uppsala, Sweden

With 5 Figures

Twenty-six patients were treated by daily intravenous or intramuscular injections of L-asparaginase (Bayer A) in doses of 200 IU/kg body weight or, in three cases, 1000 IU/kg. Treatment usually lasted for a period of 28 days. Twenty patients (14 children and 6 adults) had acute leukemia and the remaining patients had different types of solid tumors. Among the children with leukemia eight achieved complete remission and three partial remission. Of the remaining three children two died within 2 weeks without signs of remission and one failed to respond to 4 weeks of treatment. All adults with leukemia and all patients with solid tumors also failed to respond.

Predictive tests were performed in 18 leukemia patients using the method described by OETTGEN et al. [1] with some modifications. Thus incorporation of ^{3}H-valine was measured in cells cultivated in a medium containing L-asparagine (50 mM) either with L-asparaginase (12 IU/ml) or without the enzyme (= control). The results (Fig. 1) indicate that the test may be of predictive value only in cases where the

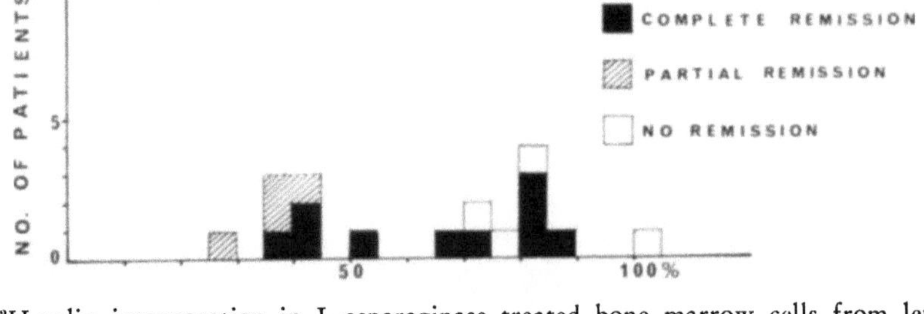

Fig. 1. ^{3}H-valin incorporation in L-asparaginase treated bone marrow cells from leukemia patients expressed in per cent of ^{3}H-valin incorporation in untreated cells. Incubation for 16 hrs. at 37°

protein synthesis of the leukemia cells decrease to less than 60% of the control by the addition of L-asparaginase.

During the course of treatment plasma samples were collected from the patients 24 hrs. after injection and stored at —20° until analyzed. L-asparaginase activity in plasma was determined by measuring the liberation of ammonia by the Berthelot reaction [2]. Incubation mixtures contained 0.1 M borate buffer, pH 8.5 and 1.0×10^{-2} M L-asparagine in a volume of 0.2 ml. Plasma (2–20 µl) was added and the mixtures incubated for 15 min at 37°. The reaction was stopped by the addition of 2.5 ml of the two Berthelot reagents (Boehringer TC UR I and II). The mixtures were then incubated at room temperature for 30 min and the absorbance at 620 nm was determined spectrophotometrically against a solvent blank. Ammonia standard curves were run with NH_4HCO_3. The presence of L-asparagine did not change the slope of the standard curve.

Antibodies to L-asparaginase were determined using a radio-immunosorbent technique [3—6]. L-asparaginase was coupled to "ultrafine" sephadex (Pharmacia, Uppsala) or "microcrystalline" cellulose particles (Merck, Darmstadt) activated with cyanogen bromide. The enzyme-coated particles were then mixed with plasma samples. A simplified scheme of the reaction when antibodies are present is shown in Figs. 2 and 3. To detect the antibodies a "sandwich" principle was used. One part of the particle suspension was exposed to ^{125}I-labelled L-asparaginase (Fig. 2) and the

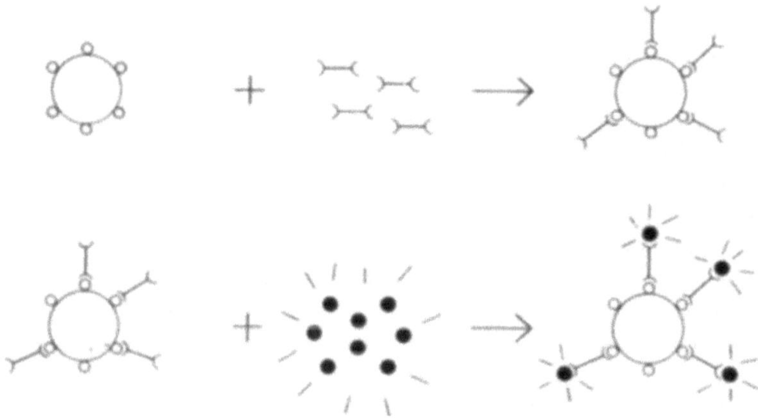

Fig. 2. Reaction between L-asparaginase (small open circles) on a polysaccharide particle (big open circle) and "bivalent" antibodies (top) to which ^{125}I-labelled L-asparaginase (small filled circles) then is bound (bottom)

other to ^{125}I-labelled antibodies to IgE (Fig. 3). Antibodies reacting with labelled L-asparaginase possessed two or more binding sites for L-asparaginase. Reagins, i. e. antibodies of the IgE type, seemed to behave as functionally monovalent antibodies in this system (Fig. 3). Finally the particles were washed thoroughly and the radioactivity was measured in a gamma counter.

Plasma from 12 of 21 patients contained antibodies on one or several occasions. Six patients had reagins and 3 patients "bivalent" antibodies. The remaining 3 patients had antibodies of both types. In this study we were not able to quantitate the antibodies. Instead an arbitrary scale based on counts per minute using 5+ as the strongest reaction was adopted for comparison.

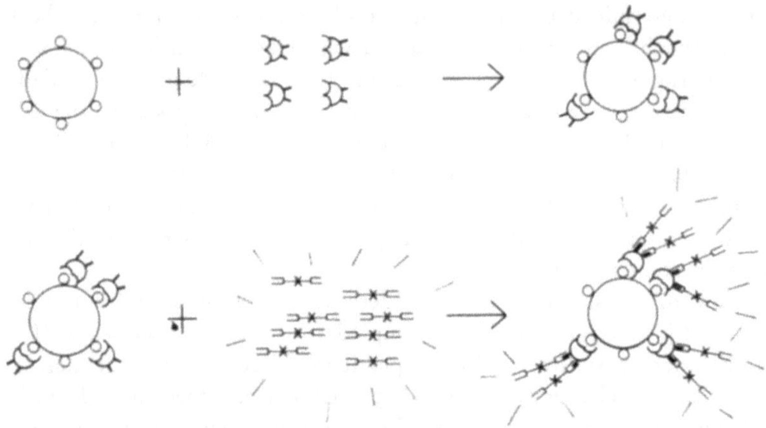

Fig. 3. Reaction between L-asparaginase (small open circles) on a polysaccharide particle (big circle) and "functionally monovalent" antibodies (top) to which ^{125}I-labelled antibodies to IgE then are bound (bottom)

The results of antibody studies on 5 patients are shown in Table I. Patients A.S-n and M.J-n exhibited the highest antibody levels. A.S-n did not show any allergic reactions and enzyme activity (0.7 IU/ml) was found in plasma at the same time as the high reagin titres. However, M.J-n exhibited a strong anaphylactoid reaction immediately after the 28th injection of L-asparaginase. A blood sample collected 24 hrs. later showed a very high antibody titer and no enzyme activity. After treatment for two weeks the patient S.-L-u suddenly developed auricular fibrillation and hypotension during the injection of L-asparaginase. A few days later a bone marrow specimen revealed unchanged lymphoblastic leukemia and pronounced plasmocytosis not present at the beginning of therapy. The relatively high titer of antibody demonstrated on the day after the reaction was unchanged two weeks later, no therapy being given in between. Patient O.W-g, having both reagins and "bivalent" antibodies, had an anaphylactoid reaction on the 27th day of treatment. At that time no enzyme activity could be demonstrated in plasma. Patient G.S-s also showed both types of antibodies in plasma. However, no allergic reactions was noted.

In this series, 5 of 21 patients showed acute anaphylactoid reactions during or within 30 min after injection of L-asparaginase. Two of these patients had only "bivalent" antibodies and two had both types of antibodies. All these reactions were noted during the first course of treatment. The fifth patient had such a reaction at the beginning of his fourth course of treatment with no detectable antibody present. Antibody analyses in patients with both types of antibodies indicated that reagins might be the first to appear during treatment. After cessation of therapy the reagins seemed to disappear earlier than the "bivalent" antibodies.

L-asparaginase activities in plasma samples with and without antibodies are shown in Fig. 4. The overlapping was considerable but the results suggested that the

Table 1. *Antibody formation during L-asparaginase treatment*

Patient (sex and age)	Date 1969	L-asparaginase bound antibodies reacting with ^{125}I-labelled anti-IgE	L-asparaginase
A.S-n	April 9 [a]	—	—
girl	May 21	+++++	—
9 years	June 6 [b]		
	12	+	—
M.J-n	April 18 [a]	—	—
girl	22	—	—
4 years	May 14 [b]		
	15	—	+++++
S.L-u	April 8 [a]	—	—
man	14	—	—
60 years	21	—	++++
	May 12 [b]	—	++++
O.W-g	May 2 [a]	—	—
boy	19	++	+
4 years	29	++	++
	30 [b]	+++	+++
	June 25	—	+++
	July 17	—	++
G.S-s	May 12 [a]	—	—
girl	14	—	—
5 years	28	+	—
	June 9	+	—
	16	+	—
	July 7 [b]		
	Sept. 25 [a]	++	+
	Oct. 1	++	++
	8	+	++

[a] Start of L-asparaginase treatment.
[b] End of L-asparaginase treatment.

occurence of antibodies, in particular of the "bivalent" type, was associated with lower enzyme activities. Reagins did not appear to be associated with any marked changes in enzyme activity in plasma.

In eight patients without detectable antibodies the mean asparaginase activity in plasma 24 hrs. after intravenous injection was 1.2 IU/ml (8 patients). In 6 patients receiving the enzyme intramuscularly the corresponding value was 0.9 IU/ml. It can thus be concluded that the different routes of administration resulted in similar final plasma enzyme levels.

Plasma levels of asparaginase during the course of treatment of five patients are shown in Fig. 5. The enzyme activity was relatively constant in patients 2 and 3, the latter having reagins in plasma. In patients 4 and 5, who both had anaphylactoid reactions, the enzyme activity decreased to zero. Patient 4 had "bivalent" antibodies

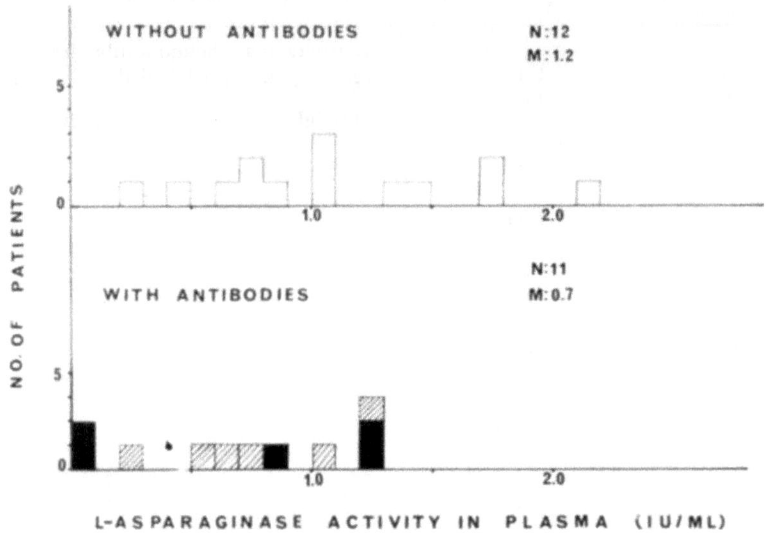

Fig. 4. L-asparaginase activities in plasma samples containing no antibodies and plasma with antibodies of reagin type (hatched bars) and "bivalent" antibodies alone or in combination with reagins (solid bars)

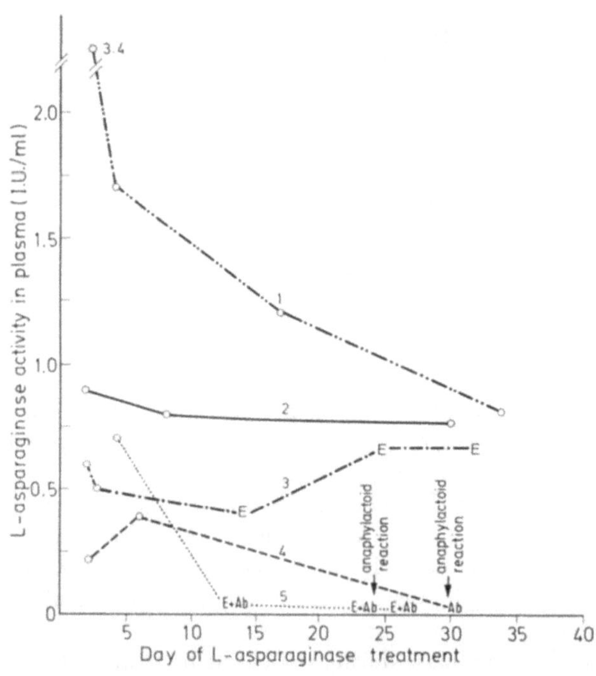

Fig. 5. L-asparaginase activities and presence of antibodies in plasma during course of treatment of 5 patients (200 IU/kg). o = no demonstrable antibodies; E = reagins; Ab = "bivalent" antibodies

alone and patient 5 having reagins as well. Thus antibodies in plasma may be associated with anaphylactoid reactions and inactivation of the asparaginase. However, as exemplified in patient 1, decreasing enzyme activity in course of treatment may also occur in the absence of antibodies.

Conclusions

The *in vitro* predictive test, the occurence of antibodies and the assay of L-asparaginase activity in plasma were investigated in a series of 26 L-asparaginase treated patients. This test was found to be of limited predictive value. Antibodies of two types were found in about half of the treated patients. Reagins, i. e. IgE antibodies, seemed to appear earlier and to disappear more rapidly than other types antibodies. Only the latter were associated with markedly depressed L-asparaginase activity in plasma and with anaphylactoid reactions.

Acknowledgements

These studies were supported by grants from the Cancer Society, Stockholm, the Swedish Cancer Society remove and the Swedish Medical Research Council (grant 16X-637).

References

1. Oettgen, H. F., Old, E. A., Boyse, E. A., Campbell, H. A., Philips, F. S., Clarson, B. D., Talal, L., Leeper, R. D., Schwarz, M. K., Kim, J. H.: Inhibition of Leukemias in Man by L-Asparaginase. Cancer Rec. **27**, 2619 (1967).
2. Fawcett, J. K., Scott, J. E.: A rapid and precise method for the determination of Urea. J. clin. Path. **13**, 156 (1960).
3. Wide, L., Porath, J.: Radioimmunoassay of proteins with the use of Sephadex-coupled antibodies. Biochin. biophys. Acta (Amst.) **130**, 257 (1966).
4. — Axén, R., Porath, J.: Radioimmunosorbent assay for proteins. Chemical couplings of antibodies to insoluble dextran. Immunochemistry **4**, 381 (1967).
5. — Bennich, H., Johansson, S. G. O.: Diagnosis of allergy by an in-vitro test for allergen antibodies. Lancet **II**, 1105 (1967).
6. — Radioimmunoassays employing immunosorbents. Acta endocr. Supplement **142**, 207 (1969).

Part VII
Clinical Effects and Side Effects

Treatment of Acute Leukemia with L-Asparaginase[1]

Ellen Loeb, J. M. Hill, N. O. Hill, A. MacLellan, A. Khan, T. R. Alexander, and M. Adachi

From the Granville C. Morton Cancer and Research Hospital of the Wadley Institutes of Molecular Medicine, Dallas, Texas, U.S.A.

With 1 Figure

The Wadley Institutes of Molecular Medicine are now in the third year of clinical investigation and treatment with the first known enzyme capable of depriving tumor cells of their vital nutrition, asparagine.

The requirement of asparagine for growth of leukemic and other tumor cells in culture as well as the metabolic differences from normal cells was established by the work of Broome [12], Broome and Schwartz [13], and McCoy and Maxwell [14]. The anti-tumor activity of asparaginase was shown in small animals by Kidd [15] and in dogs by Hill [16], and Old et al. [17]. The discovery by Mashburn and Wriston [18] that asparaginase from bacteria *(E. coli)* had antilymphoma activity and the investigation of methods of production and purification by Whelan and Wriston [19], Cedar and Schwartz [20], and Roberts et al. [8] opened the way for extensive animal studies and ultimately clinical trials. The results in animals (6C3HED leukemia in mice) with asparaginase therapy were and still are a challenge to the clinician, in spite of the obvious difference of species, size, transplantable versus spontaneous leukemia, and other factors. In the mouse, cure has been obtained in these animals by the single injection of asparaginase intraperitoneally a day or two before anticipated death. The animal recovers in about 10 days and lives out its life expectancy or shows no sign of disease at autopsy at about one-half life.

The present report is concerned with the clinical experience in the treatment of 68 patients with L-asparaginase in acute leukemia. Asparaginase now appears destined to play a worthwhile role in the treatment of leukemia as a good, and at times, very rapid remission inducing agent which can be employed at any stage of the disease. The lack of cross-resistance with other forms of therapy, the speed of response in sensitive cases, and the freedom from bone marrow depression of normal cell lines

---

[1] Read before the Symposium on Experimental and Clinical Effects of L-asparaginase at Wuppertal-Elberfeld, Germany — from October 24 to 26, 1969, by Ellen Loeb, M.D.

are advantages in the effective treatment of late phases of the disease, as well as an initial therapy. A number of side effects, mostly of mild to moderate degree, can now be attributed to asparaginase since endotoxin-free material has become available. A more serious possible complication or side effect in patients treated with asparaginase is suggested by the report of HASKELL et al. [10], who noted that pancreatitis occurred in 5 out of 49 patients in their series. Likewise, HILL et al. [11] have found three patients who developed pancreatitis on asparaginase therapy, out of 65 patients receiving such treatment. On the other hand, TALLAL et al. [5], reporting on asparaginase therapy in 111 children with leukemias and solid tumors, did not report any incidence of pancreatic involvement.

Materials and Methods

Asparaginase used in these clinical trials was prepared as previously described until November, 1968. Since that time, the development of a human leukocyte sensitivity or immobilization test [9] has made it possible to test for endotoxin down to 10^{-12} grams per 0.01 ml, and to reject any material for human use not meeting these standards. The chick embryo test as described by MILNER and FINKELSTEIN [21] and NARAINE [22] with a sensitivity down to 10^{-9} grams per 0.01 ml was not sensitive enough to assure freedom from endotoxic reactions in humans, but was useful in the validation of the human leukocyte tests for endotoxin down to these levels and by dilution of known endotoxin down to 10^{-12} grams per 0.01 ml of asparaginase preparation. The use of animals for testing effectiveness and for attempts to determine an LD_{50} has been described previously [1, 11]. The asparaginase, as routinely prepared in our laboratory since November, 1968 for intravenous use in batches of 10 to 40,000,000 IU were preserved deep frozen or for longer storage, were freeze dried. It had a specific activity over 300 IU per mg of protein. It could not be purified further with repeated ethanol precipitations. Preparative acrylamide gel electrophoresis of a production batch also failed to show an increase in specific activity (333 IU per mg protein vs. 337 IU per mg protein).

Amino acid levels on patient's serum samples were determined on a Phoenix automatic amino acid analyzer. The serum was deproteinized with 6% sulfosalicylic acid. The acid and neutral amino acids were determined by the method of BENSON, GORDON and PATTERSON [24], using lithium citrate buffer. Basic amino acids were determined by the method of MOORE and STEIN [25], using sodium citrate buffer.

Plan of Treatment

Initially, dosage was limited by the patient's tolerance to the impurities, probably chiefly endotoxin in the preparation. Emphasis was on desensitization. Later, as relatively pure material became available, we attempted to give all patients 1000 IU or more per kg daily, for at least twenty days. Patients continuing to respond to therapy were treated until remission or failure to improve further (rarely over 28 days total), while those showing no improvement or excessive side effects had asparaginase therapy discontinued. The patients obtaining remission went into other protocols, e. g. maintenance on twice weekly administration, or combination therapy. The asparaginase was given intravenously once daily and occasionally divided doses were given when patients exhibited more than a mild reaction to the material. Base line determinations prior to therapy, during, and after therapy included kidney and liver function studies, proteins, and coagulation functions. Bone marrow examinations were taken prior to therapy at least once during treatment and at the end of treatment. During the first few days of treatment where uric acid renal tubular obstruction could become a problem, the urine pH was kept alkaline with sodium bicarbonate and rarely uric acid precipitation was noted.

Results

As shown in Table 1, a good therapeutic response (complete and partial remission) in acute lymphocytic leukemia was obtained in 23 out of 28 patients receiving asparaginase, or 82%. In the lymphocytic group all were children except 4 patients over 14 in the complete remission category and 3 patients in the partial remission group. The number of patients receiving no specific therapy other than asparaginase at any time were 10 patients, 5 obtained a complete remission; 4 obtained a partial remission, and 1 showed no response.

A good response (complete and good partial remissions) to the enzyme treatment was seen in 20 out of 40 patients (50%) in acute granulocytic leukemia. Eleven of these obtained complete remission (27.5%). A significant clinical improvement or fair remission was seen in 7 additional cases. It should be noted that of the 11 complete remissions, 8 were in patients less than 14 years of age, and 4 in the partial remission group were in this category. The number of new patients previously

Table 1. *L-asparaginase therapy in acute leukemia*

Diagnosis	Total	Complete remission No.	%	Partial remission No.	%	Fair remission No.	%	Poor response No.	%
Acute lymphatic leukemia	28	14	50.0	9	32.1	2	7.1	3	10.7
Acute granulocytic leukemia	40	11	27.5	9	22.5	7	17.5	13	32.5
Total	68	25	36.8	18	26.5	9	13.2	16	23.5

Table 2. *L-asparaginase therapy in acute leukemia. Treatment for at least 20 days at 1000 IU/kg/day or more*

Diagnosis	Total	Complete remission No.	%	Partial remission No.	%	Fair remission No.	%	Poor response No.	%
Acute lymphatic leukemia	11	11	100.0						
Acute granulocytic leukemia	21	10	47.6	7	33.3	2	9.5	2	9.5
Total	32	21	65.6	7	21.9	2	6.3	2	6.3

untreated receiving asparaginase as the only specific therapy were 11 with 4 complete remissions, 3 partial remissions, 3 fair remissions, and 1 poor response.

Table 2 represents the smaller group of patients receiving adequate therapy (1000 IU per kg daily for at least 20 days). In this group, the complete remission rate was 47.6% for granulocytic and 100% for lymphocytic leukemia. Combining good partial remissions with complete remissions [2] gave rates of 80.9% in the granulocytic leukemias.

Three cases of acute leukemia treated with asparaginase were not included in the above tables because the asparaginase was given during a remission previously induced by conventional agents.

Tables 3 and 4 give a condensed summary of all patients who achieved a complete remission with asparaginase therapy. Shown in these tables are the following: age, sex, total dose administered, dose to induce remission, days to obtain remission and remission length in weeks, as well as a designation of the patient's status at time of tabulation. Only one case in the granulocytic series received combined therapy. In this instance, conventional therapy was continued along with asparaginase treatment, even though such therapy had apparently failed to induce remission over a three month period of time. The mean value for total dosage administered to the acute granulocytic leukemia patients was 2,603,581 IU. The mean dose to induce remission in IU per kg per day was 2473. The mean of the number of days to achieve remission was 26.3 and the mean lengths of remission was 16.8 weeks for this group. In the case of acute lymphocytic leukemia, the mean total dosage per patient for the group was 2,468,500 IU, the mean dose to induce remission in IU per kg per day was 1423, while the mean days to obtain remission was 19.6 and the mean length of remission in weeks was 14.6.

In Table 5, side effects associated with asparaginase therapy have been listed. It should be noted that these figures are taken from our total experience, covering not only leukemia but other malignant diseases. The side effect of nausea and vomiting was divided into the severe group requiring discontinuance of the therapy either temporarily or permanently and in the mild to moderate group, where the symptoms did not require even temporary discontinuance.

Table 6 summarizes the more extensive coagulation factor studies which were performed before and during asparaginase therapy in a number of patients treated with the heavy dosage schedules and receiving highly purified asparaginase believed to be endotoxin-free. It should be mentioned that none of the patients in this group, nor in our entire series, developed bleeding or other significant clinical findings (excluding acute pancreatitis) related to coagulopathy induced by the enzyme therapy.

An interesting statistic relating both to the depression of coagulation factors and the elevations of SGOT and serum Bilirubin mentioned in Table 5 was the finding of fatty metamorphosis of the liver in 32 out of a total of 44 post mortem examinations performed on patients who had received asparaginase therapy.

---

[2] *Complete remission*—clearing of leukemic blasts from marrow and blood that persists at least two weeks; patient well by standard clinical criteria. *Partial remission*—clearing of blasts in peripheral blood without complete clearing of marrow; improvement in clinical status. *Fair remission*—significant improvement in laboratory and clinical findings not qualifying as partial remission. *Poor results*—failure to reach above criteria.

Table 3. *L-asparaginase therapy—complete remissions in acute lymphatic leukemia*

Case No. sex—age initials	Total dose IU	Dose to induce remission IU/kg/day	Days to obtain remission	Remission length in weeks
67 ALL 305 F – 4 yrs. D.C.	2,133,000	1503	8	20 [a]
66 ALL 324 M – 17 yrs. D.H.	4,220,000	1483	19	5 [b]
68 ALL 330 M – 12 yrs. S.S.	2,070,000	2000	26	27 [c, d]
68 ALL 327 F – 15 yrs. M.C.J.	4,323,000	2000	18	17 [c]
66 ALL 300 M – 9 yrs. F.H.	213,000	171	39	4 [b]
66 ALL 302 M – 13 yrs. D.B.	302,424	236	13	6 [b]
68 ALL 316 F – 7 yrs. L.W.	3,715,750	2057	18	12 [b]
68 ALL 319 M – 24 yrs. W.M.H.	3,055,000	1405	30	10.5 [b]
68 ALL 320 F – 2 yrs. S.F.	3,806,000	1080	9	18 [a]
65 ALL 288 M – 6 yrs. R.L.	2,690,000	2347	18	21.5 [c, d]
69 ALL 332 F – 3 yrs. M.E.H.	625,500	1377	18	20.5 [c, d]

[a] Out of remission, living. [b] Dead. [c] Still in remission. [d] Maintenance on other Rx.

Table 7 shows the dosage, the number of days of therapy with asparaginase, and other specific prior therapy in 7 patients in the late stages of leukemia and other neoplasms found to have acute pancreatitis. In 6 of the patients, the diagnosis was made clinically; in one, only at autopsy. Three of the clinical diagnoses were confirmed at autopsy. The 3 patients diagnosed clinically without autopsy confirmation all showed definite hypotension, epigastric pain, nausea, and vomiting, abdominal distention with marked increase in blood amylase or blood sugar or both.

In addition to the patients listed in Table 7 the study of post mortem findings in 44 patients coming to autopsy out of these series of 104 cases, indicated focal areas

Table 4. *L-asparaginase therapy—complete remissions in acute granulocytic leukemia*

Case No. sex—age initials	Total dose IU	Dose to induce remission IU/kg/day	Days to obtain remission	Remission length in weeks
68 AGL 552 M – 17 yrs. J.L.F.G.	4,710,500	2234	34	5 [a]
68 AGL 561 F – 5 yrs. R.M.	2,869,300	2676	14	23 [a]
68 AGL 562 F – 3 yrs. L.L.S.	545,000	1804	12	21 [a, b]
68 AGL 557 F – 35 yrs. R.T.	5,986,500	3862	35	6.5 [a, c]
66 AGL 497 M – 4 yrs. M.L.	3,470,930	3325	44	15 [d]
68 AGL 565 F – 8 yrs. E.P.	1,150,000	2362	23	24 [d]
65 AGL 449 F – 8 yrs. C.S.	1,991,000	2000	28	11 [d]
68 AGL 566 M – 7 yrs. O.C.	1,280,000	2362	[e]	27 [a]
69 AGL 574 M – 8 yrs. H.T.	1,420,000	1633	21	20 [f, g]

[a] Dead.
[b] Mongoloid—chromosome 21 trisomy.
[c] Major erythroleukemia component.
[d] Out of remission, living.
[e] Received conventional treatment with L-asparagine to obtain and maintain remission.
[f] Still in remission.
[g] Maintenance on other Rx.

of pancreatic or fatty necrosis in 7 additional patients. These lesions varied from microscopic areas of fatty necrosis to pancreatic abscess and necrosis of the head of the pancreas. In this category were 3 multiple myelomas (of the 5 treated), one Hodgkin's disease, 3 additional acute myelogenous leukemias, and one carcinoma of the breast. A comparison review of 32 autopsies of patients with acute leukemia not treated with asparaginase revealed no findings of acute diffuse pancreatitis; however, there were two cases of pancreatic fat necrosis. Twenty-eight of these patients, or 93%, had had steroid therapy. Incidentally, 6 examples of fatty metamorphosis of the liver were found in this series of autopsies.

Table 5. *Side effects observed in asparaginase therapy. 104 cases leukemia and other malignant disease*

Side effects		Total cases No.	%
Hyperglycemia		13	12.5
5% or more weight loss		14	13.5
Allergic reactions		14	13.5
Serum bilirubin elevation above 2.5 mg-%		19	18.3
Mental confusion (mild to moderate, none severe)		25	24.0
SGOT (persistent increase over 60)		39	37.5
Chills and fever		65	62.5
Vomiting:	mild to moderate	64	61.5
	severe	18	17.3

Table 6. *Coagulation factor changes during L-asparaginase therapy*

	No. of patients studied	Abnormal	Mean values for each group Initial level	Maximum abnormality	Change %
A.H.G. (VIII)	14	3	100.00% N	92.04% N	7.95
Proconvertin (VII+X)	5	3	83.75% N	67.91% N	15.83
Quick's prothrombin	18	11	91.93% N [a]	68.5 % N	23.43
P.T.C. (IX)	14	9	97.27% N	67.19% N	30.08
P.T.A. (XI)	14	6	99.09% N	67.42% N	31.67
Proaccelerin (V)	5	3	98.33% N	57.08% N	41.25
Prothrombin (II)	5	5	95.00% N	53.33% N	41.67
P.T.T.	18	15	39.96 sec	101.23 sec	61.26
Fibrinogen (I)	21	21	373.71 mg-%	126.31 mg-%	247.4

[a] %N (percent of normal control plasma).

Table 8 summarizes the findings in 5 patients with leukemic meningitis who were given intravenous asparaginase therapy. All patients received substantial amounts of the enzyme, the smallest dose being 1000 IU per kg per day in this group. All but one case showed excellent response with reduction of spinal fluid cell counts from levels above 500 to normal or near normal levels. One patient with acute granulocytic leukemia, in the terminal stage of the disease, showed no improvement.

Serum amino acid determinations were made on several patients with acute leukemia before, during and after asparaginase therapy. In general, amino acid levels in the patients with leukemia were moderately depressed (10—20% below lower limits of normal). With the exception of asparagine and glutamine, the amino acids rose to the normal range during asparaginase therapy. On discontinuance of the enzyme, the amino acids fell to pre-treatment levels or a little below. Fig. 1 shows the changes in a white male, age 22, with acute granulocytic leukemia in serum amino acid levels before, shortly after, during and following cessation of asparaginase therapy, together with a determination of the asparaginase levels in the blood stream. Also shown are the reciprocal patterns of change in the serum glutamate and aspartate, products of enzymatic destruction of asparagine and glutamine. At the dosage

Table 7. *7 patients in late stage of leukemia and other neoplasms. Developing acute pancreatitis on L-asparaginase and steroid therapy*

Code No. sex—age name	Days asparaginase Rx prior to acute pancreatitis	Asparaginase Rx before pancreatitis	Other Rx prior to asparaginase	G.I. symptoms prior to asparaginase	Blood sugar	Amyl-ase	Comment
68 AGL 548 M – 40 yrs. R.B.	5	5000 IU/kg/day	6-MP, Steroids, AME, VCR	Upper abdominal pain	740	1120	Autopsy. Pancreatitis—old
68 ALL 329 F – 33 yrs. A.I.	10	2000 IU/kg/day	Steroids, & VCR	Nausea, vomiting, headache	385	1650	No autopsy. Pancreatitis improved prior to death from leuk.
68 AGL 540 F – 35 yrs. J.J.	10	2000 IU/kg/day	Massive Steroids & VCR [a]	Upper abd. pain diarrhea	—	536	Autopsy—Acute pancreatitis
68 AGL 547 M – 13 yrs. R.A.	4	2000 IU/kg/day	AME, 6-MP, VLB, Steroids	No specific symptoms	155	632	No autopsy. Exp. leukemic meningitis
69 ALL 334 M – 8 yrs. D.S.F.	5	2000 IU/kg/day	Ara.C., 6-MP, & Steroids	No specific symptoms	824	353	No autopsy. Pancreatitis improved prior to death from leuk.
63-353 M – 48 yrs. C.E.O. Lymphosarcoma	15	1000 IU/kg/day	P-32, Steroids, Urethane Cyclophos.	Nausea, vague abdominal pain	150	830	Autopsy—pancreat. duct obstruction with acute pancreatitis
68-54 M – 65 yrs. J.A.C. Ca.	3	800 IU/kg/day	Steroids	No specific symptoms	—	—	Dx. at autopsy, acute pancreatitis

[a] Patient also received vincristine concomitantly with asparaginase.

Table 8. *CNS leukemia treated with I.V. asparaginase*

Case No. sex—age initials	Previous asparaginase treatment	Previous treatment	Spinal fluid cell count Initial	Final	Days to maximum clearing of spinal fluid	Average dose IU/kg/day
65 AGL 449 F-9 C.S.	No	AME, MP, VCR, Steroid	1105	0	7	2100
68 ALL 312 M-13 J.M.B.	Yes	AME, MP, VCR, Steroid	5050	15	29	2000
68 ALL 329 F-33 A.I.	No	Steroid, MP, AME, VCR, Cyclophos.	680	42	10 days Rx.	2000
68 AGL 540 F-35 J.J.	No	Steroid, AME, VCR, Cyclophos.	500	450	10 days Rx. Pt. expired	1350
67 ALL 310 M-14 R.L.G.	Yes	AME, MP, VCR, Steroid	1000	1	13	1000

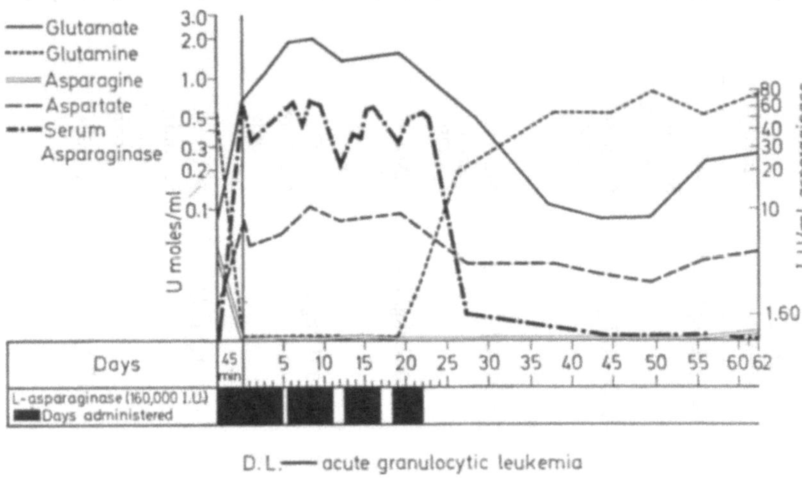

Fig. 1. Serum amino acid levels during L-asparaginase therapy

of 2000 IU per kg per day, asparagine and glutamine values are already down to undetectable levels at 45 minutes after administration. Asparagine remained at undetectable levels for around 55 days. However, the much smaller glutaminase component of the asparaginase preparation is reflected in the return to normal or near normal glutamine levels shortly after cessation of therapy.

Discussion

Asparaginase seems to compare favorably with the well established conventional agents for the induction of remission, especially in acute granulocytic leukemia. The unusual response in our adequately treated acute granulocytic leukemia patients may relate in part to the high proportion of patients under 14 years of age (8 out of 11 complete remissions and 4 out of 9 good partial remissions). Of interest was the complete remission obtained by the 35-year-old patient with a major erythroleukemia component, resistant to conventional treatment.

Asparaginase remissions seem to be considerably shorter than those obtained with standard antimetabolite therapy. For example, the mean length of remission of 16.8 weeks for the granulocytic group and 14.6 weeks for the lymphocytic group is not outstanding but appears to be very worthwhile in view of the fact that such remissions can be obtained in patients otherwise resistant to all former therapies. Further treatment with asparaginase does not adversely influence results with subsequent conventional agents. In our own series, the majority of patients who achieved remissions with asparaginase were also given maintenance therapy. Although we have given up to 17,000 IU per kg per day of asparaginase, it is our impression that 1000 IU per kg per day may be all that is required to achieve optimum results. Certainly, little more effect could be expected from giving a larger dose than that required to deplete glutamine as well as asparagine down to undetectable levels in the patient's serum. A more convenient schedule of treatment such as two or three times weekly is suggested by our amino acid studies in the blood of patients under therapy, along with consideration of the fairly long half-life of asparaginase in the blood stream (our mean—18 hours). Ohnuma et al. [26] have studied the effect of single intravenous injections of asparaginase with doses repeated several days later. One patient in their report with acute myelogenous leukemia attained complete remission after a single dose of 1000 IU per kg.

In addition to its high remission inducing rate, this enzyme at times has achieved remission in a very short period; for example, 8 days to clear the marrow. In general, it appears to be intermediate between steroids or vincristine and antimetabolites in speed of action.

Another advantage to asparaginase therapy is its effectiveness in patients suffering from leukemic meningitis. Although asparaginase does not pass from the blood to the spinal fluid [27], apparently the depletion of asparagine in the blood sets up a gradient for depletion in the spinal fluid. Tan and Oettgen [27] administered asparaginase intrathecally with a response in some patients with CNS leukemia.

Some revision in our concept of the effect of asparaginase on normal versus malignant tissues may be necessary in view of some adverse reactions and side effects now known to occur in patients. The purest asparaginase preparations which we have used contain around one per cent glutaminase activity, which was shown capable of the depletion of glutamine, as well as asparagine. This dual enzymatic action must be taken into account with respect to therapeutic results, as well as adverse reactions. The earlier, rather simplistic concept that a clear-cut difference in the nutritional requirement of normal and certain neoplastic cells could be exploited to give an entirely safe, yet very effective therapy of malignant disease no longer seems entirely tenable. Recently, Astaldi et al. [28] and Ohno [29] have shown that asparaginase inhibits the blastic transformation of lymphatic cells under the influence of phytohemagglutinin. Much more information concerning the special amino acid requirements of different normal tissues and their ability to synthesize asparagine and glutamine might help to explain some of the adverse reactions observed clinically.

The two most common side effects were mild to moderate nausea and vomiting, and chills and fever approximating 60% of the cases treated. However, these symptoms tended to disappear with continuing therapy and were considered acceptable for the results expected, although distressing to the patient. However, an additional 17% of patients had sufficiently severe nausea and vomiting to require temporary or permanent discontinuance of therapy. Mental confusion seen in 24% of treated patients was considered mild to moderate only, and was observed only in adults, and was reversible. No discontinuance of therapy was necessary on this basis. Some evidence of liver disfunction was commonly seen. The SGOT with persistent increase over 60 was seen in 37.5% of cases, while serum Bilirubin elevation above 2.5% was observed in only 18.3%. These changes were related to the fatty metamorphosis found on liver biopsy or at autopsy (80% of cases so examined). Depression of serum albumin levels was seen in about 40% of our cases. This effect we believe is definitely associated with depletion of asparagine and/or glutamine. However, the intravenous administration of plasma, albumin and other human protein products, as well as prior chronic debilitating disease, makes this figure somewhat uncertain. Weight loss of significant degree was relatively uncommon. One 17-year-old boy with acute leukemia lost 18 pounds of body weight on asparaginase therapy. However, the therapy was continued and no further weight loss occurred. Around 13% of the patients showed a weight loss of 5% or more. Although coagulation factors were depressed during asparaginase therapy, particularly the fibrinogen, clinical hemorrhage has not been an associated problem in our series.

The role of asparaginase therapy in pancreatitis is difficult to evaluate. However, our experience seems to indicate some causal relationship. Nevertheless, it should be recognized that acute pancreatitis can occur as a complication of leukemia and has been reported with some frequency associated with steroid therapy [32]. In our series (Table 8), there were 7 patients who developed acute hemorrhagic pancreatitis out of 104 patients treated. It may be significant that all of these were late in the disease, had received prior conventional therapy, and were on, or recently had steroid administration. Seventeen new, previously untreated, patients with acute leukemia did not show any incidence of pancreatitis. It should be noted that 4 of the 7 patients with acute pancreatitis improved on symptomatic therapy and died later of their disease.

Of the 3 patients who died with pancreatitis, the patient with lymphosarcoma was found to have duct obstruction in the pancreas due to the tumor lesions.

The etiology of acute diffuse pancreatitis is obscure and any explanation of the relationship of asparaginase therapy to pancreatitis would be premature. However, in this connection, the work of KHAN et al. [33] and de ALMEIDA and GROSSMANN [34] may be relevant. KHAN et al. were unable to produce pancreatitis or significant, observable pathologic changes in the pancreas of rabbits treated with a single large dose of asparaginase.

Hyperglycemia resulted in the majority of animals receiving 2000 IU per kg or more. A significant reduction (75% reduction in required dose) in the dosage of asparaginase required to produce hyperglycemia was seen when a single dose of Prednisolone (1 mg per kg) was administered intravenously at the same time the asparaginase was given [35]. De Almeida and Grossmann [34] gave ethionine, the ethyl analog of methionine, to dogs, cats and monkeys, with the production of acute pancreatitis accompanied by elevation in the blood amylase and lipase.

Until more is known about the etiology of pancreatitis and its possible relationship with asparaginase therapy, we believe it would be worthwhile to have the patient in good nutritional status, especially to have normal serum protein levels with special reference to albumin. Measures should also be taken, insofar as possible, to have the patient free of infection and coagulation defects. During enzyme therapy, the blood sugar should be followed carefully and the patient observed for any of the earliest clinical signs of pancreatitis, which should be used as an indication for blood amylase determinations. Upon diagnosis of pancreatic involvement, the asparaginase should be discontinued and in addition to symptomatic treatment, we have found plasmaphoresis and replacement of the patient's cells suspended in normal, platelet-rich plasma worthwhile [36]. Such therapy not only replaces depleted asparagine and glutamine but could remove the assumed split products resulting from pancreatic destruction.

Asparaginase therapy of acute leukemia has now had sufficient clinical trials to establish its value, along with conventional agents. Especially recommending its use are its good remission rate, a fairly rapid speed of response, its effectiveness in central nervous system leukemia, and its lack of cross-resistance with other agents. The results in acute granulocytic leukemia seem promising in our own rather small group. The unfavorable aspects such as a fairly short remission and most of the side effects, seem quite acceptable for the results obtained. It is hoped further studies will clarify and perhaps solve the problem of pancreatic involvement. More important, even than these results, may be the opening of a new field of enzyme therapy through depletion of amino acids or nutritional factors.

Summary

Intravenous administration of the enzyme L-asparaginase used as an agent for the treatment of acute leukemia now appears to have a well established place. A total of 116 patients have received intravenous asparaginase for a variety of conditions at the Wadley Institutes of Molecular Medicine. Sixty-eight of these patients were treated for acute leukemia. In the adequately treated group of patients with acute leukemia, receiving at least 1000 International Units per kilogram daily for at least 20 days, there were 10 complete remissions out of 21 patients with acute granulocytic leukemia for 47.6% complete remission rate, and out of 11 patients with acute lymphocytic leukemia for 100% complete remission rate.

Many of the characteristics of the highly purified asparaginase produced by an original method in our laboratories are given. The material had approximately 1% glutamine activity. Serum amino acid studies indicated that doses of 1000 IU per kg per day, or more, resulted in undetectable levels of asparagine and glutamine. The level of asparagine remained depressed up to 50 or more days, while the glutamine remained at undetectable levels for only 5 days or less.

Seven patients, all in the late, previously treated group receiving steroid therapy, developed acute pancreatitis. Side effects included nausea and vomiting, chills and fever, depression of serum albumin, decrease in fibrinogen and to a lesser extent, prothrombin accelerators, increased SGOT and serum Bilirubin levels, mental confusion (reversible and in adults only), weight loss and hyperglycemia. The chief advantages of asparaginase were high incidence of remission, freedom from cross-resistance with other agents, effectiveness in

CNS leukemia, and fairly rapid response to treatment. The disadvantages, in addition to side effects and the possible relationship to pancreatitis, were fairly short remissions averaging 16.8 weeks in the acute granulocytic group and 14.6 weeks in the acute lymphocytic group.

Acknowledgment

This work was supported by grants and donations from the following: W. W. CARUTH, JR., through the Community Chest Trust Fund; the Leland Fikes Foundation; Mr. and Mrs. E. E. FOGELSON; the Hillcrest Foundation; H. L. Hunt Foundation; Merck, Sharp & Dohme Research Laboratories, of Rahway, New Jersey; Southwest Medical Foundation; and the Wadley Leukemia Association.

Technical Acknowledgment

The technical assistance of Salvador Comparini in the production of the Asparaginase used in this project is gratefully acknowledged.

References

1. HILL, J. M., ROBERTS, J., LOEB, ELLEN, KHAN, A., MACLELLAN, A., HILL, R. W.: L-asparaginase therapy for leukemia and other malignant neoplasms. J. Amer. med. Ass. 202, 882—888 (1967).
2. OETTGEN, H. F., OLD, L. J., BOYSE, E. A., CAMPBELL, H. A., PHILLIPS, F. S., CLARKSON, B. D., TALLAL, LISA, LEEPER, R. D., SCHWARTZ, M. K., KIM, J. H.: Inhibition of leukemias in man by L-asparaginase: Presented at American Society of Hematology meeting from Sloan-Kettering Institute for Cancer Research and Memorial Hospital for Cancer and Allied Diseases, New York, N. Y., December 1967.
3. HILL, J. M., LOEB, ELLEN, ROBERTS, J., MACLELLAN, A., KHAN, A., HILL, N. O.: L-asparaginase therapy of leukemia: Presented at International Society of Hematology meeting from Wadley Institutes of Molecular Medicine, New York, N. Y., September 1968.
4. BURCHENAL, J. H., KARNOFSKY, D. A., MURPHY, M. L., OETTGEN, H. F.: Presented at International Society of Hematology meeting from Sloan-Kettering Institute for Cancer Research and Memorial Hospital for Cancer and Allied Diseases, New York, N. Y., September 1968.
5. TALLAL, L., TAN, C., OETTGEN, H., MCCARTHY, M., HELSON, L., MURPHY, L.: L-asparaginase in 111 children with leukemias and solid tumors: Presented at 60th Annual Meeting of American Association for Cancer Research, San Francisco, Calif., March 1969.
6. JAMRA, M., CUNHA, LUCIANA, PATTO, G., LORENZI, THEREZINHA F.: Emprego da L-asparaginase em leukemia aguda: Presented at II Congresso Nacional, Colegio Brasileiro de Hematologia, Sao Paulo, Brazil, May 1969.
7. HILL, J. M.: Treatment of acute leukemia with L-asparaginase: Presented at II Congresso Nacional, Colegio Brasileiro de Hematologia, Sao Paulo, Brazil, May 1969.
8. ROBERTS, J., BURSON, G., HILL, J. M.: New procedures for purification of L-asparaginase with high yield from *Escherichia coli*. J. Bact. **95**, 2117—2123 (1968).
9. HILL, J. M., PENNINGTON, KAREN: A new method for determining toxicity of *E. coli* L-asparaginase preparations: From Wadley Institutes of Molecular Medicine, May 1969. To be published.
10. HASKELL, C. M., CANELLOS, G. P., LEVENTHAL, B. G., CARBONE, P. P.: L-asparaginase toxicity, Cancer Res. **29**, 974—975 (1969).
11. HILL, J. M., LOEB, ELLEN, MACLELLAN, A., KHAN, A., ROBERTS, J., SHIELDS, WILMA F., HILL, N. O.: Enzyme therapy of acute leukemia: Response to Highly Purified L-asparaginase. Cancer Res. 1969.

12. BROOME, J. D.: Studies on the mechanism of tumor inhibition by L-asparaginase. Effects of the Enzyme on Asparagine Levels in the Blood, Normal Tissues, and 6C3HED Lymphomas of Mice: Differences in Asparagine Formation and Utilization in Asparaginase. Sensitive and Resistant Lymphoma Cells. J. exp. Med. **127**, 1053—1080 (1968).
13. — SCHWARTZ, J. H.: Differences in the production of L-asparagine in asparaginase-sensitive and resistant lymphoma cells. Biochim. biophys. Acta (Amst.) **138**, 637—639 (1967).
14. MCCOY, T. A., MAXWELL, M., KRUSE, P. F., JR.: The amino acid requirements of the Jensen sarcoma *in vitro*. Cancer Res. **19**, 591—595 (1959).
15. KIDD, J. G.: Regression of transplanted lymphomas induced *in vivo* by means of normal guinea-pig serum. I. Course of Transplanted Cancers of Various Kinds in Mice and Rats Given Guinea Pig Serum, Horse Serum, or Rabbit Serum. J. exp. Med. **98**, 565—582 (1953).
16. HILL, J. M.: Advances en el tratamiento de las neoplasias de tejido linfoiedo: Read before the 17th National Assembly of Surgeons, Mexico City, DF, November 14, 1966.
17. OLD, L. J.: Treatment of Lymphosarcoma in the Dog With L-asparaginase. Lancet **1967 I**, 447—448.
18. MASHBURN, L. T., WRISTON, J. C., JR.: Tumor inhibitory effect of L-asparaginase from *Escherichia coli*. Arch. Biochem. **105**, 451—452 (1964).
19. WHELAN, HELEN A., WRISTON, J. C., JR.: Purification and properties of L-asparaginase from *Escherichia coli B*. Fed. Proc. **27**, 586 (1968). Abstract.
20. CEDAR, H., SCHWARTZ, J. H.: Production of L-asparaginase II by *Escherichia coli*. J. Bact. **96**, 2043—2048 (1968).
21. MILNER, K. C., FINKELSTEIN, R. A.: Bioassay of endotoxin: Correlation between pyrogenicity for rabbits and lethality for chick embryo. J. infect. Dis. **116**, 529—536 (1966).
22. NARAINE, M.: The developing chick embryo as an experimental model for the bioassay of endotoxin in *E. coli:* Thesis. The Graduate Research Institute of Baylor University, and Wadley Institutes of Molecular Medicine, Dallas, Texas, 1968.
23. LIU, Y. P.: Isolation, purification, and characterization of *E. coli* L-asparaginase: Ph. D. Thesis. The Graduate Research Institute of Baylor University, and Wadley Institutes of Molecular Medicine, Dallas, Texas, 1969.
24. BENSON, J. V., JR., GORDON, M. J., PATTERSON, J. A.: Accelerated chromatographic analysis of amino acids in physiological fluids containing glutamine and asparagine. Analyt. Biochem. **18**, 228—240 (1967).
25. STEIN, W. H., MOORE, S.: The free amino acids of human blood plasma. J. biol. Chem. **211**, 915—926 (1954).
26. OHNUMA, T., HOLLAND, J. F., FREEMAN, A., SINKS, L.: Studies of asparaginase and asparagine in acute leukemia: Presented at 60th Annual Meeting of American Association for Cancer Research, San Francisco, Calif., March 1969.
27. TAN, C., OETTGEN, H.: Clinical experience with L-asparaginase administered intrathecally: Presented at 60th Annual Meeting of American Association for Cancer Research, San Francisco, Calif., March 1969.
28. ASTALDI, G., ERIDANI, S., PONTI, G. B., VALENTINI, R., GIANGRANDE, A.: Influence of antiblastic agents applied either *in vivo* or *in vitro* on human lymphocyte transformation in cell culture. Blut Band XIX, Heft 1, pp. 8—16, April 1969.
29. OHNO, R.: Inhibition of lymphocyte blastogenesis by L-asparaginase (LA): Presented at 60th Annual Meeting of American Association for Cancer Research, San Francisco, Calif., March 1969.
30. KHAN, A., HILL, J. M.: Neutralizing precipitin in the serum of a patient treated with L-asparaginase. The J. Lab. clin. Med. **73**, 846—852 (1969).
31. — — Steroid-Induced pancreatitis. From Wadley Institutes of Molecular Medicine. To be published elsewhere.
32. RIEMENSCHNEIDER, T. A., WILSON, J. F., VERNIER, R. L.: Glucocorticoid-Induced pancreatitis in children. J. Pediat. **41**, 428 (1968).
33. KHAN, A., ADACHI, M., HILL, J. M.: Diabetogenic effect of L-asparaginase. From Wadley Institutes of Molecular Medicine, Dallas, Texas. To be published elsewhere.

34. De Almeida, A. L., Grossman, M. I.: Experimental production of pancreatitis with ethionine. Gastroenterology 20, 554—577 (1952).
35. Khan, A., Hill, J. M.: Potentiation of the diabetogenic effect of L-asparaginase by prednisolone. From Wadley Institutes of Molecular Medicine, Dallas, Texas. To be published elsewhere.
36. Hill, J. M.: Acute pancreatitis associated with asparaginase therapy: Treatment With Plasmaphoresis. From Wadley Institutes of Molecular Medicine, Dallas, Texas. To be published elsewhere.

Clinical Experience with L-Asparaginase[1]

H. F. Oettgen, Lisa Tallal, Charlotte C. Tan, M. L. Murphy, B. D. Clarkson, R. D. Golbey, I. H. Krakoff, D. A. Karnofsky, J. H. Burchenal

From the Sloan Kettering Institute for Cancer Research and the Memorial Hospital for Cancer and Allied Diseases, New York, N. Y., U.S.A.

With 3 Figures

Inhibition of acute leukemia in man by L-asparaginase was first reported in 1967 [7, 10]. As larger enzyme supplies became available, clinical trials have been conducted by several groups of investigators, and the therapeutic activity as well as toxic effects have been evaluated in patients with many types of neoplastic disease [1—8, 10—17]. This report is an account of the experience gained over a period of $2^1/_2$ years at the Memorial Hospital in New York.

A total of 390 patients, 219 adults and 171 children (patients under 15 years of age), was treated in 440 trials. Enzyme preparations from the following sources were used: Worthington Biochemical Corporation, Freehold, New Jersey; Squibb, The Institute for Medical Research, New Brunswick, New Jersey; Farbenfabriken Bayer, Wuppertal, Germany; Merck, Sharp and Dohme Research Laboratories, West Point, Pennsylvania. The specific activity of the more than 60 different batches ranged from 35 IU per mg protein in the beginning to 350 IU per mg protein during the past year. The enzyme preparation was administered at a daily dose of 10, 50, 200, 1000 or 5000 IU/kg body weight. This resulted in mean plasma levels of 0.4 to 70 IU/ml during maintenance therapy. Asparaginase was given by straight intravenous injection to most patients; only a few were treated by the intramuscular or intrathecal route. Adult patients treated with doses of 1000 or 5000 IU/kg/day received the enzyme in 50—200 ml of saline as intravenous infusion over a period of 1 hour. Although most patients were treated for a four week period, in others treatment had to be discontinued earlier because of limited supplies, severe side effects or progressing disease. Seventeen patients were treated over longer periods, ranging from 2 to 8 months. Only 30 of the 50 patients receiving a daily dose of 5000 IU/kg—and this includes only 5 of the 23 adult patients—could be treated at this dose for a period of 3—4 weeks. The treatment of the remaining 20 patients was discontinued earlier because of toxicity, progressing disease or death.

Therapeutic Effects

The group of patients whose disease responded most often to treatment with asparaginase were the children with acute lymphoblastic leukemia. Of the total number of

[1] Supported by grants CA08748 and CA05826 of the National Cancer Institute.

96 children with this disease who received asparaginase, 78 were treated for 2 weeks or longer. In only 15 of these had the diagnosis of leukemia been made one month or less before asparaginase therapy. Twentynine patients were treated during the first year and 32 patients during the second year of their illness. The remaining 17 patients had been ill for more than 2 years (Table 1). Only 11 of the 78 patients had no chemotherapy before they were treated with asparaginase. All of the remaining 67 patients had received prednisone previously, many had been treated with methotrexate, vincristine and 6-mercaptopurine, and about one third had received daunomycin or arabinosyl cytosine (Table 2). Thirtytwo of the 78 patients achieved

Table 1. *Children, acute lymphoblastic leukemia. Duration of disease before L-asparaginase therapy*

Total number		91
Treated for 2 weeks or longer		78
Duration of disease (from diagnosis)		
< 1 month	15	
1— 6 monts	5	
7—12 months	9	
1— 2 years	32	
2—3 years	13	
> 3 years	4	

Table 2. *Children, acute lymphoblastic leukemia. Chemotherapy preceding L-asparaginase trial*

Total number	78
Previous chemotherapy	67
Prednisone	67
Methotrexate	61
Vincristine	60
6-Mercaptopurine	53
6-Thioguanine	2
Daunomycin	29
Ara-C	17

complete remissions (M1, H1, P1, S1; see appendix). In 10 additional patients the bone marrow rating was M1 but they did not qualify for a complete remission because their hemoglobin levels were not in the normal range. The total number of patients whose bone marrow was rated M1, i. e. normal with respect to both cellularity and differential count, was 42 of 78 patients treated, or 54 per cent. As far as these small figures go, there was little difference in remission rate between the groups treated at a dose of 10, 200, 1000 or 5000 IU/kg/day (Table 3). Unhappily, all remismions were temporary. Their duration ranged from less than three weeks to more than one year. The median was 60 days for patients who received 10 or 200 IU/kg/day and 120 days for patients who were treated with 1000 or 5000 IU/kg/day (Table 4). Although suggestive, these figures do not necessarily indicate that the

Table 3. *Children, acute lymphoblastic leukemia. Incidence of remissions associated with L-asparaginase therapy*

Dose IU/kg/day	Number of patients	Number of CR	Number of GPR-M1	Per cent remissions
10	12	4	1	42
200	28	13	5	64
1000	22	12	0	55
5000	16	3	4	44
Total	78	32	10	54

CR Complete remission
GPR-M1 Good partial remission with M1 bone marrow rating

Table 4. *Children, acute lymphoblastic leukemia. Duration of remissions obtained with L-asparaginase therapy*

Therapy Dose IU/kg/day	Duration	Remission Number	Duration (days) Range	Mean	Median
10	Maintained	5	38—145	79	61
200 → 50	Maintained	5	28—247	98	50
200	28 days	6	19—104	67	64
200	Maintained	4	40—104	67	63
1000	28 days	12	58—403+	154+	122
5000	28 days	7	20—158	98	129

Table 5. *Children, acute lymphoblastic leukemia. Correlation of duration of remission and duration of disease before L-asparaginase therapy*

Duration of disease	Number of patients	Number of remissions (per cent)	Duration of remissions (days) Range	Mean	Median
1 mo.	15	10 (66)	20—403+	162+	142
1 yr.	14	7 (50)	19—247	85	58
2 yrs.	32	13 (40)	38—179	84	63
2 yrs.	17	12 (70)	42—158	100	114

higher dose is likely to produce a longer lasting remission. This becomes evident when we examine the correlation between the duration of asparaginase-induced remissions and factors other than asparaginase therapy. The duration of the disease prior to therapy is one of these factors. The median duration of remissions was 142 days for patients who had been ill for one month or less, 60 days for patients whose disease had lasted from one month to 2 years (calculated from the time of diagnosis), and 114 days for patients who had leukemia for more than 2 years (Table 5). Seven of the 10 remissions in the first group were obtained by treatment with 1000 IU/kg/day. A related, though not identical factor that can be considered is the number of chemotherapeutic agents used prior to asparaginase therapy. The median duration was 138 days for untreated patients, 102 days for patients who had been treated previously with prednisone, vincristine, methotrexate and 6-mercaptopurine and 71 days for those who had received daunomycin, arabinosyl cytosine and cytoxan in addition (Table 6). There was an interesting correlation between the time necessary for the induction of a remission with asparaginase and the duration of this remission. In Fig. 1, the time that elapsed from the beginning of therapy to an M1 bone marrow rating is plotted on the ordinate, and the time from M1 to M3,

Table 6. *Children, acute lymphoblastic leukemia. Correlation of duration of remission and number of chemotherapeutic agents used before L-asparaginase therapy*

Previous therapy	Median duration disease (months)	Number of patients	Number of remissions	Median duration remission (days)
None	—	10	9	138
Pred, VCR, MTX, 6-MP	18	10	5	102
Pred, VCR, MTX, 6-MP (TG), Dau, Ara-C, Cy	21	40	20	71

Pred = Prednisone; VCR = Vincristine; MTX = Methotrexate; 6-MP = 6-mercaptopurine; TG = 6-Thioguanine; Dau = Daunomycin; Ara-C = arabinosyl cytosine; Cy = Cytoxan.

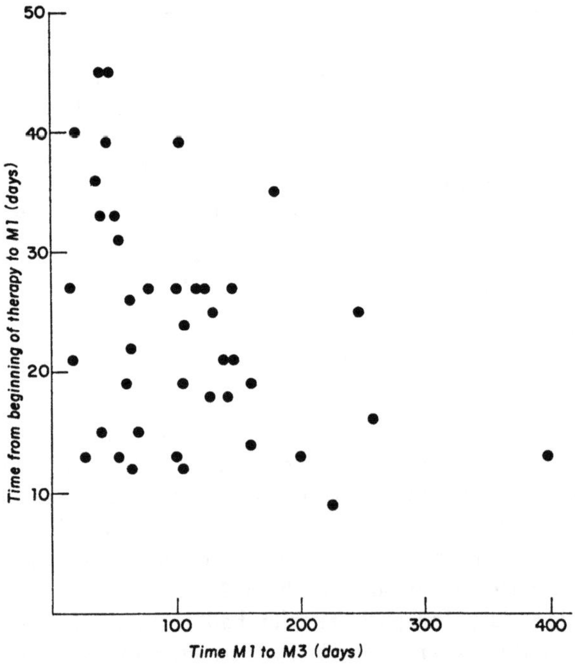

Fig. 1. Correlation of duration of remission induction with duration of remission in children with acute lymphoblastic leukemia

i. e. the duration of remission, on the abscissa. It is evident that no patient with a long induction phase achieved a remission of long duration (there was no obvious relation between the time needed for remission induction and the duration of the disease prior to asparaginase therapy). In Fig. 2, the induction time is plotted for each dose level. It was shorter at 1000 IU/kg/day (median 18 days) than at the other dose levels. Clearly, the question of what is the optimal dose and schedule of asparaginase administration in acute lymphoblastic leukemia can only be answered by comparing the results obtained in larger groups of closely matched patients.

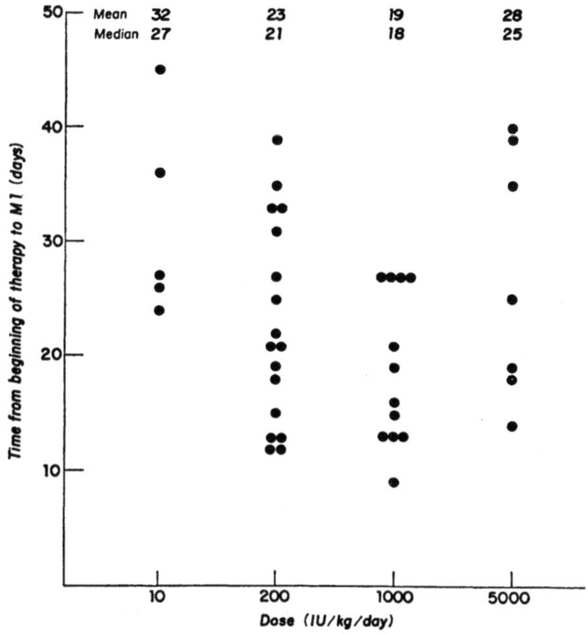

Fig. 2. Correlation of duration of remission induction with dose administered

Eight children received a second course of L-asparaginase, preceded by desensitization with intravenous injections at 10 min intervals, starting with 1 IU and doubling the dose for each of the subsequent injections. In Table 7 the duration of the first remission, the duration of the interval, the drugs used during the interval, and the duration of the second remission are listed. Only in one patient (L. E.) can we be certain that two separate remissions were induced by L-asparaginase. The two other patients who experienced a remission had been given their first course of asparaginase therapy at the beginning of a remission induced by other drugs. In four patients, after an initial asparaginase-induced remission, a second remission could not be induced. A second attempt also failed in a patient who had not responded to the first course of therapy.

Six children were treated at the beginning of a remission induced by other drugs. The duration of the disease, the drugs given previously to these patients, and the duration of the remission are listed in Table 8. Three of these remissions have now

Table 7. *Children, acute lymphoblastic leukemia. Results of a second course of L-asparaginase therapy*

Patient	Duration first remission (days)	Interval (days)	Drugs used during interval	Duration second remission (days)
L. D.	152 [a]	156	—	58
L. E.	103	90	—	114
A. F.	108 [a]	101	—	25
S. R.	62	90	—	—
P. W.	99	100	—	—
M. C.	57	365	Ara-C, VCR, Pred, Cy	—
A. P.	102	281	Pred, MTX, Dau	—
J. Y.	—	146	Dau, Pred, Ara-C, TG	—

[a] Remission induced by other drugs; L-asparaginase given at beginning of remission.

Table 8. *Children, acute lymphoblastic leukemia. Treatment with L-asparaginase during remission induced by other drugs*

Patient	Dose IU/kg/day	Duration of disease (months)	Drugs used previously	Duration of remission (days)
M. F.	200	3	Dau, Pred, MTX	240
L. D.	1000	29	Pred, 6-MP, VCR, Cy, MTX	152
D. I.	1000	3	Pred, VCR, Ara-C, TG	458+
A. F.	1000	20	Pred, 6-MP, MTX	108
D. C.	1000	42	Pred, 6-MP, MTX, VCR	401+
E. L.	1000	33	Pred, VCR, MTX	367+

lasted longer than one year without maintenance chemotherapy, and relapse has not yet occurred.

In 7 of 14 asparaginase-sensitive cases meningeal infiltrates responded to intravenous asparaginase administration as documented by an improvement of spinal fluid abnormalities. In 9 cases asparaginase was given intrathecally. Although this was tolerated and effective, it cannot yet be considered to be a superior method of treating meningeal leukemia with asparaginase.

In 13 children with other types of acute or chronic leukemia and in 22 children with solid tumors only one response to L-asparaginase therapy was seen. It occurred in one of 4 patients with Hodgkin's disease and lasted less than one month.

In adults we observed a remission in 5 of 12 adequately treated patients with acute lymphoblastic leukemia—a remission rate close to that observed in the children. By contrast, only 4 of 27 adequately treated patients with acute myeloblastic leukemia achieved a complete remission.

The results of therapeutic trials in 105 adult patients with 22 different types of solid tumors were rather disappointing (Table 9). There were 2 relatively large groups: 21 patients with lymphosarcoma or reticulum cell sarcoma and 31 patients with malignant melanoma. A significant response was observed in 2 patients of the lymphosarcoma group and in one patient with disseminated malignant melanoma. Although a decreased urinary excretion of chorionic gonadotrophin was observed in three women with choriocarcinoma, the measurable metastatic lesions did not decrease in size. No effect on the disease was seen in any of the patients with other types of solid tumors. The number of cases is much too small, of course, to allow the conclusion that these neoplasms are generally not responsive.

Recently, an additional group of 24 children with acute lymphoblastic leukemia was treated with a combination of asparaginase and other agents. The protocol is shown in Fig. 3. Asparaginase and prednisone were given over a period of 4 weeks. Four injections of vincristine were given at the start and after 1, 2 and 3 weeks.

Table 9. *Adults, solid tumors. Incidence of response*

Tumor	Number of patients	Number of responses	Tumor	Number of patients	Number of responses
Lymphosarcoma	21	2	Cancer head and neck	6	0
Hodgkin's disease	8	0	Thyroid	2	0
Malignant melanoma	31	1	Lung	2	0
Choriocarcinoma	3	0	Large bowel	4	0
Osteogenic sarcoma	1	0	Breast	5	0
Ewing sarcoma	2	0	Ovary	1	0
Embr. Rhabdomyosa.	2	0	Cervix	1	0
Spindle cell sarcoma	2	0	Kidney	2	0
Leiomyosarcoma	2	0	Liver	3	0
Microglioma	1	0	Prostate	1	0
Neuroblastoma	2	0	Testis	3	0

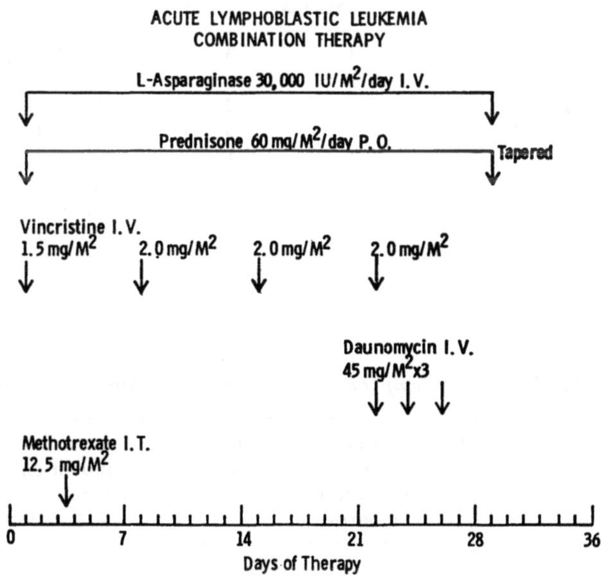

Fig. 3. Acute lymphoblastic leukemia: combination therapy

Daunomycin was given 3 times on alternating days during the third week. At some time during the first week methotrexate was given intrathecally. This regimen produced severe toxicity (bone marrow depression and neuropathy) in many patients. Therefore, the last three patients received only 2 injections of 1.0 and 1.5 mg/M^2 of vincristine, 3 injections of 30 mg/M^2 of daunomycin and 6.0 mg/M^2 of methotrexate.

Untreated cases of acute lymphoblastic leukemia were seen infrequently. Therefore, children with a variety of "drug-backgrounds" were treated according to the combination protocol and many of them had received one or more of the drugs of the combination previously. The patients are listed in Table 10, grouped according to their previous drug therapy. There are only four untreated cases in this group of 24 patients. The number of cases in each group is quite small and half of the patients have not yet relapsed. One can certainly not say what the data seem to imply, namely, that neither the incidence nor the duration of the remissions appears to decrease as the number of the drugs of the combination that were used previously increases. Without doubt, the incidence of remissions was higher—18 of 21 cases—in the group receiving combination therapy than in the group that was treated with 1000 IU/kg/day of asparaginase alone—12 of 22 cases (Table 11). This one would expect. It is also not unexpected that the induction time was generally longer in the group receiving combination therapy, if one considers the myelosuppressive effect of methotrexate, vincristine and daunomycin. Only 5 of 18 patients achieved a complete remission in less than one month, which was the rule for the patients receiving asparaginase alone. The median duration of the remissions in this heterogeneous group was not longer than in the group treated with asparaginase alone.

Table 10. *Children, acute lymphoblastic leukemia. Combination chemotherapy*

Previous therapy	Number of patients	Number of remissions	Duration (days)
None	4	3	33, 29+, 20+
Pred	3	3	110+, 78+, 59
Pred, MTX	2	2	92, 85+
Pred, VCR, MTX	5	3	172+, 103, 56
Asp	1	1	132+
Pred, Asp	1	1	104
Pred, Asp, VCR, MTX	2	2	97, 60
Pred, Asp, MTX, Dau	2	2	139+, 71+
Pred, Asp, VCR, MTX, Dau	1	1	125

Asp = L-asparaginase

Table 11. *Children, acute lymphoblastic leukemia. Combination chemotherapy*

Asparaginase 1000 IU/kg/day ×28	Number of patients	Median duration of disease (months)	Number of remissions	Remission induction time < 1 month	Median duration of remissions (days)
Alone	22	7	12	12	121
Combination	21	8	18	5	104 or less

For patients with acute myeloblastic leukemia, a protocol combining L-asparaginase, arabinosyl cytosine, thioguanine, vincristine and methotrexate was adopted. The results cannot yet be evaluated. It has become clear, however, that the doses of arabinosyl cytosine, thioguanine, vincristine and methotrexate that can be tolerated are smaller when L-asparaginase is given at the same time.

Toxic Effects

L-asparaginase therapy produced a number of side effects which are listed in Tables 12 and 13. An immediate febrile response, nausea and vomiting were expected endotoxin effects and were observed in about 50 per cent of the patients. More than half the patients showed a loss of weight, the mean loss being 10 per cent of the pre-treatment weight after 4 weeks of therapy. The degree of the weight loss at the different dose levels is shown in Table 13. Generalized edema associated with hypoproteinemia was observed in less than 10 per cent of the cases. One third of the patients developed signs of depressed cerebral function such as somnolence, lethargy or even confusion, sometimes associated with an abnormal electronencephalogram. These were most severe at a dose of 5000 IU/kg/day. Allergic reactions, most often urticaria, were observed in one third of the patients. No fatal anaphylactic reaction

Table 12. *Side effects of L-asparaginase therapy*

Side effect	Children		Adults	
	Number of cases evaluated	Per cent abnormal	Number of cases evaluated	Per cent abnormal
Fever				
Anorexia, nausea, vomiting	147	49	156	59
Weight loss	108	61	113	76
CNS-depression	147	33	156	46
Edema	137	7	130	5
Hypersensitivity	120	35	127	33

Table 13. *Weight loss during L-asparaginase therapy*

	Dose IU/kg/day	Body weight (per cent of pre-treatment weight) Weeks of therapy			
		1	2	3	4
Children	10	97.7	97.3	98.8	98.3
	200	96.4	95.5	93.8	93.1
	1000	96.5	94.9	94.3	93.5
	5000	96.5	95.5	96.4	90.8
Adults	10	96.2	95.7	94.5	92.8
	200	97.1	95.9	96.0	95.4
	1000	97.5	97.4	96.6	94.6
	5000	94.0	94.3	93.8	91.3

was seen. Antibodies to the enzyme preparation were demonstrated in the serum of most patients. A serum sickness syndrome was observed in 3 cases.

Biochemical determinations revealed abnormalities in serum lipids, serum proteins, serum calcium, liver function tests and blood urea nitrogen (Table 14). A few examples may suffice. The changes in serum cholesterol are shown in Table 15. The patients are grouped according to the dose administered. The largest decrease of serum cholesterol occurred during the first week of therapy, and the nadir was reached after two weeks. The degree of hypocholesterolemia was not dose-dependent. The changes in the serum levels of phospholipids, triglycerides and total lipids closely paralleled the pattern of the cholesterol levels.

Table 14. *Biochemical abnormalities during L-asparaginase therapy*

	Children		Adults	
	Number of cases evaluated	Per cent abnormal	Number of cases evaluated	Per cent abnormal
Decrease of serum cholesterol	97	85	124	82
Decrease of serum albumin	82	71	62	82
Decrease of serum fibrinogen	—	—	33	97
Decrease of serum calcium	57	37	99	60
Increase of serum alkaline phosphatase	114	31	126	47
Increase of serum GOT	121	46	123	63
Increase of serum bilirubin	85	29	105	51
Increase of serum 5′-nucleotidase	55	15	108	26
Increase of BSP-retention	99	57	25	84
Increase of blood urea nitrogen	137	34	146	88

Table 15. *Hypocholesterolemia during L-asparaginase therapy*

Dose IU/kg/day	Serum cholesterol levels (mg/100 ml, mean) Weeks of therapy				
	0	1	2	3	4
10	161.4	105.6	88.8	105.2	109.7
200	183.0	96.7	88.2	103.7	114.7
1000	172.5	118.5	86.1	100.1	106.0
5000	158.9	88.1	89.3	90.0	100.0

After the initial episode of hypolipidemia, two adult patients developed a remarkable degree of hyperlipidemia, their serum having the appearance of cream. The total lipid level of one of the patients reached a peak of 7000 mg/100 ml serum. When a low fat diet was started while the patient was still on asparaginase therapy, the lipid levels had already begun to decline and continued to do so. Shortly afterwards the patient was in relapse, asparaginase was discontinued and treatment with another agent was started. The biochemical pattern was that of the mixed (exogenous and endogenous) hyperlipidemia or type V hyperlipoproteinemia. It is not clear in which way L-asparaginase was related to this episode.

Eighty per cent of the patients developed hypoalbuminemia without proteinuria. Table 16 shows the pattern of serum protein levels as it was followed by means of paper electrophoresis. Albumin, α_2-and β-globulin levels decreased to the end of the second week of therapy and did not change during the third and fourth week. The gamma globulin levels increased continuously throughout the period of therapy. These changes were further investigated by assaying sera for individual proteins by means of the quantitative radial immunodiffusion technique. The concentration of IgM, IgA and IgG increased. Least affected were α-acid glycoprotein, α_2-macroglobulin and α-antichymotrypsin. The levels of α-antitrypsin, ceruloplasmin, haptoglobin, transferrin, β_2-glycoprotein I, β_{1a}-globulin (C'3), β-lipoprotein, α_2-antithrombin, β_2-glycoprotein II, β_2-glycoprotein III, hemopexin, α_1-lipoprotein and anti-Gc-globulin decreased.

Table 16. *Serum proteins during L-asparaginase therapy (Paperelectrophoresis)*

Weeks of therapy	Serum levels of protein fractions (per cent of pre-treatment levels) Albumin	α_1-Glob.	α_2-Glob.	β-Glob.	γ-Glob.
0	100.0	100.0	100.0	100.0	100.0
1	85.1	96.5	77.8	78.5	130.8
2	77.8	94.4	67.8	72.3	145.6
3	75.8	93.2	67.2	76.1	162.9
4	75.6	97.1	67.8	75.9	173.1

A decrease in plasma fibrinogen levels was noted in most patients, with some values of 50 mg/100 ml or less. In order to determine whether this was due to increased consumption or decreased production, the survival of autologous ^{131}I-fibrinogen was studied in patients with solid tumors. Asparaginase therapy was started several days after the labelled autologous fibrinogen had been administered. Although the total plasma fibrinogen level fell during therapy, the rate of decrease of the labelled fibrinogen was not altered by L-asparaginase therapy. This indicates that, at least in this type of patient, the decrease of plasma fibrinogen levels was due to decreased synthesis rather than increased consumption. Factor V, VIII, euglobulin lysis time, thrombin time, prothrombin time and partial thromboplastin time showed no changes in these patients [1].

When the serum calcium levels were plotted against the total serum protein concentration according to the nomogram described by McLean and Hastings [9], half of the seemingly subnormal levels fell within the normal range. The other half was just below the lower limit of normal. If one considers that the hypoproteinemia was mostly due to a decreased concentration of serum albumin (the immunoglobulin levels actually increased) and that the nomogram is not corrected for this particular constellation, the low calcium levels can probably be explained on the basis of the serum protein changes alone. (Most of the protein-bound calcium is bound by the albumin fraction.) Serum phosphorus was not elevated.

In order to examine the possibility that the azotemia was caused by uric acid nephropathy due to the destruction of neoplastic tissue, the levels of blood urea nitrogen were recorded separately for the patients who responded to therapy and for those who did not respond (Table 17). It is evident that the blood urea nitrogen level rose in all groups within the first 24 hours of asparaginase administration, whether or not there was a response to therapy. In most patients, beginning with the second day of treatment, the blood urea nitrogen levels gradually declined although therapy was continued. A return to pretreatment levels was seen by the end of the second or third week of therapy. In some adult patients (both responders and non-responders), however, blood urea nitrogen levels remained abnormally high between 20 and 40 mg/100 ml serum.

Table 17. *Blood urea nitrogen during L-asparaginase therapy*

Type of patient	Blood urea nitrogen (mg/100 ml, mean) Days of therapy									
	0	1	2	3	4	5	6	7	14	28
Children, responders	10.6	19.9	18.4	17.0	13.2	15.7	11.1	13.7	13.6	11.0
Children, non-responders	10.5	16.6	14.5	15.1	14.6	13.9	12.4	13.2	11.4	10.5
Adults, responders	14.8	30.4	30.1	23.6	22.6	21.5	20.6	22.2	19.7	18.9
Adults, non-responders	13.4	24.3	27.1	23.3	23.0	24.8	23.6	21.3	19.9	17.6

Transient proteinuria of a slight degree, usually lasting only a few days, was observed in 12 of 147 trials in children (8 per cent) and in 19 of 156 trials in adults (12 per cent). Of 68 adult patients, 13 (19 per cent) had abnormally high plasma glucose levels on occasion. One patient developed clinical diabetes without ketonuria. Transient glucosuria, usually limited to one day, was seen in 5 of 147 trials in children (3 per cent) and in 5 of 156 trials in adults (3 per cent). Ketonuria was not observed.

L-asparaginase therapy had remarkably little effect on normal hematopoietic cells. In a number of patients with acute leukemia approaching complete remission a delayed return to normal of the hemoglobin levels was observed, although a high proportion of erythroid percursor cells was seen in the bone marrow and an increased number of reticulocytes in the peripheral blood. A decreased white blood cell count was observed in 5 of 27 children (19 per cent) and in 24 of 89 adults (27 per cent) with solid tumors. The incidence of leukopenia was not dose-dependent. Counts below 2000 per mm^3 were seen only occasionally. The nadir was reached after 2 weeks of therapy and was followed, in most cases, by a slow increase while treatment was continued. Both granulocytes and lymphocytes were affected. A decreased platelet count was found in 2 of the 27 children (7 per cent) and in 12 of the 89 adults (13 per cent) of this group. The incidence of thrombocytopenia was not dose-dependent. Platelet counts below 50,000 per mm^3 were quite exceptional. The nadir was reached after $2^1/_2$ weeks of therapy, and from then on the platelet count rose in most patients although therapy with L-asparaginase was continued.

At autopsy, fatty metamorphosis of the liver was recorded in 40 of 55 cases (73 per cent). A slight degree of fatty metamorphosis of the liver is not an infrequent finding in any autopsy series. Two factors, however, suggest strongly that fatty metamorphosis in these cases was related to the administration of L-asparaginase. First, the incidence was highest (33 of 37 cases) in the group that had received the enzyme preparation for at least one week, and where death had occurred within less than two weeks after treatment had been discontinued. None of 7 patients who had been treated for less than one week, and only 6 of 10 patients who died more than one month after treatment had been discontinued showed some degree of fatty metamorphosis. Second, severe fatty metamorphosis, sometimes with necrosis of hepatocytes, was only seen in 21 of the 33 cases of the first group but not in the other groups. At the dose of 10, 200 or 1000 IU/kg/day the incidence and severity of fatty metamorphosis were the same. (The number of cases treated with 5000 IU/kg/day was too small to assess the incidence in this group.) Focal necrosis and inflammation of the pancreas was also noted only in the group of patients (6 of 37 cases) who had been treated for at least one week and who died less than two weeks after treatment had been discontinued. Again, no dose-dependence was found.

The clinical significance of asparaginase toxicity can best be assessed by asking how often the sum of the various side effects caused sufficient concern so that treatment was either discontinued or continued at a lower dose. This was considered necessary in 7 children and 30 adult patients. In the children, hypersensitivity to the enzyme preparation was the reason to discontinue therapy in 6 cases. In the seventh case, the dose was reduced from 5000 IU/kg/day to 1000 IU/kg/day because of fever and lethargy. In the adults, the reasons for discontinuing therapy or reducing the dose were as follows: Nausea and vomiting in 7 cases, impaired hepatic function in 10 cases, hypofibrinogenemia in 4 cases, hemorrhage in 2 cases, lethargy or confusion in 12 cases, edema in 1 case and hypersensitivity in 5 cases. (In some patients more than one of these manifestations of toxicity was observed.) It is to be noted that, excepting the 3 patients with severe hypersensitivity reactions, not one of the adult patients received less than 1000 IU/kg/day. The dose of 5000 IU/kg/day could be maintained only rarely over a period of four weeks in adult patients.

To summarize, asparaginase therapy was certainly not without side effects. However, the type of toxicity differed from that observed with many other agents in several respects. First, the bone marrow was not the most affected organ, and the toxicity seemed to be centered in other organ systems. Second, the biochemical abnormalities were usually not progressive throughout the period of therapy but tended to maintain a plateau after the second week of treatment or even to become somewhat less pronounced. This could indicate that adaptive mechanisms come into play, such as for instance a compensatory increase of asparagine synthetase levels in normal cells. The sum of the side effects seen at a dose of 5000 Units/kg/day represents a clear hazard for many adults. That children fared somewhat better at this dose may again indicate the importance of adaptive mechanisms.

Conclusions

What, then, are our conclusions as to the present and possible future value of asparaginase in the treatment of human cancer? At present, it is often useful as a temporarily effective agent in patients with acute lymphoblastic leukemia, less commonly in patients with acute myeloblastic leukemia and more rarely still in patients with other types of cancer. As for the future, the initial hope that higher doses might be more effective has to be abandoned because the highest doses that have been used did not give better results and produced a level of toxicity which clearly prohibits the administration of yet higher doses. Efforts are now underway to determine whether the combination of asparaginase with other agents will give better results. In these studies it has been noted that patients receiving L-asparaginase are more susceptible to the toxic effects of vincristine, and perhaps also to those of arabinosyl cytosine, thioguanine and daunomycin as well. Two possible explanations come to mind: First, the catabolism of cytotoxic agents might be depressed in a liver that is affected by L-asparaginase. If this were so, effective blood and tissue levels could be maintained with lower doses of these agents. Second, the metabolic demands made on normal tissues by an asparagine deficiency might make them more susceptible to the toxic effects of cytotoxic agents. In this case, the therapeutic index of these agents would be reduced and the patients might actually be deprived of some of their therapeutic activity. Whatever mechanism is involved, a course of L-asparaginase after therapy with other agents appears more attractive than simultaneous combination therapy. In the small number of responsive patients with severe hypersensitivity reactions the usefulness of asparaginase therapy might be extended if preparations with different antigenic properties were available. Some hope may be held—in terms of increasing the spectrum of responsive tumors and for obtaining more prolonged remissions—for attempts to modify the enzyme molecule so that its distribution throughout all intercellular compartments becomes more favorable. This could be of importance particularly if one considers that, in the body tissues, one type of cells could provide a microenvironment containing asparagine for another asparagine-dependent cell type. It is doubtful that the theoretically crucial condition, namely isolation of each and every neoplastic cell in the body from an extra-cellular source of asparagine within a period short enough to preclude adaptation has ever been achieved. In view of our ignorance as to whether acquired resistance is selective or adaptive, we must recognize that the potential value of asparagine deprivation may not really have been tested and possibly cannot be tested adequately with present L-asparaginase therapy.

References

1. Bettigole, R. E., Himelstein, E. S., Oettgen, H. F., Clifford, G. O.: Hypofibrinogenemia due to L-asparaginase: Studies using ^{131}I-fibrinogen. Clin. Res. **17**, 399 (1969). (Abstr.)
2. Canellos, G. P., Haskell, C. M., Arseneau, J., Carbone, P. P.: Hypoalbuminemic and hypocholesterolemic effect of L-asparaginase (NSC-109, 229) treatment in man—a preliminary report. Cancer Chemother. Rep. **53**, 67—69 (1969).
3. Capizzi, R. L., Peterson, R., Cooney, D. A., Creasey, W. A., Handschumacher, R. E.: L-asparaginase therapy of acute leukemia: Biochemical and clinical observations. Proc. Amer. Ass. Cancer Res. 10, 12 (1969). (Abstr.)
4. Clarkson, B. D., Krakoff, I. H., Burchenal, J. H., Karnofsky, D. A., Golbey, R. B., Dowling, M. D., Oettgen, H. F., Lipton, A.: Clinical results of treatment with E. coli L-asparaginase in adults with leukemia, lymphosarcoma and solid tumors. Cancer (in press).
5. Gralnick, H. R., Henry, P. H.: L-asparaginase induced coagulopathy. Proc. Amer. Ass. Cancer Res. 10, 32 (1969). (Abstr.)
6. Haskell, C. M., Canellos, G. P., Leventhal, B. G., Carbone, P. P., Serpick, A. A., Hansen, H. H.: L-asparaginase toxicity. Cancer Res. **29**, 974—975 (1969).
7. Hill, J. M., Roberts, J., Loeb, E., Khan, A., MacLellan, A., Hill, R. W.: L-asparaginase therapy for leukemia and other malignant neoplasms. J. Amer. med. Ass. **202**, 882—888 (1967).

8. Lash, E., Schwartz, M. K., Tallal, L., Oettgen, H. F.: Serum lipids in patients receiving L-asparaginase. XII Congress, International Society of Hematology, New York 1968. (Abstr.)
9. McLean, F. C., Hastings, A. B.: Clinical estimation and significance of calcium-ion concentration in the blood. Am. J. med. Sci. 189, 601—619 (1935).
10. Oettgen, H. F., Old, L. J., Boyse, E. A., Campbell, H. A., Philips, F. S., Clarkson, B. D., Tallal, L., Leeper, R. D., Schwartz, M. K., Kim, J. H.: Inhibition of leukemia in man by L-asparaginase. Cancer Res. 27, 2619—2631 (1967).
11. — — — Schwartz, H. K.: Therapeutic effects of L-asparaginase on asparagine-dependent neoplasms; laboratory and clinical studies. J. clin. Invest. 47, 74 a (1968).
12. — Schulten, H. K.: Hemmung maligner Neoplasien des Menschen durch L-asparaginase. Klin. Wschr. 47, 65—71 (1969).
13. — Stephenson, P. A., Schwartz, M. K., Leeper, R. D., Tallal, L., Tan, C. C., Clarkson, B. D., Golbey, R. B., Krakoff, I. H., Karnofsky, D. A., Murphy, M. L., Burchenal, J. H.: The toxicity of E. coli L-asparaginase in man. Cancer (in press).
14. Schmidt, C. G., Gallmeier, W.: Zur Enzymtherapie der Leukämien. Dtsch. med. Wschr. 48, 2299—2309 (1968).
15. Tallal, L., Tan, C., Oettgen, H. F., Wollner, N., McCarthy, M., Helson, L., Burchenal, J., Karnofsky, D., Murphy, M. L.: E. coli L-asparaginase in the treatment of leukemia and solid tumors in 131 children. Cancer (in press).
16. Tan, C., Oettgen, H. F.: Clinical experience with L-asparaginase administered intrathecally. Proc. Amer. Ass. Cancer Res. 10, 92 (1969). (Abstr.)
17. Whitecar, J. P., Jr., Harris, J. E., Bodey, G. P., Freireich, E. J.: Host effects of L-asparaginase treatment. Clin. Res. 17, 408 (1969).

Appendix

Criteria for Evaluating Chemotherapy in Acute Leukemia

(J. S. Hewlett, J. D. Bettle, Jr., R. C. Bishop, W. M. Fowler, S. O. Schwartz, P. S. Hagen, J. Louis: Cancer Chemother. Rep. 42, 27, 1964)

I. Criteria for Rating Categories

Qualitative or quantitative changes which appear to be the operation of normal homeostatic mechanism, or physiologic responses of the patients to non-leukemic stimuli rather than a part of the disease, should not be considered abnormalities (eg. secondary to medication or the normoblastic hyperplasia seen in early phases of remission, etc.).

1.1. Bone Marrow (Category M)

1.1.1. Ratings for Parameters

Type leukemia PARAMETER Parameter rating	All Blast cells [b]	Lymphocytic [a] Lymphocytes+ blast cells [b]	Granulocytic+other types Leukemic+blast cells [b]
1	0—5	0—40	0—5
2	6—25	41—69	6—39
3	25	69	39

[a] Include childhood undifferentiated leukemia with the lymphocytic group. Percentage values given for Parameter Rating represent percentage of all marrow elements.

[b] This term includes blast cells as well as all cells which cannot be classified as either blast cells or more mature *normal* elements, and includes "leukemic cells", "pathologic lymphocytes", and "stem cells".

1.1.2. Ratings for Category M

Rating of this category will be determined by the most abnormal parameter found. Bone marrows qualifiying for M1 ratings must contain qualitative and quantitative normal erythropoiesis, granulopoiesis, and megakaryopoiesis.

1.2. Hemogram (Category H)

1.2.1. Ratings for Parameters

Rating	Hemoglobin Child <2	>2	Adults M	F	Neutrophilic granulocytes	Blasts [a]	Platelets
1	10	11	12	10	1500	0	100,000 (phase) or normal
2					500 to 1499	< 5%	< 100,000 or decreased
3	<7				< 500	> 5%	< 25,000 or 25% of normal

[a] This term includes blast cells as well as cells which cannot be classified as either blast cells or more mature normal elements, and includes "leukemic cells", "pathologic lymphocytes", and "stem cells".

1.2.2. Ratings for Category H

The rating for category H is determined by the sum of the ratings for all of the parameters (hemoglobin, neutrophilic granulocytes, blast [a] cells, and platelets. Ratings indicating improvement in this category must not be ascribable to transfusion of any blood elements. Mononuclear cells must not exceed 7000 cells/cu. mm. (10,000 for <2 years) for an H1 rating. The appearance of 1—2% blast cells on an isolated count will not preclude an H1 rating.

Rating		Sum of parameter ratings
1	=	4
2	=	8
3	=	> 8

1.3. Category P—Physical Findings

1.3.1. Ratings for Each Parameter

Each physical finding constitutes a measurable parameter. The degree of abnormality for each parameter will be rated as follows:

a. *Liver*

1 = within normal limits for age
2 = definite enlargement (to umbilicus)
3 = enlargement below umbilicus

b. *Spleen*

1 = within normal limits for age
2 = definite enlargement (to umbilicus)
3 = enlargement below umbilicus

c. *Lymph Nodes*

1 = within normal limits
2 = definite enlargement
3 = massive enlargement (grossly visible)

d. *Other Leukemic Organ Involvement*

(If present, note and score separately: skin, CNS, kidney, lungs, etc.)

1 = none
2 = definite
3 = marked

1.3.2. Ratings for Category P

The final rating for Category P is based on the sum of the numerical values given to each Parameter.

Category P rating		Sum of parameter rating
1	=	4
2	=	5—8
3	=	> 8

1.4. Category S—Symptoms

Rating for category S is determined by the performance activity of the patient ratings listed below:

1 = Asymptomatic and normal activity
2 = Symptomatic with normal or limited activity but less than 50% of normal waking hours in bed.
3 = Symptomatic with more than 50% of time in bed.

II. Criteria for Rating Disease Status

A. *No Evident Disease:*	A rating of one in all categories (M1, H1, P1, S1)
B. *Moderate Disease:*	A rating of 2 in one or more categories, but no rating of 3 in any category.
C. *Extensive Disease:*	A rating of 3 in one or two categories.
D. *Extreme Disease:*	A rating of 3 in more than two categories.

III. Terms for Describing the Response to Therapy

A. *Complete Remission* (CR):	Improvement to disease status A.
B. *Good Partial Remission* (GR):	Improvement to disease status B.
C. *Poor Partial Remission* (PR):	Improvement to disease status C.
D. *No Remission* (NR):	No change in any status.
E. *Progressive Disease* (PD):	Deterioration from initial disease status, or if initially in status D, documented deterioration in any category.

Clinical Experience with L-Asparaginase

P. P. CARBONE [1], C. M. HASKELL [1], BRIGID G. LEVENTHAL [1], J. B. BLOCK [2], and O. S. SELAWRY [1]

The administration of L-asparaginase has resulted in reports of beneficial effects in patients with acute leukemia [1—5]. The initial clinical and laboratory studies indicated that L-asparaginase selectively inhibits cancer cells dependent on the non-essential amino acid L-asparagine and offered the promise that L-asparaginase would not be harmful to normal cells. However, later clinical reports dispelled hope for a broad spectrum antitumor effect and also revealed unexpected forms of toxicity [1—7]. Evaluation of the several clinical studies indicates that while the antitumor responses are unique and reproduceable in acute lymphocytic leukemia of children, toxicities are often not consistent in one report compared to another. These differences might be attributable to problems in preparing large quantities of a bacterial protein, and the inclusion of contaminants like endotoxin. In addition it is now possible to obtain L-asparaginase from other species [8] as well as in crystalline form [9] although no major studies have been reported with these preparations. Thus one can only evaluate the relative merits and toxicities of specific preparations, because no comparative clinical trials of the various materials are available.

This report from the Chemotherapy Area of the National Cancer Institute summarizes our experience with *E. coli* L-asparaginase in a variety of malignancies [6] including Burkitt's tumor [10]. It also includes results from a preliminary study of the combined use of L-asparaginase and azaserine, a glutamine antagonist in acute lymphocytic leukemia of childhood [11].

Materials and Methods

E. coli L-asparaginase was obtained as a dry powder from Merck Sharp and Dohme (specific activity of 321—363 IU/mg protein) or from Squibb (specific activity 121—231 IU/mg protein). The dry preparation was stable at 5° C for several months and at 25° C in normal saline for several days. The dosage and days on treatment are shown in Table 1. The drug was administered intravenously as a single dose by infusion over 20 to 40 min. Azaserine (NSC-742) was obtained from the Cancer Chemotherapy National Service Center and given in schedules shown in Table 2.

[1] Medicine Branch, National Cancer Institute, National Institutes of Health, Bethesda, Maryland 20014, U.S.A.

[2] Baltimore Cancer Research Center, National Cancer Institute, National Institutes of Health, Baltimore, Maryland 21205, U.S.A.

Two clinical trials were conducted. The first involves 24 patients with a variety of disseminated solid tumors, 20 patients with adult chronic and acute leukemia, and 11 children with acute lymphocytic leukemia (ALL) treated with asparaginase alone, evaluated primarily for toxicity but also for antitumor response (Table 3). In addition 16 children with ALL received asparaginase and azaserine and were compared to the 11 children with ALL treated with asparaginase alone. All children had received prior therapy and were in relapse with 40—60% abnormal cells in the marrow. The starting dose of azaserine was 60 mg/m² on regimen 2 and 90 mg/m² on the high dosage schedule (regimen 3). These patients were randomly allocated to 1 and 2 and then 1 and 3. The groups were comparable in age, prior therapy and initial status.

Table 1. *Patients treated with L-asparaginase alone*

Maximum dose (IU/kg)	Number of patients	Days of maximum dose treatment Median	Range
50—100/day	6	8	3—20
200/day	36	24	3—120
400—1000/day	6	15	3—23
> 1000/day	4	6	4—15
1000 twice weekly	1	13	—
1500/week	2	—	12, 12

Table 2. *28 day drug regimens*

Regimen 1	Asparaginase 6000 IU/m² I.V. 3 days of 4
Regimen 2	Asparaginase 6000 IU/m² I.V. 3 days of 4 Azaserine p. o. in 6 divided doses 60 mg/m² day 4, 8 75 mg/m² day 12, 16 90 mg/m² day 20, 24
Regimen 3	Asparaginase 6000 IU/m² I.V. 3 days of 4 Azaserine p. o. in 6 divided doses 90 mg/m² day 4, 8 120 mg/m² day 12, 16 150 mg/m² day 20, 24

Eight patients with advanced lymphosarcoma, 6 with Burkitt's tumor were treated at the NCI-Makerere University Lymphoma Treatment Center in Kampala, Uganda.

A complete response was defined as disappearance of measurable tumor masses and a partial remission as ≧ 25% decrease in the sum of the product of 2 diameters. In the patients with acute leukemia a complete remission was defined as < 5% abnormal cells in the marrow and return of peripheral blood picture to normal. A partial remission was defined as decrease in peripheral blood or bone marrow blasts by 25% or more. A complete response in patients with chronic leukemia was defined as a decrease in organs and abnormal cells in the peripheral blood to normal size or levels. All the patients were hospitalized and were observed clinically and with laboratory tests for toxicity.

Table 3. *Patients treated with L-asparaginase alone*

Disease	Number of patients	Partial response	Complete response
Melanoma	5	1	
Undifferentiated carcinoma	2		
Breast carcinoma	1		
Myeloma	1		
Bronchogenic carcinoma	1		
Teratocarcinoma	1		
Osteogenic sarcoma	1		
Hypernephroma	1		
Burkitt's tumor	1		
Hodgkin's disease	3		
Lymphosarcoma	7	3	1
Chronic granulocytic leukemia	2		1
Chronic granulocytic leukemia, blast crisis	3	1	
Chronic lymphocytic leukemia	1		
Acute granulocytic leukemia—acute myelomonocytic leukemia	6		1
Acute lymphocytic leukemia—adult	8	2	2
Acute lymphocytic leukemia—children (under 15 years)	11	1	3
Total	55	8	8

Results

The spectrum and details of the tumor response to L-asparaginase alone is shown in Table 3 and 4. For the American patients with solid tumors significant but incomplete response occurred in three of seven patients with lymphosarcoma. A complete remission lasting 27 weeks was achieved in one patient with malignant lymphoma. In the six patients with chronic leukemia, one patient with chronic granulocytic leukemia achieved a good response. A very dramatic response occurred in an adult patient with acute granulocytic leukemia that lasted for nine weeks. Five of 19 patients with ALL achieved a complete remission with a median duration of nine weeks despite maintenance with 6-mercaptopurine or methotrexate (Table 4).

Of the eight patients treated with L-asparaginase in Uganda, all had been refractory to prior chemotherapy. They received doses and schedules as shown in Table 5. No responses were seen in the six Burkitt's or the two non-Burkitt's patients.

For the comparative study of L-asparaginase with or without azaserine, the response to therapy, time to remission and duration of complete remission is shown in Table 6. There was no obvious difference in the response rate of duration of remissions between the three regimens.

The bone marrow toxicity in those children with ALL who achieved a complete remission for this study is shown in Table 7. No patient treated with asparaginase alone (regimen 1) developed granulocytopenia or thrombocytopenia on therapy. Two patients on azaserine and asparaginase had a significant fall in granulocytes

Table 4. *Patients treated with L-asparaginase alone*

Diagnosis	Age	Sex	Response	Dose (IU/kg/day)	Duration treated (days)	Duration response (weeks)	Prior therapy for Cancer X-ray	Chemotherapy
Melanoma	41	F	25%	200 [a]	68	2	yes	yes
Lymphosarcoma	71	M	complete	200 [a]	31	1	no	no
Lymphosarcoma	49	M	25%	200 [a, b]	47	2	yes	yes
Reticulum cell sarcoma	53	F	75%	200 [a]	28	27	no	yes
Lymphoma and CLL	54	M	25—50%	400 [b]	6	2	yes	yes
CGL	26	M	complete	200 [b]	3	2	no	no
CGL, blast crisis	18	M	PB Imp.	100 [a]	10	1	no	yes
AGL	51	M	complete	1500 [b]	15	9	no	yes
ALL	24	M	complete	200 [a]	120 [e]	9 [e]	no	yes
ALL	21	M	complete	200 [a]	28	23 [c]	no	yes
ALL	47	M	PB Imp.	200 [a]	25	2	no	yes
ALL (?)	18	M	PB Imp.	200 [a]	35	2	no	yes
ALL	9	M	complete	200 [a]	35	7 [d]	no	yes
ALL	12	F	complete	200 [a] 50 [a]	34	27 [c]	no	yes
ALL	7	M	complete	50 [a]	25	5 [c]	no	yes
ALL	8	M	PB Imp.	200 [a]	30	5	no	yes

BP Imp. = Improvement in peripheral blood blast counts.
[a] = L-asparaginase obtained from Squibb and Company.
[b] = L-asparaginase obtained from Merck, Sharp and Dohme.
[c] = Patient maintained on methotrexate 25 mg/m² i. m. twice weekly.
[d] = Patient maintained on 6-Mercaptopurine 30 mg/m²/day orally.
[e] = Part of 4 month treatment course included intermittent use of L-asparaginase as maintenance therapy.

Table 5. *NCI-Uganda results with asparaginase*

No patients	Dosages	
4	1500 IU/kg weekly×2	
3	200 IU/kg daily×6	No responses
1	500 IU/kg daily×7	

Table 6. *Response to combinations of agents*

	No. Pts.	No. Imp.	No. CR	Days to CR	Days duration of CR	Maintenance ASP	MTX	6-MP	AZA
Regimen 1	11	2	5	22 (15—58)	33, 53, 64*, 162, 192 (15—58)	1	3	1	
Regimen 2	7	1	2	34 (28—41)	28, 33		2		
Regimen 3	9	1	7	18 (11—37)	17, 33, 50, 58*, 74+, 88, 133+		3	2	2

Imp. = Improved
CR = Complete remission
* = Median remission

ASP = Asparaginase 1500 IU/m² t. i. w. IV
MTX = Methotrexate 25 mg/m² b. i. w. IM
6-MP = 6-Mercaptopurine 25 mg/m² daily p. o.
AZA = Azaserine 150 mg/m² q 4 days p. o

Table 7. *Hematologic toxicity in patients treated with combinations of agents*

	Number of complete remissions	During therapy Granulocytes < 1000/cu. mm.	Thrombo-cytopenia	At M_1 Granulocytes < 1000	< 500	Platelets < 150,000
Regimen 1	5	0	0	1	1	1
Regimen 2	2	1	1	0	1	0
Regimen 3	7	1	1	2	0	2
Total	14	2	2	3	2	3

(< 1000/mm³) and one in thrombocytes (< 100,000/mm³) while on therapy for induction.

Five patients had persistent granulocytopenia and three had thrombocytopenia at the time a marrow remission was achieved. The addition of azaserine does appear to result in more bone marrow toxicity than expected from L-asparaginase alone.

Toxic Reactions

All patient charts were reviewed for toxic reactions and evaluations are reported for those patients in whom toxicity could be clearly related to L-asparaginase treatment. The major forms of drug related side effects were gastrointestinal symptoms, hypersensitivity reactions and liver dysfunction, occurring in over two-thirds of the patients, and severely limiting drug administration in about 10% of the patients. The hypersensitivity reactions all occurred days to weeks after start of therapy, and were most often urticaria with or without respiratory symptoms. Two patients developed anaphylactic shock, one a serum sickness-like reaction and one hypotension.

Limiting bone marrow toxicity was not seen, although a slight decrease in median values for WBC and platelets were noted after as compared to before therapy. A fall in hemoglobin by 2 g/100 ml was recorded in five of eight evaluable patients. Clotting abnormalities were recorded as a decrease in fibrinogen or changes in prothrombin and partial thromboplastin times. Significant clinical bleeding could not be attributed to L-asparaginase therapy in any of the patients.

Liver function abnormalities occurred in 33 of 35 evaluable patients. Disturbances in liver chemistry tests related to L-asparaginase occurred in bilirubin, alkaline phosphatase, and SGOT. Depression of serum albumin and cholesterol occurred. Liver biopsies in two patients indicated toxic hepatitis with fatty metamorphosis.

Azotemia (BUN $>$ 20 mg-%) occurred primarily as a pre-renal phenomenon in most patients, however, two patients developed severe primary renal failure and oliguria associated with intravascular coagulation in one case, and associated with hyperglycemia and renal tubular necrosis in the other.

Table 8. *Summary of L-asparaginase toxicity*

Problem	Patients evaluable	Patients with problem	Patients with serious problem
Nausea, anorexia, vomiting	50	33	6
Fever	44	30	5
Hypersensitivity	55	14	9
Anemia	8	5	0
Clotting abnormalities	20	16	1
Liver dysfunction	35	33	4
Azotemia	35	17	2
Pancreatitis	54	6	3
Central nervous system-adults only	35	18	5

An unexpected toxicity was pancreatitis occurring in six patients, three of whom had severe clinical signs and symptoms requiring drug cessation. This complication occurred at 200 IU/kg as well as higher doses and occurred in as few as three days. Four patients died within three weeks of L-asparaginase therapy and were found to have pancreatitis at necropsy. One patient had hyperglycemia without ketosis.

Another unexpected major toxicity was central nervous system dysfunction with abnormalities in the EEG, personality changes, severe depression and confusion. In two patients an acute organic brain syndrome similar to acute alcoholic delirium tremors occurred and quickly abated after L-asparaginase was stopped. These central nervous system abnormalities, although seen at 200, 400 and 1500 IU/kg/day, were somewhat dose related in that the time of onset was sooner at the higher doses.

Discussion

The present study summarizes the experience at the National Cancer Institute with two different preparations of *E. coli* L-asparaginase. Similar antitumor responses have been reported by others [2—4 and 12—16]. A high rate of response to L-asparaginase has been uniquely restricted to acute lymphocytic leukemia of childhood, less often in patients with lymphosarcoma and acute myelocytic leukemia and rarely in solid tumors. The responses are described as short, and may be reinduced subsequently in some patients. Despite the rather limited spectrum of antineoplastic activity its usefulness in childhood lymphocytic leukemia remains an important new therapeutic avenue to be explored.

The use of L-asparaginase has been primarily on a daily schedule. The results from our own studies, as well as those of OHNUMA [17] suggest that plasma L-asparagine depression following a single dose of L-asparaginase may persist up to three weeks or longer. This suggests that an intermittent schedule of administration may be as effective as daily administration.

Another approach which may improve therapy is to combine L-asparaginase with other agents. This approach is encouraging for two reasons. First, the lack of significant bone marrow depression with L-asparaginase makes it a prime candidate for use in combination with a variety of myelosuppressive drugs. Secondly, the mechanism of action and mode of resistance to L-asparaginase in animals [18—21] and human leukemia [22] are fairly well understood, and the central role of glutamine in their process has suggested the use of glutamine antagonists as a relatively specific way of enhancing L-asparaginase therapy. This notion has led to animal studies with glutamine antagonists [23—25] and to our studies with azaserine in patients with ALL [11]. Despite the fact that our results were inconclusive with azaserine, we feel that this approach warrants further study.

The organ toxicity reported here indicates a wide spectrum of effects of L-asparaginase on normal tissues. These effects are probably related to L-asparagine depletion although they may be due to the endotoxin or glutaminase content of the *E. coli* preparations used in our studies. Some of the effects of asparaginase are undoubtedly related to the inhibition of protein synthesis in the liver, pancreas and brain. The exact reason for this inhibition is not known but is most likely due to asparagine depletion, although glutaminase or endotoxin effects may also play a role. Central nervous system effects of L-asparaginase is probably a result of a combination of factors, including inhibition of amino acid incorporation in the brain, release of ammonia as well as impairment of liver function.

Summary

Escherichia coli L-asparaginase has been administered to 79 patients with neoplastic diseases at the National Cancer Institute and in Uganda. Responses were seen most often in patients with acute lymphocytic leukemia and in four of seven patients with lymphosarcoma. The addition of azaserine, a glutamine antagonist, to L-asparaginase did not offer any therapeutic advantage.

Drug related toxicity was seen in most patients and was severely limiting in 10%. Major drug toxicity included hepatic insufficiency, hypersensitivity, pancreatitis and central nervous system disturbances. Bone marrow toxicity was not apparent. Studies of combination chemotherapy with L-asparaginase and interrupted schedules are indicated.

References

1. HILL, J. M., ROBERTS, J., LOEB, E., KHAN, A., MACLELLAN, A., HILL, R. W.: L-asparaginase therapy for leukemia and other malignant neoplasms. J. Amer. med. Ass. 202, 882—888 (1967).

2. Oettgen, H. F., Old, L. J., Boyse, E. A., Campbell, H. A., Philips, F. S., Clarkson, B. D., Tallal, L., Lepper, R. D., Schwartz, M. K., Kim, J. H.: Inhibition of leukemias in man by L-asparaginase. Cancer Res. **27**, 2619—2631 (1967).
3. — Schulten, H. K.: Hemmung maligner Neoplasien des Menschen durch L-asparaginase. Klin. Wschr. **47**, 65—71 (1969).
4. Mathé, G., Amiel, J. L., Schwarzenberg, L., Schneider, M., Cattan, A., Schlumberger, J. R., Hatat, M., De Vassal, F., Jasmin, C., Rosenfeld, C.: Essai de traitement de la leucemie aigue lymphoblastique par la L-asparaginase. Presse méd. **77**, 461—463 (1969).
5. Hill, J. M., Loeb, E., MacLellan, A., Khan, A., Roberts, J., Shields, W. F., Hill, N. O.: Response to highly purified L-asparaginase during therapy of acute leukemia. Cancer Res. **29**, 1574—1580 (1969).
6. Haskell, C. M., Canellos, G. P., Leventhal, B. G., Carbone, P. P., Block, J. B., Serpick, A. A., Selawry, O. S.: L-asparaginase: Therapeutic and toxic effects in patients with neoplastic disease. New Engl. J. Med. (in press).
7. — — — — Serpick, A. A., Hansen, H. H.: Letter to the editor: L-asparaginase toxicity. Cancer Res. **29**, 974—975 (1969).
8. Wade, H. E., Elsworth, R., Herbert, D., Keppie, S., Sargeant, K.: A new L-asparaginase with antitumor activity. Lancet **1968 II**, 776—777.
9. Ho, P. K., Poore, G. A.: Experimental antitumor activity of crystalline L-asparaginase from *E. coli*. Proc. Amer. Ass. Cancer Res. **10**, 39 (1969).
10. Canellos, G. P., Carbone, P. P., Ziegler, J. L.: L-asparaginase and Burkitt's lymphoma. Lancet **1969 II**, 380.
11. Leventhal, B. G., Skeel, R. T., Yankee, R. A., Henderson, E. S.: L-asparaginase and azaserine in acute lymphocytic leukemia. Cancer Chemother. Rep. **54**, 47—51 (1970).
12. Schmidt, C. G., Gallmeier, W. M.: Zur enzymtherapie der leukamien. Dtsch. med. Wschr. **93**, 2299—2309 (1968).
13. Tallal, L., Tan, C., Oettgen, H., McCarthy, M., Helson, L., Murphy, L.: L-asparaginase in 111 children with leukemias and solid tumors. Proc. Amer. Ass. Cancer Res. **10**, 92 (1969).
14. Lipton, A., Viola, M., Tauro, G., Gee, T., Krakoff, I., Clarkson, B.: Treatment of leukemias and lymphomas in adults with *E. coli* L-asparaginase. Program of the 5th Annual Meeting of the Amer. Soc. of Clinical Oncology, San Francisco (Abstract No 23), March 22, 1969.
15. James Holland: Personal communication.
16. Emil Frei, III: Personal communication.
17. Ohnuma, T., Holland, J. F., Freeman, A., Sinks, L.: Studies of asparaginase and asparagine in acute leukemia. Proc. Amer. Ass. Cancer Res. **10**, 66 (1969).
18. Patterson, M. K., Jr., Orr, G. R.: Asparagine biosynthesis by the nivokoff hepatoma. Isolation, purification, property and mechanism studies of the enzyme system. J. biol. Chem. **243**, 376—380 (1968).
19. Broome, J. D.: Studies on the mechanism of tumor inhibition by L-asparaginase. J. exp. Med. **127**, 1055—1072 (1968).
20. Horowitz, B., Madras, B. K., Meister, A., Old, L. J., Boyse, E. A., Stockert, E.: Asparagine synthetase activity of mouse leukemias. Science **160**, 533—535 (1968).
21. Prager, M. D., Backynsky, N.: Asparagine synthetase in normal and malignant tissues; correlation with tumor sensitivity to asparaginase. Arch. Biochem. **127**, 645—654 (1968).
22. Haskell, C. M., Canellos, G. P.: L-asparaginase resistance in human leukemia: Asparagine synthetase. Biochem. Pharmacol. (in press).
23. Mashburn, L. T.: The effect of combined therapy with L-asparaginase on P1798 lymphosarcoma. Proc. Amer. Ass. Cancer Res. **9**, 45 (1968).
24. Jacobs, S. P., Wodinsky, I., Kensler, C. J., Venditti, J.: Therapy of experimental leukemias with combination of L-asparaginase and glutamine antagonists. Proc. Amer. Ass. Cancer Res. **10**, 43 (1969).
25. Tarnowski, G. S., Mountain, I. M., Stock, C. C.: Combination therapy of animal tumors with L-asparaginase and glutamine antagonists. Proc. Amer. Ass. Cancer Res. **10**, 92 (1969).

Result of a Cooperative Study with L-Asparaginase in Human Leukemias

Report of the Section "Oncology" of the Paul-Ehrlich-Society for Chemotherapy

H. GERHARTZ and H. BEGEMANN

Hämat.-onkol. Abt. Med. Klinik Westend der Freien Universität Berlin u. Med. Klinik, Krankenhaus München-Schwabing, Germany

With 4 Figures

Through the Paul-Ehrlich-Society for Chemotherapy, clinical trials of L-asparaginase[1] were conducted in three different programs (Table 1): First, in an orientation trial, an attempt was made to treat all cases of acute leukemias at a constant dose of 200 IU/kg daily intravenously for a period of 4 weeks. The second trial was an

Table 1

Program 1	All acute leukemias		L-asparaginase alone for 2—4 weeks	200 U/kg daily
Program 2	Acute myeloblastic leucemia	a)	L-asparaginase alone for 2—4 weeks	3000 U/kg daily
		b)		2×1500 U/kg daily
Program 3	Acute lymphoblastic leucemia		Dauno-rubidomycine	1,5 mg/kg on 1., 7., 14., 21. day
		a)	+Vincristine	0,05 mg/kg on 1., 7., 14., 21. day
			+Prednisone	1,5 mg/kg daily
		b)	+L-asparaginase	200 U/kg daily

attempt to produce remissions in cases of acute myeloblastic leukemias with the high dose of 3000 IU/kg of L-asparaginase per day. In a third trial we asked whether, in acute lymphoblastic leukemia, the therapeutic effect of Dauno-Rubidomycine+Vincristine+Prednisolone could be improved by the addition of L-asparaginase. Trials 1 and 2 are now finished. This report is based essentially on the first trial in

[1] The drug used exclusively was FBb 6366, Bayer-Werke, Wuppertal-Elberfeld.

a group of 120 patients from 20 different hospitals (Table 2). All patients were treated only with L-asparaginase; ten patients had to be excluded because the first examination was incomplete. 64 patients suffered from lymphoblastic leukemia (ALL), 12 from promyelocytic leukemia (APL), 30 from myeloblastic leukemia (AML), 7 from monocytic leukemia (AMOL), 5 from myeloblastic crisis in chronic myelocytic leukemia (CMLM) and 2 from erythroleukemia (EL).

Table 2.

L-asparaginase	Cases	CR	PR	IMP	F	Not to judge
ALL	64	11	13	15	20	5
APL	12	2	1	3	5	1
AML	30	0	0	8	20	2
AMOL	7	0	0	1	6	0
CMLM	5	0	0	2	3	0
EL	2	0	0	0	0	2
Total	120	13	14	29	54	10
CLL	3	0	2	0	0	1
CML	1	0	1	0	0	0

Complete *remissions* (CR) were achieved in 13 and partial remissions (PR) in 14 patients; they occurred only in cases of lymphoblastic and promyelocytic leukemia, never in a case of myeloblastic leukemia. In addition, we obtained some symptomatic improvement (IMP) in nearly one quarter of all cases of acute leukemia. The effect of L-asparaginase alone in a few cases of chronic leukemia was small and of short duration.

On a percentage basis (Table 3): in 59 cases of lymphoblastic leukemia there were 19% complete remissions and 22% partial remissions, i. e. a total of 41% remissions; in (11) cases of promyelocytic leukemia there were 18% complete and 10% partial remissions. Complete failures (F) occurred in 34% of the cases of lymphoblastic leukemia, in 45% of the cases of promyelocytic leukemia and in 73% of the cases of all other forms of acute leukemia; on the whole there were 49% failures.

When remissions were obtained, the duration of treatment was about 4 weeks on the average, but in cases with little improvement the treatment lasted only 19 days and in failures only 13 days (Table 4). The mean *dose* was 6—7000 IU/day or 185,000 IU/course. Some patients who failed to respond received a higher dose; on the average the dose was nearly twice as high in these cases.

The highest dose, 3000 IU/kg/day, given either in one or in two daily infusions did not produce better results (Table 5). In 34 patients (22 acute myeloblastic leukemias) a partial remission was seen only in one case each of acute myeloblastic and acute promyelocytic leukemia. Less than 50% of the patients were able to tolerate this dose for longer than 2 weeks. Higher doses increased the toxic but not the therapeutic effect. The optimum dose is probably less than 200 IU/kg.

As far as we can say the *combination treatment* with L-asparaginase and Dauno-Rubidomycine does not seem to improve the poor results in acute myeloblastic

Table 3. *L-asparaginase results in acute leucemia* (in % of cases)

	CR	PR	IMP	F	
ALL (59 pts.)	19	22	25	34	100%
APL (11 pts.)	18	10	27	45	100%
Others (40 pts.)	0	0	27	73	100%

Table 4

	pts.	Duration of treatment days	Dosis IU per kg per day	per day	Total
CR	13	26	200	7,240	188,200
PR	14	30	212	6,080	182,500
IMP	29	19	245	15,300	290,714
F	55	13	394	22,440	291,700

Table 5. *L-asparaginase 3000 U/kg/die*

	pts.	CR	PR	F
AML	22		1 (+Prednisone)	21
CMLM	2			2
APL	5		1	4
EL	2			2
CML	1			1
CLL	2			2
	34	0	2	32

Only 16 of 34 pat. were treated for more than 14 days

leukemia and myeloblastic crisis (Table 6). However, when using the 4 drug-combination (Table 7) we obtained a complete remission in one case of myeloblastic and one case of monocytic leukemia and 4 remissions among 7 cases of lymphoblastic leukemias.

Clinical success is clearly dependent on a sufficiently long *period of treatment* (Table 8). Complete remissions occurred earliest after 12 days, partial remissions after 10 days. However, for various reasons we were unable to treat approximately 1/3 of the patients for a long enough period. When evaluating only the cases which had been treated adequately for a period of at least two weeks (Table 9), we saw 49% remissions in acute lymphoblastic leukemia; in 22% of the cases we achieved complete and in 27% partial remissions. The number of acute promyelocytic leukemia cases is too small to allow definitive statements; apparently they respond to enzyme therapy almost as well as acute lymphoblastic leukemias. In the other types of acute leukemia we noted a reduction in symptoms in 42% of the cases, but no remissions.

Table 6. *Combined chemotherapy*

		Cases All	> 12 days treated	CR	PR	F
L-asparaginase	AML	5	3			5
+Dauno-rubidomycine	CMLM	1	0			1
	CML	1	1			1
	CLL	1	1		1	
		8	5	0	1	7

Table 7. *Combined chemotherapy*

		Cases All	> 12 days treated	CR	PR	F
L-asparaginase	ALL	9	7	1	3	5
+Dauno-rubidomycine	AML	1	1	1		
+Vincristine	AMOL	1	1	1		
+Prednisone						
		11	9	3	3	5

Table 8. *Duration of treatment*

	< 1 week	1—2 weeks	> 2 weeks	
CR	0	1	12	
PR	0	1	13	
IMP	4	7	18	
F	14	14	27	
NJ	9			
pts. total	27	23	70	120

Table 9. *L-asparaginase-results only cases more than 14 days treated*

	CR	PR	IMP	F
ALL 45 pts.	22	27	22	29
APL 5 pts.	40	20	0	40
Others 19 pts.	0	0	42	58
	in % of cases			

It appears that the rate of remissions is dependent on the *age* of the patient. For example, (Table 10) we found remissions in 49% of the children under 10 years of age and in 29% of the patients of 11—20 years of age. Remissions were seen in only 9% of the adults. In order to take into account that in children the more often responsive lymphoblastic leukemia is much more common and in adults the less often responsive myeloblastic leukemia, we compared the number of remissions only in the cases of lymphoblastic and of promyelocytic leukemia. None the less we saw that children under 10 years of age (53% remissions) and patients from 11—20 years of age (44%) responded more frequently than adults (only 23%). 67% of the patients in remissions were under 10 years, only 18% over 20 years of age.

Table 10. *% remissions in acute leucemia*

Years	ALL+APL	Refer to all cases
0—10	53	49
11—20	44	29
> 20	23	9

Table 11. *Dependence on pretreatment*

	Remissions	Failures
Pretreated	74%	84%
Not pretreated	26%	16%
	100%	100%

Table 12. *Dependence on initial value of leukocytes*

Leukocytes	Remissions 27 pts.	Failures 83 pts.	Total 120 pts.
< 4,000	33	31	32
4—10,000	33	25	26
> 10,000	33	44	42
	100%	100%	100%

The clinical results depended apparently little on the duration of illness: among the remissions the percentage of not pretreated early cases was 26, among the failures 16, that means of small difference only (Table 11).

Clinical success was only in small measure related to the number of *leukocytes* at the beginning of treatment (Table 12): leukocyte counts under 4000 were somewhat more frequent among the patients achieving remissions and leukocyte counts in the normal range were considerably more common in that group than in the patients who failed to respond and who had high leukocyte counts more frequently. Leukocyte counts above 50,000 were twice as frequent among the failures as among the remissions.

For each of the 4 result groups we calculated the mean leukocyte counts every other day. Leukocytes (Fig. 1) decreased markedly in approximately the same way in cases of complete remission, partial remission and also in cases of improvement, during the first 4 days of treatment. The complete remissions reached a value of 2—3000 on the 6th day; the cases of partial remission reached this value on the 12th day. These values remained constant. Interestingly, values of 5—7000 were reached among the cases of improvement between the 10th an 24th day. Among those who failed to improve, the initial decrease in leukocytes was only suggestive.

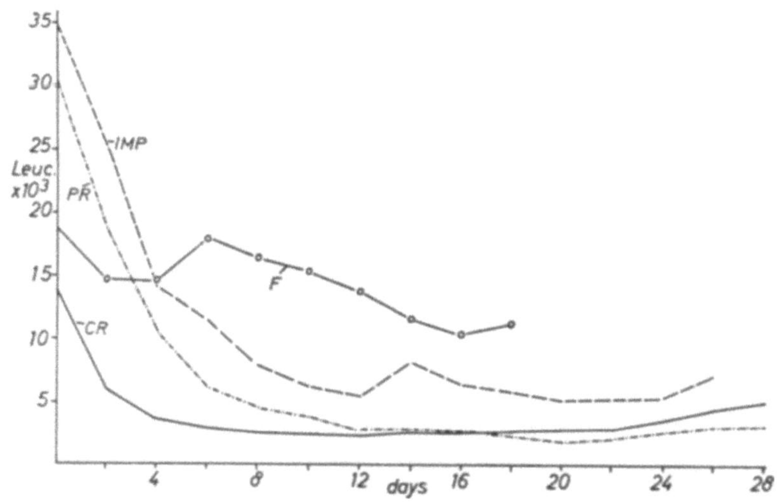

Fig. 1. Mean value of leucocytes in acute leucemia, L-asparaginase.
CR = 13 Patients
PR = 14 Patients
IMP = 29 Patients
F = 54 patients

However, from the 6th day on there was a slight but continuous decrease of leukocytes by about 40% in these cases. With treatment period of medium length (for the failures 13 days and for the cases which improved 19 days) the decrease in leukocytes was detectable for at least 5 days after discontinuation of therapy. A leukocyte count of less than 2,000, directly related to therapy, was observed in 43% of all patients. The intensity of the initial decrease of leukocytes hardly allows any conclusions as to how successful therapy will be. However, reaching a leukocyte count of below 4,000 seems to be a prerequisite for the achievement of a remission.

If one looks at the percentage of *leukemic cells* in the blood (Fig. 2), one sees that a decrease in cases of improvement occurs generally only at the beginning and in the cases of partial remission to a small degree as late as during the 3—4th week of treatment. On the other hand, in cases of complete remission the percentage of leukemic cells decreases almost arithmetically during the entire period of treatment, from a value of 76% to 26%. (It has to be noted here that in cases of lymphoblastic leukemia it was often impossible to separate leukemic cells from lymphocytes, so that both groups were counted together; thus the leukemic cell group also contains the lymphocytes.) Apparently one can expect successful therapy, if the percentage of leukemic cells continues to decrease after the 10th day of treatment.

The number of *erythrocytes,* due to the transfusions which were often necessary, increased during the first two weeks of therapy (Fig. 3). In the cases where remission occurred, however, there was a clear increase during the 3rd and 4th week of treatment; in the case of failure, on the other hand, a gradual decrease was apparent

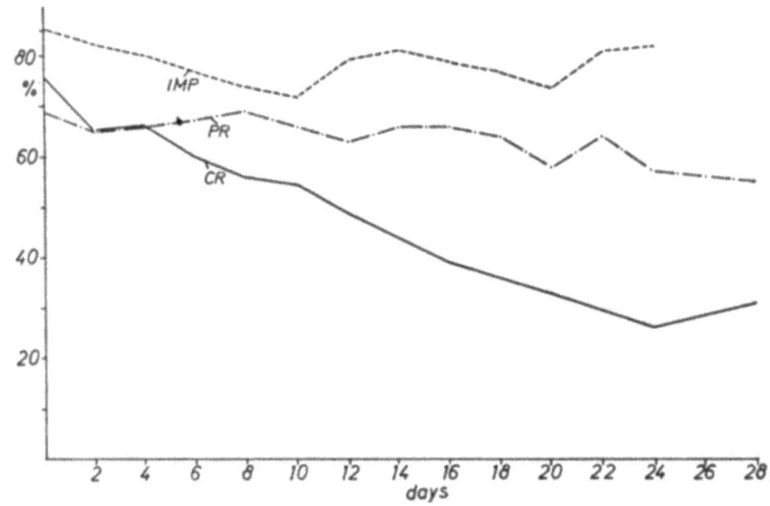

Fig. 2. Percent leucemic cells in blood under treatment with L-asparaginase in acute leucemias (in lymphoblastic leucemias lymphocytes are included)

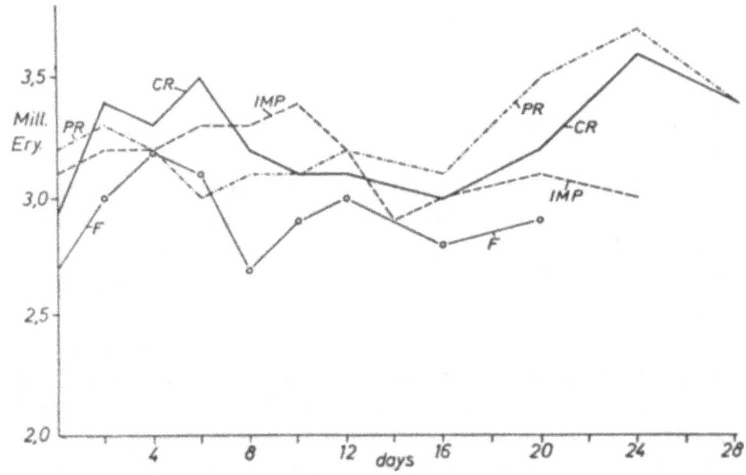

Fig. 3. Changes of erythrocytes in acute leucemia, L-asparaginase, mean values

at that time. Signs of hemolysis were observed in 9% of the patients. In 31% the hemoglobin decreased to less than 7%.

The number of *thrombocytes* was hardly lower in the patients who failed to respond than in those who achieved a complete remission (Fig. 4). Between the 2nd and 10th day a slight decrease occurred in all groups. While in cases of failure, the thrombocytes continued to decrease during further treatment, in cases of complete remission a steep and distinct increase was seen from the 6th day on.

In cases of partial remission there was a noticeable increase in thrombocytes beginning in the 3rd week, but this increase was not as marked as in cases of

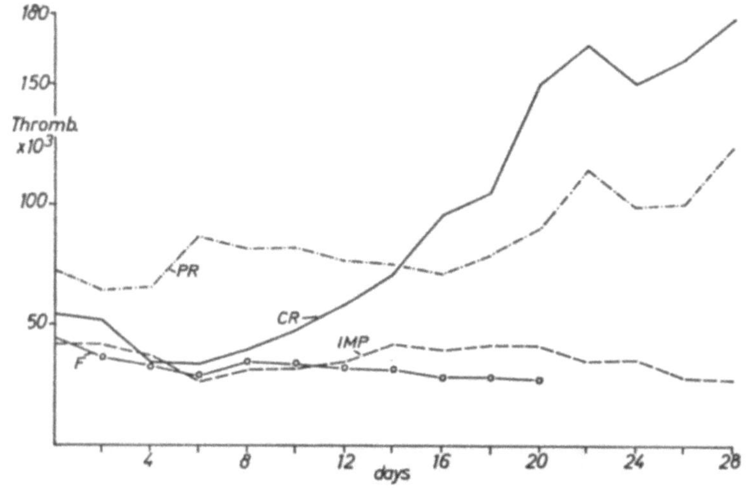

Fig. 4. Thrombocytes in acute leucemia, L-asparaginase, mean values

complete remission. A decrease in thrombocytes to less than 25,000 due to therapy, occurred in 14% of the patients. A hemorrhagic diathesis, including primary thrombopenia, was observed in 49% of all cases. Occasionally we saw more serious localized hemorrhages, especially in the digestive tract.

Serial *bone marrow* smears were available for 66 patients so that a comparison could be made of the findings before therapy and after 2 and 4 weeks of therapy (Table 13). In the case of failure there was no meaningful change: however, in the cases which "improved" (as indicated) there was some increase in erythropoietic and decrease in leukemic cells. In the cases of complete remissions the leukemic cells decreased from 85% to 3% and in cases of partial remissions from 83% to 29%. Concurrently there was a distinct improvement in erythropoiesis and granulopoiesis. The improvement of the bone marrow, if it was achieved at all, was apparent in the first bone marrow aspirate after 2 weeks and increased only slightly thereafter.

Conclusions as to whether the enzyme therapy is likely to be successful can be drawn as early as in the 2nd week of treatment. A remission can be expected if the number of leukemic cells in the blood and bone marrow has fallen to less than 50% of the starting value, if the leukocytes in the blood have decreased to less than

Table 13

Bone-marrow	11 pts. Complete remission				14 pts. Partial remission			
	Erythro-poiesis	Normal granulo-poiesis	Leukemic cells	Lympho-cytes	Erythro-poiesis	Normal granulo-poiesis	Leukemic cells	Lympho-cytes
Before therapy	6	5	85	4	8	8	83	1
After 2 weeks	35	31	10	24	23	27	30	20
4 weeks	40	44	3	13	25	34	29	12
	13 pts. Improvement				28 pts. Failure			
Before therapy	3	16	79	2	7	10	78	5
After 2 weeks	10	23	57	10	4	10	82	4
4 weeks	12	17	61	10				

4,000 and if the thrombocytes have shown a continuous increase during the 2nd week of treatment.

Splenomegaly and *hepatomegaly* were more common among those patients who later achieved a remission than in those who did not respond. A decrease in size was achieved (Tables 14, 15) in 50% of all cases and a normalisation in 30%. Enlarged lymph nodes became normal in 50% of the cases (Table 16).

Side effects: A loss of *weight* (Table 17) was noticed in 70% of all patients, which amounted to—on the average—1.3 kg after one week and in the case of failure, 3—5 kg after 2—3 weeks. It might actually be higher because of some water retention which occurs during enzyme therapy. The loss of weight occurred more slowly in those who achieved a remission than in those who failed to respond.

Table 14. *Splenomegaly*

	Cases	Before treatment	Regression to > 2 cm	< 2 cm	Not palpable
CR	13	11			11
PR	14	9		5	4
IMP	29	16	6	4	2
F	55	26	9	2	2
Total	111	62	31	18	19
	%	57	50		30

Table 15. *Hepatomegaly*

	Cases	Before treatment	Regression to < 2 cm
CR	13	8	8
PR	14	10	6
IMP	29	11	3
F	55	26	3
Total	111	55	20
	%	50	36

Table 16. *Lymphomas*

	Cases	Before treatment	Normalised
CR	13	6	6
PR	14	5	3
IMP	29	6	4
F	55	22	6
Total	111	39	19
	%	35	49

Table 17. *Weight in kg* (L-asparaginase)

	Number of pts.	Before treatment	After weaks 1.	2.	3.
CR	12	33.9	33.0	32.6	39.0
PR	13	29.0	28.3	28.1	27.8
IMP	22	55.1	53.5	51.7	49.9
F	32	58.2	57.0	60.5	
Remissions	25	31.4	30.5	30.3	33.4
Failures	54	57.0	55.5	56.9	57.0
Together	79	48.9	47.6	45.6	

Table 18. *Sedimentation rate after 2 hours*

	Before treatment	After weaks 1.	2.	3.	4.
CR	81	32	20	16	10
PR	65	34	15	11	27
IMP	88	47	35	35	
F	103	51	35		
Together	90	45	29		

Table 19.

	Cases	Before therapy	After weeks 1	2	3
S.G.O.T.	99	21	19	26	36
S.G.P.T.	96	17	16	19	20
Fibrinogen	71	364	220	171	181
Quick's time	67	76	63	64	70
Serumprotein	62	6.6		5.3	
Gamma-globulins	60	15		26	
Cholesterol	45	189		138	

A decrease in the *erythrocyte sedimentation* rate was noticed in all groups (Table 18). During the 4 week period the ESR fell in cases with complete remission from 81 mm to 10 mm, in cases with partial remission from 65 mm to 27 mm, and in patients who improved slightly from 88 mm to 36 mm; even when treatment failed the ESR decreased from 103 mm to 35 mm.

There were distinct changes in the *serum protein* levels (Table 19): the total protein decreased from 6.6 to 5.3 g-% within 2 weeks, while the gamma globulins increased from 15% to 26%. A decrease in plasma fibrinogen to less than one half was observed in 80% of the patients. At the same time the prothrombin level decreased. The serum transaminase levels tended to increase. This, together with a decrease in the coagulation factors and an increase of the serum bilirubin in 32 out of 53 tests, the appearance of bile pigment in the urine in 18% of the patients and a decrease of serum cholesterol in 28 out of 45 tests, can be interpreted as evidence of damage to *liver* cells (Table 20). This is also indicated by the appearance of fat in liver cells and liver cell necrosis, seen repeatedly at post-mortem examination. The alkaline serum phosphatase levels were elevated in 21 of 72 tests, whereas LDH determinations showed a normalization of primarily pathological values more often than a worsening. Liver damage was evident clinically in 30% of the cases.

Table 20.

In cases	Standard	Pathol. at start of therapy	Improve under therapy	Number of course-controls	Worse at all
Serumbilirubin	< 1 mg-%	10	3	53	32
S.G.O.T.	< 12 mU/ml	59	14	99	39
S.G.P.T.	< 12 mU/ml	48	13	96	31
L.D.H.	< 200 mU/ml	41	17	27	8
Alk. phosphatasis	< 50 mU/ml	20	2	72	21
Creatinine	< 1 mg-%	18	7	48	20
Fibrinogen	250—500 mg-%	23	7	71	56
Quick's time	> 80%	34	7	67	36
Cholesterol	120—250 mg-%	7	4	45	28

Table 21. *Percent side-effects under L-asparaginase. n = 109 cases*

Nausea	64	Anemia < 7 g-% Hb	31
Vomiting	46	Haemolysis	9
Diarrhoe	18	Sec. leucopenia < 2000	43
Ulcera mouth	26	Sec. thrombopenia < 25,000	14
Intestinal	13	Haemorrh. diathesis	49
		Local bleeding	42
Central reactions	40		
Headache	23	Liver disorder	30
Cardiovascular disorder	25	Bile pigment in urine	18
Vasodepression	18	Kidney-disorder	10
EKG-disorder	6	Albuminuria	15
Neurological disorder	13	Microhaematuria	24
		Macrohaematuria	7
Thrombophlebitis	4	Haemorrh. cystitis	6
Alopecia	13	Cylindruria	2
Allergic reactions	6		
Infections	23	Weight loss	70

Not only the liver but also the kidneys may suffer damage from enzyme therapy. This is indicated by an increase in creatinine above 1 mg-% in 20 out of 48 tests by the appearance of an albuminuria in 15% of the cases, as well as by occasional cylindruria and edema.

General side effects were quite frequent (Table 21). Thus 64% of the patients experienced nausea, 46% vomiting and 18% diarrhea. Central disturbances, such as dizzyness and perspiration, appeared in 40% of the cases, headaches in 23%, disturbance of the blood circulation in 25% and a decrease in blood pressure (of more than 20 mm systolically) in 18% and temporary neurological symptoms in 13% of the cases. Allergic reactions to the heterologous enzyme protein were observed in 6% of the cases and a slight fever was seen with the first batches; later when the batches were purer, fibrile reactions were rare.

The side effects of L-asparaginase are considerable and differ from those caused by other chemotherapeutic agents.

The toxicity for haemopoietic cells is less pronounced but other cells are definitely affected as, for instance, the liver cells. The therapeutic indication is limited almost exclusively to acute lymphoblastic and promyelocytic leukemia, where the results are good. But even in these cases the rate of remissions with asparaginase as the only treatment remained below that achieved in combinations with cytotoxic drugs. Thus the clinical usefulness of L-asparaginase seems to be manifest particularly in combination with antimetabolites.

Clinical Experience with L-Asparaginase

G. HAMILTON-FAIRLEY [1, 2], J. S. MALPAS [1], and D. A. G. GALTON [3]

With 2 Figures

Three sources of L-asparaginase, two derived from E. coli (supplied by E. R. Squibb and Farbenfabriken Bayer AG), and one obtained from Erwinia carotovora (supplied by the Microbiological Research Establishment, Porton) have been made available to us and have been used in the treatment of acute myeloid leukemia, acute lymphoblastic leukemia, lymphoblastic lymphosarcoma, and malignant melanoma.

The dosage of Squibb, Bayer or Porton L-asparaginase has been kept the same for all three preparations. A dose of 1000 IU/kg/day was given initially but the dose was later based on surface area because it is known that the enzyme is virtually confined to the plasma (HALL and CAMERON, 1969). The dose per square meter is 30,000—35,000 IU/day. The daily dose is divided into two halves and given intravenously every twelve hours in about 10 ml of saline. In children where intravenous administration is not always possible it can be given intramuscularly in about 4 ml of saline.

In nearly all patients a small initial dose has been given intradermally or intravenously to determine any sensitivity. One unit is followed by 10 units and then 50 units. The full regime is then started and continued if possible for 28 days.

Acute Lymphoblastic Leukemia

In fifteen of the 23 patients with acute lymphoblastic leukemia, who were treated with various types of L-asparaginase, the immediate effect of therapy could be assessed as they had active disease at the time. The other 8 patients received Bayer L-asparaginase while in remissions induced by vincristine and prednisolone followed by 6-Mercaptopurine. In these patients L-asparaginase was used with methotrexate and folinic acid in a programme designed to reduce the total number of leukemic cells in the body still further.

Induction of remission

The results of treatment in the 15 patients in relapse are shown in Table 1.

[1] St. Bartholomew's Hospital, London, E.C. 1.
[2] Chester Beatty Research Institute and Royal Marsden Hospital, Sutton, Surrey, England.
[3] Chester Beatty Research Institute and Royal Marsden Hospital, London, S.W. 3.

Thirteen of the 15 patients had been given a considerable amount of chemotherapy previously. It can be seen that Squibb, Bayer or Porton L-asparaginase can induce partial or complete remission, where complete remission has been defined as a return to health with a normal peripheral blood count and a bone marrow examination in which the number of leukemic cells and blasts is less than 5%. The total of 5 complete and 6 partial remissions in 15 patients is similar to the experience at the Sloan-Kettering, reported here by Dr. OETTGEN.

Table 1. *Acute lymphoblastic leukemia treated in relapse with L-asparaginase*

Type of L-asparaginase	Number in complete remission	Number in partial remission	Number of failures	Total
Squibb	—	1	1	2
Bayer	3	2	3	8
Porton	1	—	1	2
Bayer and Porton	1	1	1	3
Total	5	4	6	15

All the patients who responded showed a very rapid disappearance of blast cells from the circulating blood, although clearance of the bone marrow usually occurred much later. An example of this is shown in Fig. 1 a.

A girl aged six (Case 13) with lymphoblastic lymphosarcoma, who had previously received prednisolone, vincristine, methotrexate and cyclophosphamide, was given Bayer L-asparaginase and within 72 hours the blast cell count in the peripheral blood fell from 250,000 per cu. mm. to zero (Fig. 1 a). The bone marrow still contained blast cells after 21 days of treatment, but at the end of the course these had disappeared, and a complete remission was obtained. During this period intrathecal methotrexate had to be given for cerebral leukemia, but the blood had been cleared of leukemic cells before methotrexate was used. This patient has been treated subsequently with three further courses of L-asparaginase. The second course once again produced rapid clearance of blast cells from the peripheral blood, and a slower return of the marrow to normal (Fig. 1 b). The third course acted initially in the same way, but on the seventeenth day of treatment blast cells appeared again in the blood and rose rapidly so treatment with L-asparaginase was stopped (Fig. 1 c), and a further remission was obtained with cytosine arabinoside. The fourth course once again showed a dramatic fall in the number of blast cells, but a rapid rise again as treatment continued (Fig. 1 d).

It is too early yet to assess the effect of the combination of L-asparaginase with other drugs used during periods of remission in this disease.

Acute Myeloid Leukemia

Our results using L-asparaginase in this disease have been disappointing. Out of a total of 10 patients a complete remission only occurred in one (Table 2). However, it became clear that although the remission rate was low, the enzyme was having

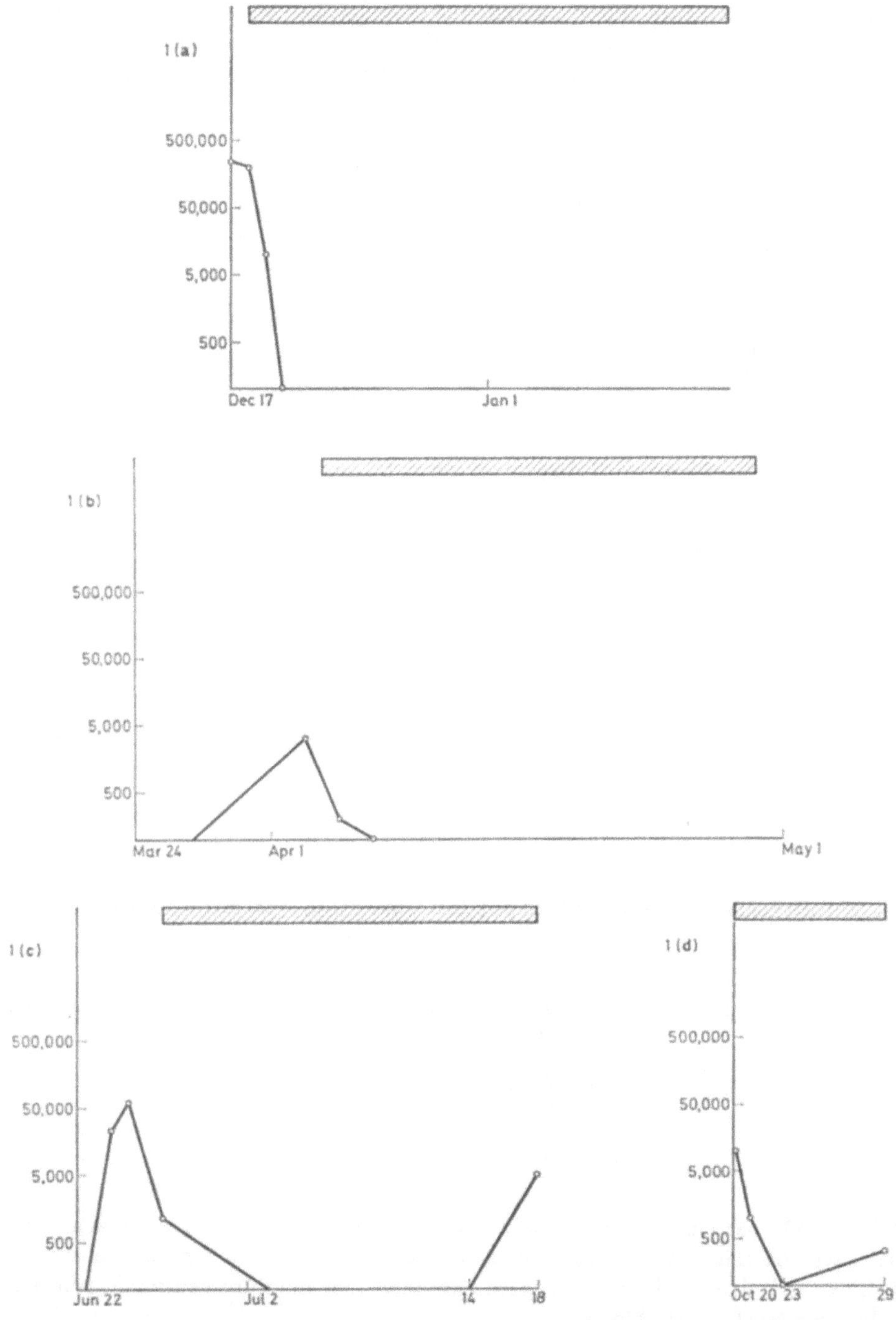

Fig. 1. Changes in the peripheral blood in a child aged 6 with lymphoblastic lymphosarcoma during 4 courses of treatment with L-asparaginase. The fourth course (Fig. 1 d) had only just started at the time of publication

some effect in that there was a marked, but short-lived, reduction in the number of circulating blast cells in 7 out of the 10 patients. This is illustrated in Fig. 2 which shows the effect of L-asparaginase on the peripheral blood of a man aged 60. The blast count initially was 143,000 per cu. mm. and the *in vitro* test showed that the cells were sensitive to the enzyme. After treatment for eight days the blast count

Table 2. *The results obtained with L-asparaginase in acute myeloid leukemia*

Type of L-asparaginase	Number in complete remission	Number in partial remission	Number of failures	Total
Squibb	—	—	1	1
Bayer	1	1	6	8
Porton	—	—	1	1
Total	1	1	8	10

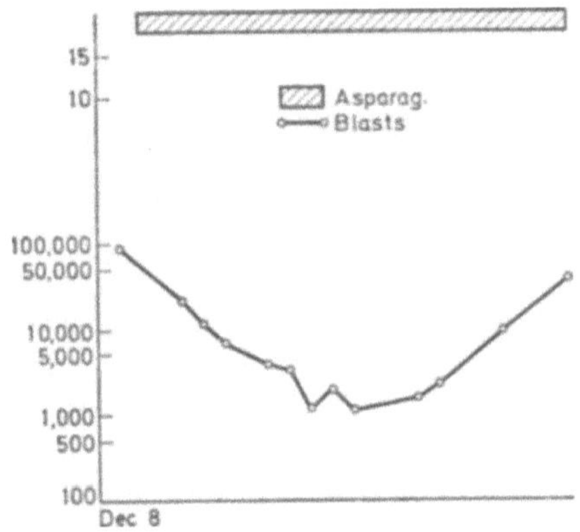

Fig. 2. Total number of circulating blast cells in a patient with acute myeloid leukemia during treatment with L-asparaginase

Table 3. *The results of using Bayer L-asparaginase in combination with cytosine arabinoside and duanorubicin in acute myeloid leukemia*

Total	Complete remission	Partial remission	Failure
10	5	1	4

fell to 1300 per cu. mm., but slowly rose again to reach 54,000 per cu. mm. after 19 days. At this time the cells were not sensitive to the action of the enzyme *in vitro*. Cytosine arabinoside was used and only after the third course did leukemic cells disappear from the blood.

For this reason we decided to use the enzyme in combination with other drugs, and have treated ten patients with Bayer L-asparaginase, cytosine arabinoside and duanorubicin. The results are summarised in Table 3. We gave L-asparaginase for

5—7 days before using the other drugs to determine whether there was any effect by the enzyme alone on the circulating blast cells. In one Patient the blood was cleared of blast cells within the first 4 days, but a complete marrow remission was only obtained after cytosine arabinoside and daunorubicin had been given.

Malignant Melanoma

Eight patients with disseminated malignant melanoma were treated with Bayer L-asparaginase and no clinical benefit was observed, despite the fact that the patients were deliberately selected because their malignant cells were sensitive to the action of the enzyme *in vitro*. However, in two patients radiotherapy was given to some of the lesions while L-asparaginase was being administered. There was definite regression of the irradiated lesions, but no effect was observed on the unirradiated lesions. This could, of course, be due to the effect of irradiation alone, but the response was unexpectedly good.

Toxicity

Using E. coli L-asparaginase (Squibb and Bayer material) nausea and vomiting, a fall in the blood levels of fibrinogen and albumin, and slight abnormalities in liver function tests have been observed. Clinical pancreatitis, as described by SCHEIN et al (1969), has not been encountered, and this may be due to the fact that they were using enzyme obtained from Merck, which clearly differs from the Bayer material. Indeed, this raises the important point that whenever the toxicity or the efficacy of L-asparaginase is discussed, it is essential to know which material is being used, as there are significant differences between the rate of clearance and toxicity of the enzyme from different sources.

Hypersensitivity has developed in several patients, and can prove troublesome. In two patients when hypersensitivity occurred we changed to using Porton L-asparaginase, and confirmed the experimental work at Porton that there is no cross-sensitivity between the E. coli and Erwinia enzymes. Antibodies raised against the E. coli enzyme do not cross-react with those raised against Erwinia (A. P. MACLENNON, 1969). Clearly, to have a second source of enzyme which is antigenically different may prove to be very useful.

Discussion

One of the major problems in the use of L-asparaginase in the treatment of human malignant disease is the development of resistance to the drug. Furthermore, it is disappointing to find that although malignant cells, particularly in myeloblastic leukemia and malignant melanoma, are sensitive to the action of the drug *in vitro*, clinical response is rare. There may be several explanations for this.

One of the most impressive effects clinically has been the rapid clearance of leukemic cells from the blood, but the very slow clearance of such cells from the marrow. This has been particularly noticeable in acute lymphoblastic leukemia where all the blast cells may disappear from the blood within 48 hours, but the marrow may not remit for 21—28 days (as shown in Fig. 1). Another interesting observation, which occurs particularly commonly in myeloblastic leukemia, is that the number of cells in the blood may fall dramatically at first but after some days reappear, and even increase in number.

One reason for the rapid clearance of cells from the blood, but the slow clearance from the marrow, could be due to the fact that after injection virtually all the enzyme remains confined to the plasma, and only trivial amounts enter the interstitial fluid compartment (HALL, 1969). Indeed, it may be that a major factor in determining the clinical response could be whether the cells pass freely from the marrow, where the concentration of enzyme is probably low, to the blood where it is certainly high. Another reason why the cells in the marrow may be less sensitive is that asparagine may pass directly from normal cells to the adjacent leukemic cells. Similar mechanisms could explain the failure of asparaginase to affect the growth of solid tumors such as malignant melanoma.

Another possibility for the development of resistance to the action of this enzyme is that from the start in human leukemia two populations of cells may exist, as we know to be the case with the L5178Y lymphoma. It may be, particularly in myeloblastic leukemia, that some cells are sensitive to asparaginase while others are not, and if the drug is used alone there is, therefore, an initial fall in the number of leukemic cells but a subsequent rise due to the growth of the resistant cell line.

Finally there is the possibility that in the presence of asparagine deprivation activation of the enzyme asparagine synthetase may occur, rendering the cells resistant to the action of L-asparaginase. However, it is difficult to explain, on this basis, how a patient may respond again once resistance has occurred, as shown in Fig. 1.

For these reasons we believe that asparaginase should be used in combination with other drugs in the treatment of acute leukemia. Although when used alone it does not produce complete remissions in myeloblastic leukemia, it still may have a role to play when used in combination, for any treatment which can reduce the number of malignant cells may be a useful agent when combined with other drugs. Similarly, the use of L-asparaginase in the treatment of malignant melanoma in combination with other forms of chemotherapy or radiotherapy has still to be elucidated.

References

HALL, J. G.: Proceedings of the meeting on L-asparaginase held at Farbenfabriken Bayer AG, Wuppertal, Germany (1969).

— CAMERON, C. B.: Personal communication 1969.

MACLENNON, A. P.: Personal communication 1969.

SCHEIN, P. S., RAKIETEN, N., GORDON, B. M., DAVIS, R. D., RALL, D. P.: Cancer Res. 29, 426 (1969).

Treatment of Acute Leukemia with L-Asparaginase — Preliminary Results on 84 Cases

CL. JACQUILLAT, M. WEIL, A. BUSSEL, J. P. LOISEL, T. ROUESSE, M. J. LARRIEU, M. BOIRON, B. DREYFUS, and JEAN BERNARD

Chemotherapy Unit, Hôpital St. Louis, 2 Place du Dr. Fournier, F-75 Paris, France

With 6 Figures

Between 1st of August 1968 and the 30th of April 1969 we treated 84 patients with L-asparaginase. This report deals with the results obtained.

Patients and Methods

Patients

The 84 patients were suffering from acute leukemia.

The first 9 patients were treated at a particularly advanced stage of the disease and death occurred before the action of the drug could be assessed. We have therefore excluded them from the rest of the study, which was carried out on 75 patients, distributed as indicated in Table 1.

Table 1. *Acute lymphoblastic leukemia—Results of treatment with L-asparaginase alone*

	L-asparaginase alone	Combinations including L-asparaginase	Total
A.L.L.	34	27	61
A.M.L.	6	8	14
Total	40	35	75

Methods

The product was supplied in vials containing 2,000 or 10,000 units. The solution was prepared immediately before use by the addition of 1 ml or 5 ml of distilled water.

Initial Treatment

L-asparaginase was administered by injection into the tubing of an intravenous drip infusion of normal saline, in one daily injection of 1,000 units/kg bodyweight. In cases of acute myeloblastic leukemia treated with L-asparaginase alone, the dose was 4,000 units/kg/day. The duration of treatment depended on the result obtained and varied from 5 to 40 days, with an average of 15 days.

Maintenance Treatment

After initial treatment, maintenance treatment with L-asparaginase was continued in some cases: a dose of 1,000 units/kg was given intramuscularly twice weekly.

All diagnostic tests were carried out in our laboratory on smears of bone marrow and blood using May Grunwald Giemsa stains. The cytological classification as acute lymphoblastic, myeloblastic or undifferentiated leukemia was made on the basis of the usual cytological criteria after panoptic staining and also by the so-called cyto-chemical techniques (P.A.S. staining of peroxydases).

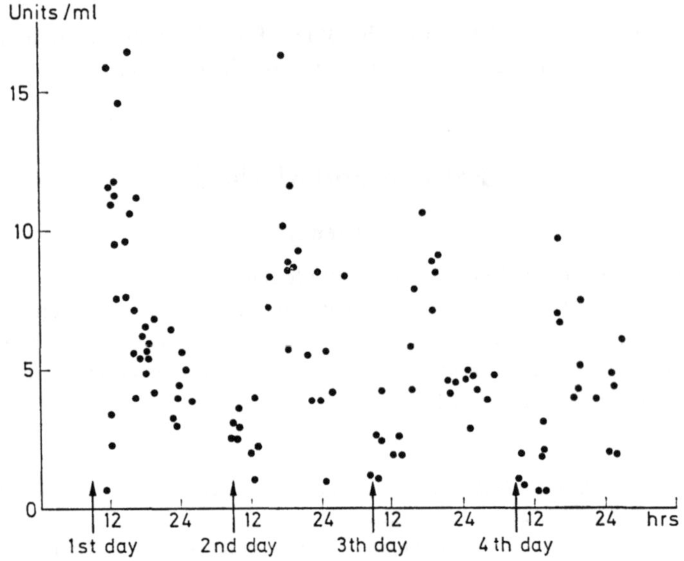

Fig. 1. Asparaginase activity in the serum. Intravenous injection of 1000 IU/kg of L-asparaginase

Special Studies

The concentration of L-asparaginase was estimated in the sera of 18 patients [1].

Fig. 1 indicates the results obtained during the first four days of treatment. The half-life of L-asparaginase appears to be of the order of 6 hours. The number of samples taken is as yet insufficient for us to be more precise.

---

[1] Concentrations of L-asparaginase were determined by MAURICE DUBOST and CLAUDE PASCAL in the Research Laboratories of the Société des Usines Chimiques Rhone Poulenc.

The sensitivity of leukemia cells in vitro was studied in 31 patients by a method very similar to that used by SOBIN and KIDD [29], KIM and OLD, and OETTGEN et al.

Suspensions of leukemia cells obtained from the bone marrow or from the peripheral blood were cultivated in the minimum essential medium of Eagle (MEM) in the absence of asparagine, in the presence of asparagine, and in the presence of asparaginase.

The incorporation of tritiated L-valine into protein was measured using a scintillation spectrometer; the number of counts per minute of the samples with asparagine was taken as 100% and the number of counts per minute of the other samples were expressed as percent of this.

Analysis of Results
Acute Lymphoblastic Leukemia Treated with L-Asparaginase Alone

Frequency of Remissions

We obtained 13 complete remissions in 34 patients (38% ± 8%).

As indicated in Table 2, this proportion appears to depend on the stage of development of the leukemia and on previous therapy. In the leukemias treated at their onset, 6 remissions were obtained in 11 cases, whereas in cases of relapse L-asparaginase produced only 7 complete remissions in 23 cases.

Table 2. *Results obtained with L-asparaginase in the treatment of acute lymphoblastic leukemia, classified according to the stage of the disease*

	1st Attack	1st Relapse	2nd Relapse	3rd Relapse	4th Relapse	Total
Complete remissions	6 [a]	2	3	2	0	13 [a]
Incomplete remissions	0	2	0	1	0	3
Partial failures	4	1	2	0	0	7
Total failures	0	2	4	2	2	10
Death during induction	1 [b]					1 [b]
Total	11	7	9	5	2	35

[a] Death occurred on the 30th day in a patient in complete remission who had undergone a total colectomy on the 20th day for multiple perforations.

[b] Death due to cerebro-meningeal hemorrhage occurring on the 6th day of treatment.

Complete Remission—Duration and Quantitative Changes

The analysis of the 13 cases of complete remission of acute lymphoblastic leukemia treated with L-asparaginase alone allowed the following observations to be made:

The establishment of a complete remission was often slow; after 5 to 10 days, the effect of treatment became evident as a decrease of the peripheral white cell count (with disappearance of circulating blast cells) and as a reduction of the cellularity of the marrow (with reduction of blasts to between 20 and 35%). A stage was often reached when the marrow was hypocellular but there remained 5 to 15% of blast cells, the nature of which was difficult to assess; between the 15th and 30th day, the peripheral blood counts were normal or subnormal, with a leucopenia of about 2,000 white cells per cu mm a neutropenia of between 30 and 40% and a thrombopenia of about 150,000 per cu mm. Treatment with L-asparaginase was then stopped. During the following week, the blood became normal, the cellularity of the marrow increased, with less than 6% of haemoblasts, and a satisfactory balance in the proportion of the cells of the red and white series and of megakaryocytes (Fig. 2).

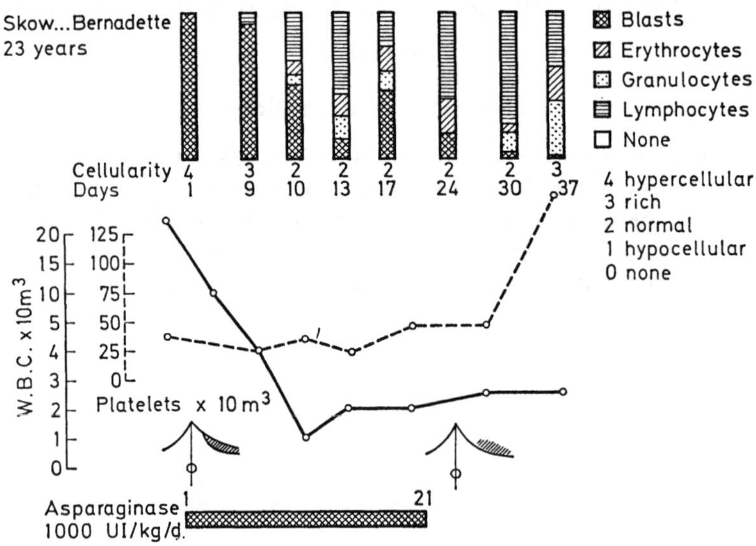

Fig. 2. Complete remission in a case of acute lymphoblastic leukemia treated with L-asparaginase alone (21 days). The bone marrow is normal, cellular and non-blastic 13 days after stopping treatment

Incomplete Remissions and Partial Failures

In a significant number of cases (10 out of 33) improvement was only partial. These were mainly cases of acute lymphoblastic leukemia resistant to all known drugs or treated unsuccessfully with several courses of poly-chemotherapy before treatment with L-asparaginase; some were suffering from aplasia induced by the leukemia or by therapy. In these cases the enlarged glands and visceral (liver, spleen, kidney) tumors disappeared and the marrow lost its cellularity and blast cells; however despite continuation of treatment 15—20% of blast cells remained in the marrow. Occasionally the marrow became normal but the remission was incomplete because neutropenia and thrombopenia persisted. In other cases (partial failures) the marrow remained blastic despite a clinical improvement (liver, spleen, lymph nodes) and a transient improvement in the blood picture.

Total Failures

In 10 cases, despite 20 to 30 days of treatment, there was no change in the blood or bone marrow. Failure to respond after the 3rd week of therapy seems to indicate resistance to asparaginase. In these cases, the first week of treatment is not characterized by a change in the size of the enlarged organs or in the blood picture (fall in white cell count and reduction of circulating blast cells).

In two cases where asparaginase treatment was completely ineffective, we observed that the triple combination of prednisone, Vincristine and daunorubicin had a remarkable effect. One month earlier the two patients were completely resistant to this triple combination.

In vitro Tests

The results obtained in the treatment of acute lymphoblastic leukemia by L-asparaginase alone, will only be considered (17 cases): In 9 cases the *in vitro* test agreed with the clinical result obtained (5 complete remissions, 4 failures). In 6 cases in which the test result was equivocal (60—70%) there were 3 complete remissions, 2 partial remissions, and 1 failure. Finally in the cases of 2 partial remissions the in vitro test was in one case positive and in the other case negative (Fig. 3).

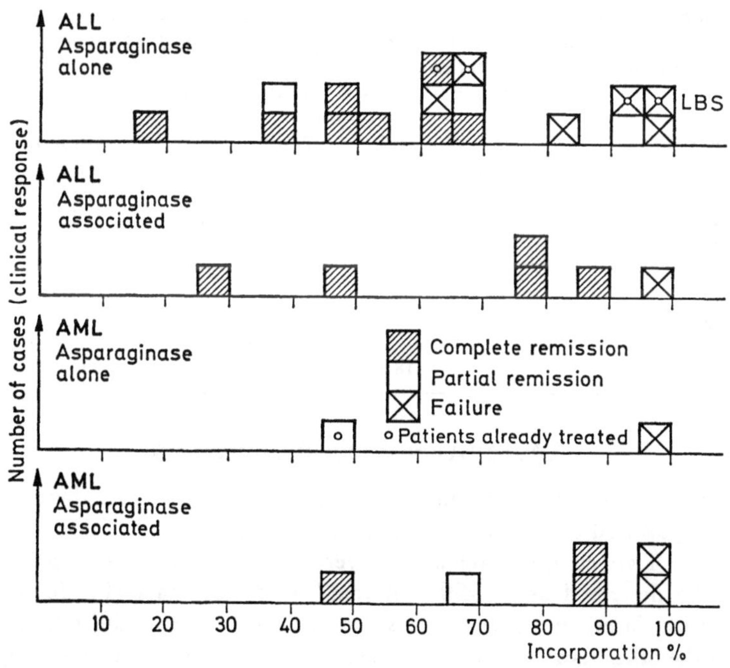

Fig. 3. Comparison of the results of the in vitro test with the therapeutic results

Acute Lymphoblastic Leukemia Treated with a Combination of L-Asparaginase—Prednisone—Vincristine—Daunorubicin

Twenty-seven cases of acute lymphoblastic leukemia in relapse were treated with combination of prednisone, Vincristine, daunorubicin and asparaginase according to the scheme shown in Fig. 4.

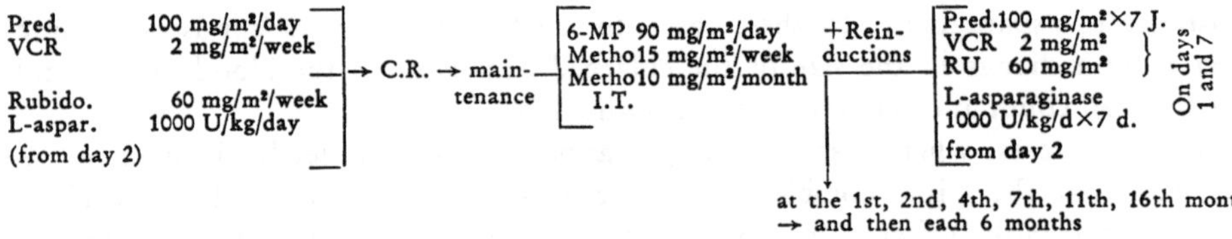

Fig. 4. Protocol of relapses of A.L.L.

Of these, 18 cases were in their first relapse and 9 cases had previous relapses. In 13 cases the patients had previously been treated according to the PARIS 06 LA 66 protocol at the onset of their diseases, that is to say they had received induction and subsequent reinduction courses of a combination of prednisone, Vincristine and daunorubicin. In 10 of these 13 cases a complete remission had been obtained rapidly. In some patients who are not included in this study, we are now conducting a controlled trial of this treatment plan in a slightly modified form at the onset of the illness.

Table 3. *Results of treatment of acute lymphoblastic leukemia with the quadruple combination: L-asparaginase, vincristine, daunorubicin, prednisone*
The figures in brackets are patients previously treated by the triple association: Prednisone-Vincristine-Daunorubicin

Number of patients	1st Attack	1st R.	2nd R.	3rd R.	4th R. or 5th R.	Total
Complete remissions		13 (6)	4 (3)	2	2 (1)	21 (10)
Incomplete remissions			1			1
Partial failures		1				1
Total failures		1 (1)				1 (1)
Death during treatment		3 (2)				3 (2)
Total		18 (9)	5 (3)	2	2 (1)	27 (13)

Acute Myeloblastic Leukemia

In 6 cases, we used L-asparaginase alone (Table 4). In 3 cases there was a rapid fall of leucocytes and blast cells in the peripheral blood and regression of the hepato-splenomegaly. Two complete remissions were obtained in cases which could most accurately be described as "undifferentiated" acute leukemia (P.A.S. reaction and negative peroxydases) in which the blasts in the bone marrow did not contain Auer bodies. On the other hand in the other three cases the marrow remained hypercellular and blastic despite high doses of 4000 units/kg/day.

Table 4. *Acute myeloblastic leukemia treated with L-asparaginase alone (4000 IU/kg/day)*

	1st Attack	1st Relapse	2nd Relapse	Total
C.R.	2			2
I.R.				
Partial failure			1	1
Total failure	1	1	1	3
Total	3	1	2	6

Table 5. *Results of treatment of acute myeloblastic leukemia with the combination of L-asparaginase, daunorubicin, methotrexate*

Number of patients	1st Attack	1st Relapse	2nd Relapse	Total
C.R.	4+1 [a]	1		5+1 [a]
I.R.				
Partial failure			1	1
Total failure	1			1
				8

[a] Died in C.R. on the 30th day after start of treatment.

In view of these disappointing results, which agreed with those of other workers, we have used an association of L-asparaginase 1,000 units/kg/day with daunorubicin 60 mg/m² and methotrexate 30 mg/m² intravenously on alternate days. The results obtained are given in Table 5; five complete remissions were obtained in eight cases. This study is still in progress and it is difficult to interpret the results because of the small number of cases (Fig. 5).

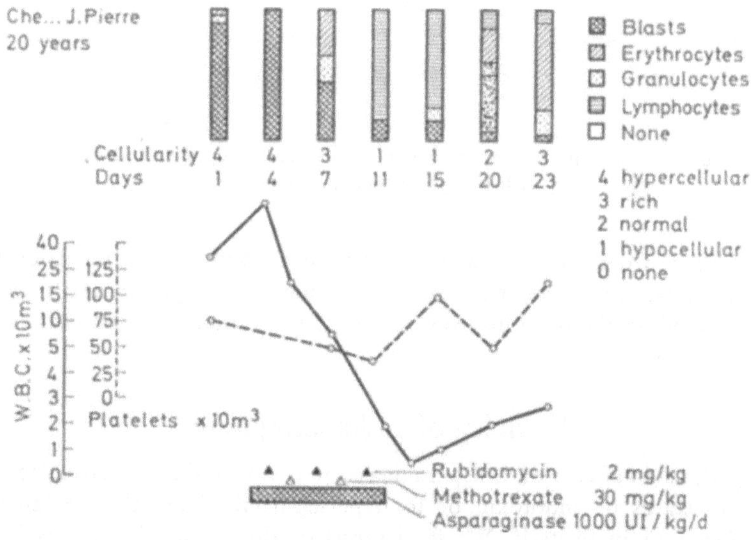

Fig. 5. Complete remission in a case of acute myeloblastic leukemia treated with the triple combination of L-asparaginase, methotrexate and daunorubicin

The Action of L-Asparaginase on Lesions in the Central Nervous System and Meninges

L-asparaginase given by the normal route, is capable of causing meningeal involvement to regress. This effect is not due to a direct action of the drug (which does not pass through the meningeal barrier) but depends on equilibration of the concentrations of asparagine in the blood and cerebrospinal fluid.

We treated five cases of acute leukemia with meningeal involvement with asparaginase by the normal route. Asparaginase failed in the case of a patient with subacute blastic leukemia without meningeal pleocytosis. A partial and brief improvement of the C.S.F. blast count was obtained in a child without any improvement of the signs of increased intracranial pressure. On the other hand, we obtained a complete remission in 3 patients with a return to normal of the C.S.F. in one week. One of these relapsed during the second month despite maintenance treatment with asparaginase; the other had an ascending polyradiculitis which regressed completely clinically; a relapse has not yet occurred after two months (Fig. 6).

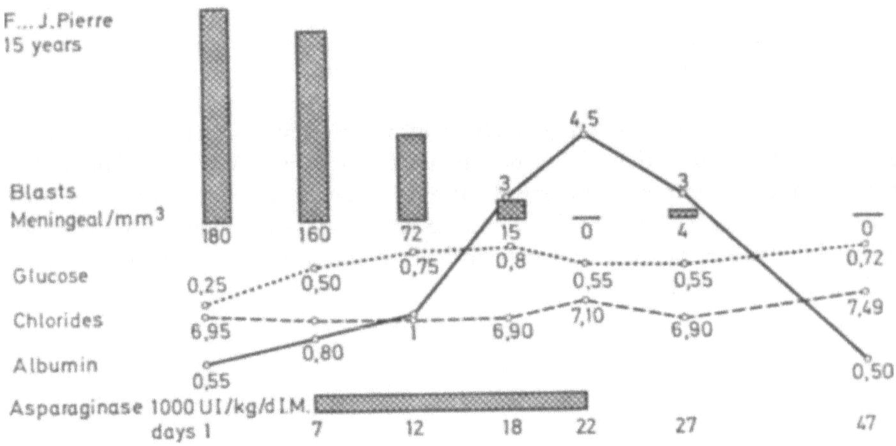

Fig. 6. Cytological and chemical improvement in the cerebro-spinal fluid during 22 days of treatment with L-asparaginase injected intravenously

Finally, in two patients with acute lymphoblastic leukemia in remission brought about by asparaginase alone, we noticed a meningeal relapse during maintenance treatment, preceding the bone marrow relapse, by two months in one case and by a month in the other.

Toxicity of L-Asparaginase

Among the side-effects of L-asparaginase, it is not a simple matter to separate those due to traces of endotoxin or to hypersensitivity from those related to the action of L-asparaginase itself. We shall therefore divide the side-effects into those appearing early and those appearing later during treatment, the latter being hepatic disorders in our experience.

Early Reactions

A slight fever (between 37° and 38°) was noted in 30% of the cases during treatment. It is difficult to attribute such a fever to the asparaginase, since acute leukemia is often accompanied by pyrexia before treatment. Three patients showed allergic reactions; urticaria in one case and angioneurotic edema in the other two; these manifestations did not reappear when treatment was recommenced with another batch of asparaginase. In one patient an intradermal injection of one unit of asparaginase in 0.1 ml of distilled water produced a local reaction after 24 hours.

More serious reactions having the appearance of protein shock were noted in 4 patients. These appeared in 3 cases when asparaginase treatment was restarted after an interval of one to four weeks, e. g. reinduction. The reactions appeared half-an-hour after injection (pyrexia of 39°—40°, shivering with cyanosis of the extremities, tachycardia with a fall of blood pressure of not more than 8 mm of mercury). These symptoms disappeared in one half to two hours under treatment with cortisone, given intravenously.

In three out of four patients the intradermal skin reaction to asparaginase was strongly positive half an hour after the injection. (One should note here that two of these patients presented with similar manifestations after injection of one of the first trial batches of asparaginase. This batch had proved to be pyrogenic in the rabbit at a dose of 200 U/kg.)

Nevertheless, treatment could be restarted in these patients, using the batches of material which are currently supplied, without reappearance of the allergic manifestations.

Because of these allergic manifestations we adopted the following therapeutic plan: the reaction to an intradermal injection of asparaginase was tested before treatment and then weekly during treatment. At every reinduction the asparaginase injections are started 48 hours after giving corticotherapy at a dose of 3 mg/kg, even when the skin test is negative.

Hepatic Disorders

An effect on the liver was seen frequently (60% of cases); it was, without doubt, responsible for a part of the marked loss of weight noted in many patients. This necessitated regular careful surveillance during the entire course of treatment: bilirubin direct and indirect, cholesterol total and esterified, SGPT, alkaline phosphatase, electrophoresis of serum proteins, fibrinogen, factors X, VII and V, need to be estimated before treatment and at least at intervals of one week during the course of treatment.

The effects of asparaginase on hepatic function are summarized in Table No. 6, which shows the various anomalies observed in 47 patients. For technical reasons, an adequate number of tests was not performed in some of the patients.

The most frequent anomaly encountered was decrease in cholesterol, occasionally as low as 0.8 g/l, but usually between 1.5 g/l and 1 g/l. High indirect bilirubin, a rise in the serum alkaline phosphatase and low albumin levels were frequently associated, the hypoalbuminemia being marked (below 20 g/l in 50% of the cases. An increase of the transaminase was less common and less important. Signs of hepato-cellular toxicity were seen more frequently when L-asparaginase was combined with other hepatotoxic drugs (in particular with daunorubicin and methotrexate) and were noted invariably when there were pre-existing signs of deranged hepatic function.

In chronological order, the first manifestation was a decrease in the cholesterol, noticed most frequently at the end of the first week, whereas the alkaline phosphatase became progressively elevated in parallel with the diminution of the serum albumin level [13].

Table 6. *Changes in the results of liver function tests during treatment with L-asparaginase*

Cholesterol	≧ 1.50	1.50—1	1—0.80	≦ 0.80
g/l	13 (28%)	25 (53%)	6 (13%)	3 (6%)
Bilirubin Indirect	≦ 5	5—10	10—20	20—50
mg/l	25 (53%)	14 (30%)	7 (15%)	1 (2%)
Transaminases S.G.P.T.	≦ 50	50—100	100—200	200—500
(U. WROBLEWSKI)	30 (64%)	14 (30%)	1 (2%)	2 (4%)
Alkaline Phosphatase	≦ 10	10—20	20—30	30—50
(U. KING)	23 (50%)	10 (21%)	9 (20%)	5 (9%)
Serum albumin	≧ 35	35—25	25—20	≦ 20
g/l	19 (40%)	8 (17%)	12 (26%)	8 (17%)

The development of signs of hepatotoxicity was usually not alarming, since all the changes returned to normal within two weeks after termination of treatment with asparaginase. In a certain number of patients we were able to restart the drug, as maintenance treatment, without the reappearance of signs of toxicity. In two cases, however, hepatic failure was responsible for death.

The first was a 60 year old man treated with L-asparaginase for acute lymphoblastic leukemia at its onset. His liver function tests were normal and he showed no hemorrhagic tendency before the beginning of treatment. Six days after the beginning of the injections, totalling 8500 U/kg of asparaginase, a syndrome of hemorrhagic jaundice appeared. The results of liver function tests performed at this time were: Bilirubin 25 mg/l (10 mg indirect), cholesterol 0.55 g/l, transaminase 98 U/Wroblewski, alkaline phosphatase 8 U/King, albumin 18 g/l, β-globulin 38 g/l and γ-globulin 42 g/l. At the same time there was a hypofibrinogenemia of 0.5 g/l without increase in the degredation products of fibrin, and a diminution in the level of factors V, VII and X respectively to 13%, 27% and 36%. Because of a misinterpretation of the results intravascular coagulation was suspected and the patient was treated with heparin. Death occurred 48 hours later, with pulmonary oedema and hemorrhage. An autopsy was not performed.

The second patient was a 12 year old child from the Cameroons suffering from acute lymphoblastic leukemia of recent onset. The child had not yet been treated.

After 11 days of treatment with asparaginase in high doses (4000 U/kg/day), the child developed a peritonitis secondary to necrotising colitis which necessitated a total colectomy. The histological examination of the surgical specimen showed numerous ulcerations resulting from leukemic infiltration. After an interruption of 48 hours following the operation, treatment with asparaginase was restarted at the same dose, because of a persistent blastic infiltration of the bone marrow. Eight days after the operation, the bowel function was normal, the general condition was satisfactory and a complete remission had been obtained. Asparaginase was then stopped. Five days later jaundice of increasing intensity appeared while the general condition of the patient deteriorated rapidly and a hemorrhagic tendency with progressive disruption of the colectomy scar occurred. The child died in a hemorrhagic and cachectic state one month after the beginning of treatment. On the day before death the bilirubin was 120 mg/l (6 mg indirect bilirubin), the total cholesterol 1.3 g/l, the transaminase 56 U/Wroblewski, the alkaline phosphatase 15 U/King, and albumin 17.5 g/l. The Quick test was 35% (70% factor V, 14% factor VII, 20% factor X), while the fibrinogen was normal at 3 g/l. It is probable that in this case malabsorption played a part in the biological anomalies which were observed, particularly those concerning the fall in factors VII and X and in the hypoalbuminemia. Autopsy showed massive liver lesions consisting of fatty degeneration and parenchymatous degeneration, with considerable cholestasis in the biliary canaliculi which was interpreted as a direct toxic effect of asparaginase on the hepatic cells. There was, in addition, leukemic infiltration of the spleen and of the mesenteric lymph glands.

Coagulation Defects

A diminution of circulating fibrinogen appears to be frequent. It was noticed in 90% of the cases which were followed in this respect. The mechanism of this hypofibrinogenemia is still not completely clear: it is only occasionally associated with circulating fibrinolytic activity (1 case out of 27), even when the fibrinogen level is very low (0.3 g/l).

It does not appear to be due to intra-vascular coagulation, since it is more frequently encountered in the absence of changes in prothrombin and factor VIII, which are frequently raised in these patients. It is also unlikely because of the constant absence of the degradation products of fibrinogen in the serum at the time. It does not appear to represent a known molecular anomaly of fibrinogen, since there was a direct concordance between the fibrinogen levels measured by both biological and by immunological techniques. On the other hand when the hypofibrinogenemia was severe, it was associated with a diminution of the circulating plasminogen level, even in the absence of detectable fibrinolytic activity. Both anomalies corrected themselves simultaneously when treatment was interrupted (Table 7). Variations in the prothrombin complex were usually moderate except in one of the two reported observations (Table 8).

Renal Insufficiency

In contrast to other authors [13] we did not observe an elevation of the blood urea due to L-asparaginase. However we have noted a severe uric acid nephropathy

Table 7. PRON. *Philippe. Changes in the results of tests concerned with hemostasis during treatment with L-asparaginase. Marked reduction of fibrinogen and plasminogen without significant change in the prothrombin factors*

	20/3/69	28/3/69	1/4/69	8/4/69
Asparaginase 1000/kg	//////////////	//////////////	//////////////	
Oncovin	△	△		
Cerubidin	▽	▽		
Platelets/mm³	240,000	320,000	120,000	120,000
Factor V (%)	90	90	> 100	
Factor VII+X (%)	68	59	> 100	
Factor II (%)	77	48	80	
Factor VIII (%)	104		160	
Factor IX (%)	102		106	
Fibrinogen (g/l)	2.8	0.7	0.3	3
Euglobulin lysis		> 4	> 4	> 4
Degredation products of fibrinogen (γ/ml)	4	38.4	8	32
Plasminogen (%)	100	5		75
Bilirubin indirect (mg/l)	9	11		
Cholesterol total (g/l)	2.15	2.30		
Transaminase (U.W.)	21	38		
Alkaline phosphatase (g/l)	22	30		
Albumin (g/l)	41	45		
γ-globulin (g/l)	12	14		

Table 8. CHE. *Emile. Changes in the results of tests concerned with hemostasis during treatment with L-asparaginase*

	27/12/68	8/1/69	9/1/69	10/1/69
Asparaginase	//////////////	//////////////		
Platelets/mm³	80,000	50,000		19,000
Quick test time (%)	65	20		18
Factor V (%)	> 100	13		30
Factor VII+X (%)	86	55		27
Factor II (%)	100	66		36
Thrombin time (sec)	18/14	24/14		21/16
Fibrinogen (g/l)	3.35	0.50	1	1
Euglobulin lysis	> 3		> 3	
Degradation products of fibrinogen (γ/ml)			1.8	3.6
Factor VIII (%)			80	
Bilirubin indirect (mg/l)	5	10	19.5	
Cholesterol (g/l)	1.60	0.55	0.75	
Transaminase	10	98	56	
Alkaline phosphatase	7	8	8	
Albumin	24	18.5	21	
γ-globulin	24.5	38.5 (β γ)	42.5 (β γ)	

in one case, due to the rapid lysis of leukemia cells caused by polychemotherapy (daunorubicin, vincristine, prednisone, L-asparaginase) started from the outset in large doses. Lysis caused by asparaginase can be severe and the usual precautions, such as the use of allopurinol and forced diuresis, should be observed.

In contrast to other authors [13, 25, 26] we did not observe pancreatic or neurological toxicity, except for a state of somnolence in certain small children which we have attributed to the invariable and sometimes considerable elevation of blood ammonia (600 to 800 γ-N: 50 to 200 γ).

Discussion

The activity of asparaginase in experimental leukemias and tumors allows one to predict a certain specificity of action. Only certain forms of leukemia appear to be sensitive to L-asparaginase. In these cases the majority of the malignant cells were destroyed, the normal cells being spared.

The results obtained in acute lymphoblastic leukemia (the most favourable indication for L-asparaginase) show that it is only in about one half of the cases that a clear-cut response occurs. Our experience agrees with that of other authors.

In the majority of cases the published papers deal with acute lymphoblastic leukemia in relapse, often in the third or even the fourth age of development. It is difficult in these conditions to state exactly what constitutes a complete remission and an incomplete remission or "good partial remission". When they considered these two groups together, TALLAL et al. [30], in a recent analysis of 61 cases of acute lymphoblastic leukemia in children, observed an M1—bone marrow rating in 36 cases. The remissions lasted from 1—8 months in 21 cases, and 15 patients were still in remission. The dose varied from 10—5000 U/kg/day.

In Germany, the dose has been smaller but in a narrower range, varying from 200—500 U/kg/day during a minimum of 15 days. In 23 cases of acute lymphoblastic leukemia, we observed 9 complete remissions and 7 incomplete remissions. The results of HILL [14] are similar; those published recently by G. MATHÉ [22] are also of the same order.

The majority of these studies do not include a sufficiently large number of patients to determine the proportion of cases that are sensitive to this treatment. Partial remissions are possible; one can therefore postulate that in one individual subject only a fraction of the blast population may be sensitive to L-asparaginase. Remissions induced and maintained by asparaginase do not last very long; it can be that the initial fall in blast population is of little importance, or that the intermittent dosages of asparaginase given during the maintenance period are insufficient to control the development of blast cells. The resistance of these cells appears to be due to compensatory mechanisms that allow the synthesis of L-asparagine.

These remarks apply equally to acute myeloblastic leukemia, where sensitivity to asparaginase is unusual without being exceptional. We have observed two complete remissions in 6 patients. The leukemia, in these instances, was of poorly differentiated type. HARRIS and FREIREICH have observed only one remission in 10 patients [11].

Is L-asparaginase active against only a fraction of malignant population? Does it spare the normal cells?

One recalls that L-asparaginase experimentally inhibits the first wave of mitosis of the normal liver and spleen, in animals subjected to a partial hepatectomy; in vitro incubation for 7 days with asparaginase destroys 70% of lymphoblasts and 34% of normal lymphocytes [26]; finally, L-asparaginase administered to New Zealand white rats on the 8th and 9th days of gestation increases the percentage of foetal resorptions and congenital malformations. In the chapter on toxicity we have commented on the hepatic disorders caused by L-asparaginase in numerous patients; fatal liver damage was observed in two patients at the beginning of our own study; actually earlier interruption of treatment has shown us that in the others the hepatic changes were always reversible.

Unlike other authors, we have never observed either pancreatic toxicity nor, more especially, a cerebral toxic effect. This difference can be due to the different methods of purification of L-asparaginase.

From this study, one must conclude that L-asparaginase used alone as induction and maintenance treatment is only partially efficacious; and that it may be toxic. Its future, apart from its theoretical interest, appears therefore to lie in its use in combination with other agents.

Experimental [18] and clinical studies have been conducted with combinations of L-asparaginase and other anti-leukemic agents. Among the glutamic acid antagonists, azaserine and azatomycine have not proved interesting. On the other hand, DON (6-diazo-5-oxonorleucine) has shown an additive effect with L-asparaginase on experimental tumors.

In acute leukemia in relapses we have used a simultaneous combination of corticotherapy, weekly injections of vincristine, daunorubicin, and asparaginase. With this we have seen more frequent and more rapid remissions than those obtained in analogous circumstances with the same combination without L-asparaginase. Other combinations, of a sequential nature, are possible and are under study in various centres.

The protein nature of L-asparaginase makes one think that asparaginase can never be used for maintenance treatment because of the immunological reactions which it evokes. Can asparaginase be used for reinduction treatment? Although intermittent treatment creates favourable conditions for immunisation, we have actually been able to give reinduction therapy including L-asparaginase to 27 patients suffering from acute lymphoblastic leukemia in relapse.

Hypersensitivity was observed in 3 patients. Putting off the start of administration of asparaginase for 48 hours in relation to the start of corticotherapy or even in relation to the first infusion of vincristine or daunorubicin, appears to be sufficient to prevent these incidents.

Our experience is too preliminary, however, to assess the potential of L-asparaginase for reinductions.

The present treatment of acute myeloblastic leukemia is accompanied by a high mortality during induction, because of the frequency and severity of aplasia caused in this form of disease by active treatment, particularly with daunorubicin. The combination with daunorubicin of a drug whose bone marrow depressing activity is less marked would be of interest; finally it may be that the granular blast cells are not totally independent of asparagine in the majority of cases. Our present experience does not allow us to come to any conclusion in this matter.

In conclusion: L-asparaginase does not only constitute an advance of great biological interest, but it also represents an important approach to the treatment of acute leukemia. The results of studies going on at present will help to define the best way of using L-asparaginase.

Summary

Study of 84 cases of acute leukemia treated with L-asparaginase.

In acute lymphoblastic leukemia, asparaginase given alone induced complete remissions in 13 of 34 patients. The combination of L-asparaginase, prednisone, vincristine and daunorubicin, given to patients with acute lymphoblastic leukemia in relapse, produced remissions in 10 of 13 cases.

In acute myeloblastic leukemia treatment with L-asparaginase alone resulted in a complete remission in two of six cases. The combination of L-asparaginase, daunorubicin and methotrexate gave remissions in 5 of 8 cases.

Regression of areas of involvement in the central nervous system and meninges was obtained in three cases when asparaginase was given intravenously. Liver functions were disturbed frequently, the liver function tests have to be followed carefully. A fall in the level of circulating fibrinogen was found in 90% of the cases where fibrinogen was determined.

It would seem that asparaginase should be given in combination with other chemotherapeutic agents, but the details of combination therapy with L-asparaginase are still under debate.

References

1. Adamson, R. M., Fabros: Antitumor activity and other biologic properties of L-asparaginase, a revue. Cancer Chemother. Rep. **52**, 6 (1968).
2. Bernard, J., Boiron, M., Jacquillat, Cl., Najean, Y., Weil, M., Thomas, M.: Traitement des leucémies aigues lymphoblastiques de première atteinte par une association de Prednisone-Vincristine-Rubidomycine. Colloque International sur la Rubidomycine et la Daunomycine Paris Hôpital Saint-Louis 11, mars 1967. Path. et Biol. **15**, 915—920 (1967).
3. Boiron, M., Jacquillat, Cl., Weil, M., Tanzer, J., Bernard, J.: L-asparaginase. Presse. méd. **76**, 44, 2095—2101 (1968).
4. Broome, J. D.: Evidence that the L-asparaginase activity of Guinea Pig Serum is responsible for ills antilymphoma effects. Nature (Lond.) **191**, 1114—1115 (1961).
5. — Factors which may influence the effectiveness of L-asparaginase as Tumor inhibitors. Brit. J. Cancer **XXII**, 595 (1968).
6. Burchenal, J. H., Oettgen, H. F.: Present states of L-asparaginase. Med. News (N. Y.), June 1968.
7. Canellos, G. P., Haskell, C. M., Arseneau, J., Carbone, P.: Hypoalbuminemic and hypocholesterolemic Effect of L-asparaginase (NSX-109229) Treatment on man: a preliminary report. Cancer Chemother. Rep. (in press).
8. Dolowy, Coll: Toxic and antineoplastic effects of L-asparaginase. Cancer Res. **19**, 1813—1819 (1966).
9. Gralnick, H. R., Henry, P. H.: L-asparaginase induced coagulopathy. Proc. Amer. Ass. Cancer Res. **123**, 32 (1969).
10. Grundmann, E.: L-asparaginase und Leukämie. Klin. Wschr. **2**, 61—64 (1969).
11. Harris, J. E., Whitecar, J. P., Bobey, G. P., Freireich, E. J.: L-asparaginase (ASP) in the treatment of adult acute leukemia. Proc. Amer. Ass. Cancer Res. **136**, 35 (1969).
12. Haskell, C. M., Canellos, G. P.: Mechanisms of L-asparaginase resistance: asparagine synthetase in animal and human neoplasma. Proc. Amer. Ass. Cancer Res. **142**, 36 (1969).
13. — — Leventhal, B. G., Carbone, P.: L-asparaginase toxicity. Cancer Res. **29**, 974—975 (1969).

14. Hill, J. M., Loeb, E., Roberts, J., MacLellan, A., Khan, A., Hill, N. O.: L-asparaginase therapy of Leukemia. Program of the XII Congress of the International Society of Hematology New York, (Abstract) 8 (1968).
15. — Robert, J., Loeb, E., Khan, A., MacLellan, A., Hill, R. W.: L-asparaginase therapy for leukemia and other malignant neoplasma. J. Amer. med. Ass. **202**, 882—888 (1967).
16. Ho, D. H., Frei, E.: Clinical Pharmacologic studies of L-asparaginase. Proc. Amer. Ass. Cancer Res. **151**, 39 (1969).
17. Kidd, J. G.: Regression of transplanted lymphomas induced in vivo by means of normal guinea pig serum: I. Course of transplanted cancers of various kinds on mice and rats given guinea pig serum, horse serum or rabbit serum. J. exp. Med. **98**, 565—582 (1953).
18. Jacobs, S. P., Wodinsky, I., Kensler, C. J., Venditti, J., Little, A. D.: Therapy of experimental leukemias with combinations of L-asparagine and glutamine antagonists. Proc. Amer. Ass. Cancer Res. **168**, 43 (1969).
19. Lash, E., Schwartz, M. K., Tallal, L., Oettgen, H. F.: Serum lipids in patients receiving L-asparaginase. Program of the XII congress of International Society of Hematology. New York (Abstract) 10, 1968.
20. Leventhal, B. G.: Asparaginase plus Azaserine in Acute lymphatic leukemia. Proc. Amer. Ass. Cancer Res. **193**, 49 (1969).
21. Mashburn, L. T., Wriston, J. C., Jr.: Tumor inhibitory effect of L-asparaginase from Escherichia coli. Arch. Biochem. **105**, 451—452 (1964).
22. Mathé, G., Amiel, J. L., Schwartzenberg, L., Schneider, M., Cattan, A., Schlumberger, J. R., Hayart, M., de Vassai, F., Jasmin, C., Rosenfeld, C.: Essai de traitement de la leucémie aigue lymphoblastique par la L-asparaginase. Presse méd. **77**, 461—463 (1968).
23. Oettgen, H. F.: Inhibition of leukemias in man by L-asparaginase. Cancer Res. **27**, 2619—2631 (1967).
24. — Plasma levels of L-asparaginase. Cancer Res. **27**, 2630 (1967).
25. — Therapeutic effects of L-asparaginase on asparagine-dependent neoplasmas laboratory and clinical studies. J. Clin. Invest. **47**, 74 a (1968).
26. — Schulten, H. K.: Hemmuning maligner neoplasien des Menschen durch L-asparaginase. Klin. Wschr. **2**, 65—71 (1969).
27. Ohnuma, T., Holland, J. F., Freeman, A., Sinks, L.: Studies of asparaginase and asparagine in acute leukemia. Proc. Amer. Ass. Cancer Res. **262**, 66 (1969).
28. Schmidt, C. G., Gallmeier, W. M.: Zur Enzymtherapie der Leukämien. Dtsch. med. Wschr. **48**, 2299 (1968).
29. Sobin, L. H., Kidd, J. G.: A metabolic difference between two lines of lymphoma 6C3HED cells in relation to asparagine. Proc. Soc. exp. Biol. (N. Y.) **119**, 325—327 (1965).
30. Tallal, L., Tan, C., Oettgen, H. F., Mac Carty, M., Helson, L., Murphy, L.: L-asparaginase in 111 children with leukemias and solids tumors. Proc. Amer. Ass. Cancer Res. **394**, 92 (1969).
31. — Oettgen, H. F.: Treatment of acute leukemia in children with L-asparaginase. Proc. Amer. Soc. Cancer Res. **9**, 70 (1968).
32. Tan, C., Oettgen, H. F.: Clinical experience with L-asparaginase administrated intrathecally. Proc. Amer. Ass. Cancer Res. **365**, 92 (1969).
33. Tarmowski, G. S., Mointain, I. M., Stock, C. C.: Combination therapy of animal tumors with L-asparaginase and glutamine antagonists. Proc. Amer. Ass. Cancer Res. **366**, 92 (1969).
34. Tomas, R. A., Schwartz, M. K., Lash, E., Oettgen, H. F., Krakoff, I. H.: Blood Levels and distribution of L-asparaginase in man. Proc. Amer. Ass. Cancer Res. **371**, 94 (1969).

The Place of the L-Asparaginase in the Treatment of Acute Leukemias

G. MATHÉ, J. L. AMIEL, A. CLARYSSE, M. HAYAT, and L. SCHWARZENBERG

Institut de Cancérologie et d'Immunogénétique, Hôpital Paul-Brousse [1]
et Service d'Hématologie de l'Institut Gustave Roussy [2]

With 3 Figures

L-asparaginase has, within a few months, taken an important place in the chemotherapy of leukemias. This clinical utilisation has confirmed the interest in the drug (MATHE et al., 1969), defined its indications and also its limits; it has made it possible to discover that the enzyme is not without action on normal cells; we shall report the results obtained at Villejuif and dwell on certain secondary effects, which were not pointed out by the first users (BURCHENAL et al., 1968; HILL et al., 1967).

Methods and Patients

Methods

L-asparaginase was administered intravenously at the rate of two daily injections. The doses varied from 400 U/kg/day to 1000 U/kg/day, i. e. 32,000 U/m^2/day. The total dose was not fixed in advance; it was either the maximum tolerated dose, or a dose sufficient to obtain an optimal effect, or determined by objective signs of resistance to the treatment.

Patients

We have carried out 135 courses of treatment with L-asparaginase in 130 patients. The ages of the patients varied from 1 to 62 years. The distribution of the patients is indicated in Table 1.

Therapeutic Results

The results obtained in patients with acute lymphocytic leukemias in the visible phase are shown in Table 2.

[1] 14, Avenue Paul-Vaillant-Couturier, 94-Villejuif, France.
[2] 16 bis, Avenue Paul-Vaillant-Couturier, 94-Villejuif, France.

Table 1. *Patients treated with L-asparaginase*

				Number of patients	No. of courses of treatment
Acute lymphoblastic leukemia	In visible phase	Treated by L-asparaginase alone		28	31
		Treated by L-asparaginase in combination with prednisone, vincristine and rubidomycin		12	12
	In non-visible phase	Treated by asparaginase alone	Not in hypoplastic phase	31	31
			In hypoplastic phase	13	13
		Treated by L-asparaginase in combination with methotrexate		11	11
Acute myeloblastic leukemia	In visible phase	Treated by L-asparaginase alone		3	5
		Treated by L-asparaginase in combination with prednisone, vincristine and rubidomycin		10	10
Blastic crisis	Of chronic myelocytic leukemia			5	5
	Of polycythemia vera			1	1
	Of lymphoblastosarcoma			4	4
Melanosarcomas				12	12
				130	135

Table 2. *L-asparaginase given alone in the treatment of visible phases of acute lymphoblastic leukemia*

Patients	Courses of treatment	Complete remissions
28	31	12 [a]

[a] 3 in 2nd visible phase. 6 in 3rd visible phase. 1 in 6th visible phase. 1 in 9th visible phase. 1 in 10th visible phase.

In 31 courses of treatment in 28 patients we obtained 12 complete remissions (43%). These remissions can occur very late in the evolution of the disease, 3 in the 2nd phase, 6 in the 3rd phase, 1 in the 6th phase, 1 in the 9th phase, 1 in the 10th phase.

L-asparaginase was used in association with prednisone, vincristine and rubidomycin in 12 cases of acute lymphocytic leukemia, which had previously been shown to be resistant to the combination of prednisone and vincristine, with 6 complete remissions in late phase of the disease (4 in the 2nd phase, 1 in the 3rd phase, and 1 in the 4th phase) (Table 3).

With respect to acute myeloblastic leukemia (Table 4), we treated 3 patients with L-asparaginase alone, one of them being a baby of 8 months; this baby had

Table 3. *L-asparaginase given in combination with prednisone (40 mg/m²/d) vincristine (1.5 mg/m²/week) and rubidomycin (30 mg/m²/twice a week in children; 10 mg/m²/twice a week in adult) in acute lymphoblastic leukemia after failure of prednisone + vincristine*

Patients	Courses of treatment	Complete remissions
12	12	6 [a]

[a] 4 in 2nd visible phase. 1 in 4th visible phase. 1 in 3rd visible phase.

Table 4. *L-asparaginase in the treatment of acute myeloblastic leukemia*

	Patients	Courses of treatment	Complete remissions
L-asparaginase alone	3	5 [a]	3 [b]
L-asparaginase given in combination with prednisone, vincristine and rubidomycin	10	10	2

[a] 3 for 8 months old baby. [b] 2 for a 8 months old baby.

3 successive courses of treatment with 2 responses and finally a failure; we obtained a second complete remission in the 3rd phase of the disease in an adult.

10 patients with acute myeloblastic leukemia were treated with a combination of L-asparaginase, prednisone, vincristine and rubidomycin. We observed 2 complete remissions in the 1st phase of the disease.

We have used L-asparaginase in combination with prednisone, vincristine and rubidomycin in 10 cases of transformation into acute leukemia. We have obtained a complete remission in one out of 5 cases of acute transformation of chronic myelocytic leukemia and in 3 out of 4 cases of transformation of lymphoblastosarcoma (Table 5).

The total failure of L-asparaginase in 12 cases of melanosarcoma must be pointed out. L-asparaginase was given in combination with vincristine and methotrexate.

Table 5. *L-asparaginase given in combination with prednisone, vincristine and rubidomycin in the treatment of blastic crises in chronic myelocytic leukemia, polycythemia vera and lymphoblastosarcoma*

Blastic crises in	Patients	Courses of treatment	Complete remissions
Chronic myelocytic leukemia	5	5	1
Polycythemia vera	1	1	
Lymphoblastosarcoma	4	4	3

Secondary Effects and Complications of L-Asparaginase

We have been able to study the side effects under favourable conditions as we have given L-asparaginase alone in 44 cases of acute lymphoblastic leukemias in the non-visible phase of their disease. In 31 cases the differential blood count was practically normal at the beginning of the course of L-asparaginase; in 13 cases the patients were in a hypoplastic state at the beginning of therapy (less than 1000 polynuclear cells/mm^3), which deterred us from using antimitotic agents.

1. Tolerance of L-Asparaginase

In 8 cases we saw an anaphylactic reaction (Table 6). In 4 of these cases the anaphylactic reaction appeared during an attempt to restart treatment with L-asparaginase after a period without treatment, and in 2 cases the reaction appeared during the first course of treatment after 14 and 17 daily injections, respectively, had been tolerated well.

Table 6. *Anaphylactic reactions in asparaginase*

Courses of treatment	Anaphylactic reaction		
	To a second course of treatment	During a first course of treatment	To a first injection of asparaginase
130	4	2	2

In two cases we observed a reaction of the anaphylactic type during the *first* injection of L-asparaginase. In one of these cases the patient had a history of severe asthma during childhood.

We made 3 attempts of desensitization without success.

Nausea was noticed frequently, and once continuous fever was observed which fell when the treatment with L-asparaginase was stopped.

The important point seems to be that the appearance of an anaphylactic reaction destroys all hope of restarting the treatment.

2. Effects on Hematopoiesis

The group of patients treated with L-asparaginase alone in the non-visible phase of the disease allows to assess, in a valid manner, the effect of the preparation on hematopoiesis.

a) In 31 patients having normal blood counts at the beginning of the treatment, there was no alteration of the hemoglobin; we did not see the anemia reported by others. There was a slight decrease in platelet count, but not to a significant degree. Much more striking was the progressive decrease in total white cell count and the absolute neutrophil count. This was a consistent finding. In spite of some times marked neutropenias we did not encounter infectious complications (Table 7).

b) In 13 patients with neutropenia before the beginning of the treatment (median 1410 granulocytes/mm^3) L-asparaginase did not aggravate the pre-existing neutropenia to complete aplasia, as can be seen in Table 8.

Table 7. *Haematological studies during L-asparaginase therapy (10 days L-asparaginase) in 31 cases in remission*

	Median Before	After
Hemoglobin	13.8	14.1
Platelets	195,000	145,000
White blood cells	7,850	3,600
Absolute P.M.N. count	5,150	1,540

Table 8. *L-asparaginase during chemotherapy-induced neutropenia*

	Number of cases	Median granulocyte count Before treatment	After treatment
L-asparaginase alone	8	1410	1430
L-asparaginase + prednisone	5	1380	2050

After treatment with L-asparaginase alone the median granulocyte count was 1430. There was little overall change; most patients remained leukopenic, but they did not become more leukopenic and there were actually 5 patients in whom the neutrophil count increased slightly. Other patients received prednisone simultaneously with L-asparaginase. Here, again, we did not see infectious complications. Thus it seems that L-asparaginase can be safely used in spite of its neutropenia-producing effect, even in leukopenic patients (Table 8).

3. *Effects on Hepatic Function and Particularly on Hemostasis* (Table 9)

These studies were done in 70 patients receiving L-asparaginase alone.

Table 9. *Biochemistries during treatment of 70 patients with L-asparaginase alone*

	Median Before	After
Urea	0.32	0.42 g-‰
Cholesterol	1.97	1.93 g-‰
Alk. phosphatase	10	13 K.A.U.
Bilirub. total	5.3	6.8 mg-‰
S.G.P.T.	40	62 F.U.
S.G.O.T.	20	44 F.U.
O.C.T.	424	488 I.U.
Total serum proteins	64	57 g-‰
Albumin	34.8	28.6 g-‰
Fibrine	3.98	1.8 g-‰

The most significant point was the fall of fibrinogen levels; it was almost constant, except for the visible phase of the disease. The other factors of hemostasis were affected a much less regularly (Fig. 1).

Other hepatic functions were little or not disturbed. In our studies, there was a slight and inconstant decrease of albumin; cholesterol remained normal usually (we noted a case of severe hypocholesterolemia, the cholesterol level fell from 1.40 g/l at the beginning of treatment to 0.48 g/l after 15 days of L-asparaginase 50,000 U/day).

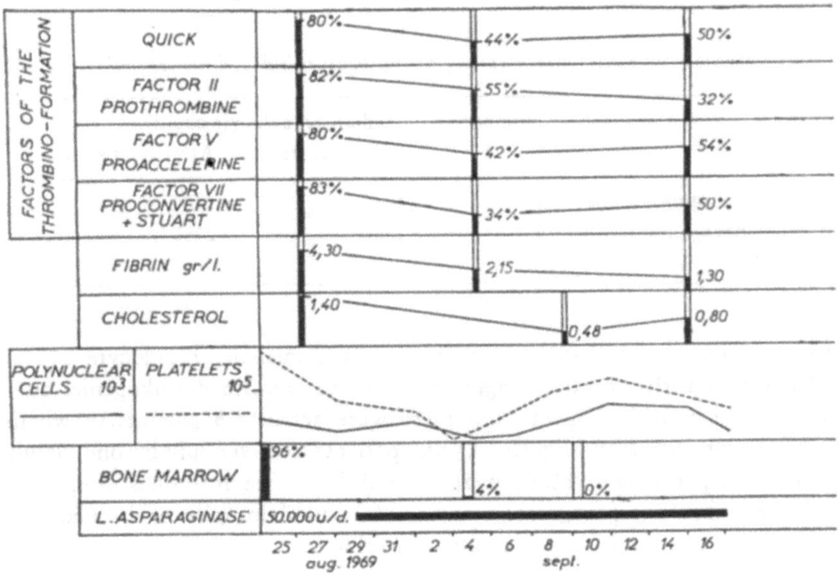

Fig. 1. Effect of L-asparaginase on various factors of hepatic function and hemostasis

4. *Effects on Immunologic Functions*

These are difficult to evaluate directly in man, even in the non-visible phase of leukemia; in fact, the treatment with L-asparaginase follows therapy with immunosuppressive antimitotic agents and the comparison of results obtained before and after treatment with L-asparaginase have therefore little significance. Therefore, we conducted a study in the mouse within the framework of the trial programs of the E.O.R.T.C.

a) Effects on the Reaction to Sheep Red Cells

18 (DBA/2×C57Bl/6)F1 female adult mice were randomised into three groups of 6 mice : A, B, C. Each mouse received 10^9 sheep red cells intraperitoneally on day 0. On day 5, the spleens were removed and the number of plaque forming cells was determined for each spleen (JERNE and NORDIN, 1963).

The mice in group A received 100 units of L-asparaginase intraperitoneally per mouse and per day on days —3, —2 and —1, those in group B on days 1, 2 and 3.

The results are summarized in Table 10.

L-asparaginase given before immunization depresses the immunological reaction; when given after the antigen it is without effect.

Table 10. *Effects of L-asparaginase on the immunologic reaction of mice against sheep red cells*

	Mean number of plaque forming splenic cells
Group A Treated with asparaginase before sheep red cells	14,900
	$P < 0.02$
Group C Controls	43,700
	NS
Group B Treated with asparaginase after sheep red cells	41,700

b) Effects on the Graft-versus-Host Reaction

23 (DBA/2×C57Bl/6) F1 mice were received total body irradiation on day 0 at a dose of 500 rads. They are randomized into two groups. 13 mice of group I received 10^7 bone marrow cells and 2.5×10^7 lymph node cells of adult C57Bl/6 donors I.V. on day 0. 10 mice of group II received the same number of cells from donors pretreated, on days —3, —2, —1, with L-asparaginase, 100 Units/mouse/day, I.P.

The mean survival time in group I was 14.6 days and in group II 19.1 days ($P < 0.05$).

c) Effects on Allogeneic Skin Grafts

15 CBA mice ($H\text{-}2^k$) were randomized into two groups. 6 mice of group I were not treated; 9 mice of group II received 100 Units/mouse/day of L-asparaginase I.P. on days —3, —2, —1. On day 0, every mouse received a skin graft from C57Br donors ($H\text{-}2^k$). The mean survival time of the grafts in the first group was 16.3 days in the second group 19.7 days. The comparison by the non-parametric test w of Wilcoxon shows that the difference is significant.

These results are in good correlation with those of Hobik (1969) showing some immunosuppressive effect of L-asparaginase on the graft-versus-host reaction in rat and mice, and with those of Ohno (1969) showing an inhibition of PHA-induced lymphocyte blastogenesis in vitro by L-asparaginase.

In conclusion our experience allows us to clarify several points.

1. L-asparaginase can induce complete remissions in acute lymphoblastic leukemias at a very late stage of the disease, when resistance to most other chemotherapeutic agents has developed.

Remissions were obtained in 12 of 28 cases, or 43 per cent.

2. L-asparaginase produces leukopenia but hardly aggravates a pre-existing leukopenia. It can therefore be used as complementary chemotherapy of acute leukemia in the non-visible phase during periods of bone marrow hypoplasia.

3. L-asparaginase, when used in combination with prednisone, vincristine and rubidomycin in the visible phase of acute leukemia, or with methotrexate in the non-visible phase, does not seem to add appreciably to the toxicity of antimitotic agents. It can therefore be integrated into the schemes of chemotherapy of acute leukemia.

4. L-asparaginase frequently induces hypersensitivity manifested as anaphylactic shock, most often during the 2nd or 3rd course of treatment, sometimes during the first course of treatment, and sometimes by the first injection. The anaphylactic shock must be distinguished from side effects like anorexia, nauseas, fever. Treatment had to be stopped. Attempts at desensitization were not effective in our experience.

5. L-asparaginase is not without effect on hepatic function. A marked decrease of fibrinogen is observed frequently; however, treatment was discontinued only once due to the hepatic toxicity.

6. L-asparaginase is immunosuppressive, as least in animals; it can not, therefore, be used at the same time as active immunotherapy (AMIEL and BERARDET, 1969).

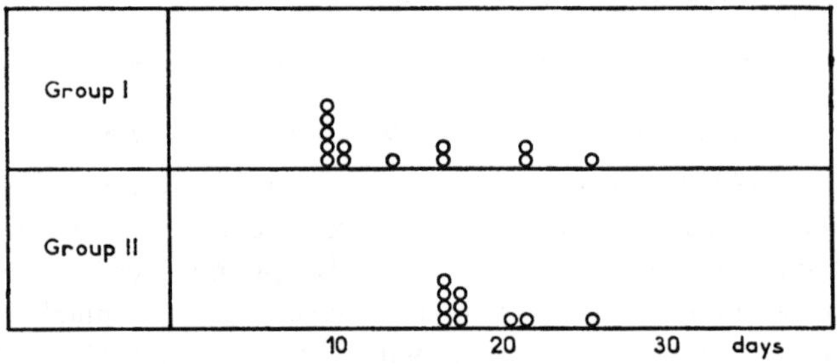

Fig. 2. Effect of L-asparaginase on the graft-versus-host reaction. (DBA/2×C57Bl/6) F1 mice irradiated with 500 rads receiving 10^7 bone marrow cells and 2.5×10^7 lymph node cells from C57Bl/6 donors. Group I: untreated donors. Group II: donors treated with L-asparaginase

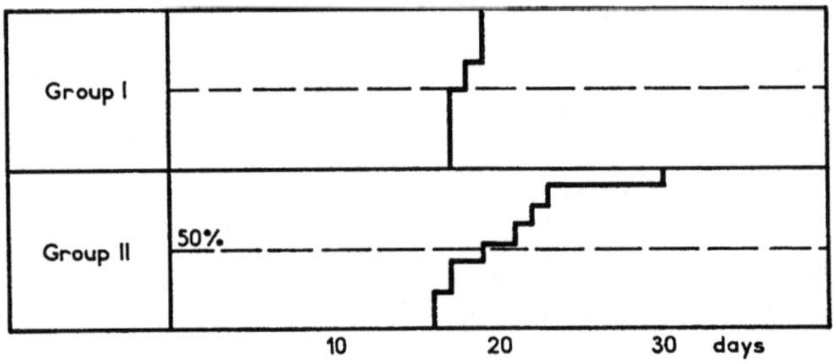

Fig. 3. Effect of L-asparaginase on the survival of allogeneic skin grafts. Recipients CBA. Donors C56Br. Group I: untreated recipients. Group II: recipients pretreated with L-asparaginase

References

AMIEL, J. L., BERARDET, M.: Essai de traitement de la leucémie E ♂ G2 associant chimiothérapie et immunothérapies actives spécifique ou non spécifique. Eev. franç Étud. clin. biol. 14, 685 (1969).

BURCHENAL, J. H., KARNOFSKY, D. A., MURPHY, M. L., OETTGEN, H. F.: Effects of L-asparaginase on leukemia and other neoplasms. In: C. R. XIIe Cong. Int. Soc. Hematol. Vol. 1, p. 7. New York 1968.

HILL, J. M., ROBERTS, J., LOEB, E., KHAN, A., HAYTON, M., HILL, R. W.: L-asparaginase therapy for leukemia and other malignant neoplasms. J. Amer. med. Ass. **202**, 882 (1967).

HOBIK, H. P.: Immunosuppressive Wirkung von L-asparaginase in der Graft-versus-Host-Reaktion. Naturwissenschaften **56**, 217 (1969).

JERNE, N. K., NORDIN, A. A., HENRY, C. C.: The agar plaque technique for recognizing antibody producing cells. In: Cell bound antibodies, p. 109. Philadelphia: Wistar Institute Press 1963.

MATHÉ, G., AMIEL, J. L., SCHWARZENBERG, L., SCHNEIDER, M., CATTAN, A., SCHLUMBERGER, J. R., HAYAT, M., DE VASSAL, F., JASMIN, C., ROSENFELD, C.: Essai de traitement de la leucémie aigue lymphoblastique par la L-asparaginase. Presse méd. **77**, 461 (1969).

OHNO, R.: Inhibition of lymphocyte blastogenesis by L-asparaginase. Proc. Amer. Ass. Cancer Res. **10**, Abstr. 261 (1969).

With Reference to Blastogenesis Inhibition by L-Asparaginase

G. R. Burgio, A. Astaldi, Jr., I. Krč [2], D. Micu [3] and G. Astaldi

The Pediatric Clinic of the University Medical School of Pavia/Italy
and
The Blood Research Foundation Center [1], Tortona Hospital/Italy

With 4 Figures

1. Introduction

The interpretation that L-asparaginase is a selective inhibitor directed only against neoplastic tissues, particularly lymphoid neoplastic tissue, does not seem to be entirely true. In fact:

1.1. Schreck [1] showed that not only leukemic but also normal lymphocytes in culture are damaged if L-asparaginase is added to the medium.

1.2. Broome [2] observed that the content of free asparagine quickly diminishes in the thymus and in the spleen of the C3H mice treated with L-asparaginase.

1.3. It appeared that some rapidly growing tissues are impaired by L-asparaginase. This effect was observed in rabbit embryos and fetuses (Adamson and Fabro [3]), and in the liver of partially hepatectomized rats (Becker and Broome [4], Grundmann [5]), as well as in the proliferation kinetics of human bone marrow in culture (Boll and Reckers [6]). Also the growth of HeLa cells in culture became highly inhibited by EC-2 asparaginase (Oerkermann and Hirschmann [7]).

1.4. Astaldi, Burgio et al. [8] showed that *E. coli* L-asparaginase intensely inhibits blastic transformation of human peripheral blood lymphocytes in the PHA-culture system.

1.5. McElwain and Hayward [9] were then able to show the same effect also when the enzyme is administered i. v., and the lymphocytes are subsequently removed and cultivated in the PHA-medium.

---

[1] Supported by "The Blood Research Foundation", Washington D.C./USA.

[2] Dr. I. Krč is Med. Assistant at the 1st Med. Clin., Univ. Medical School, Olomouc/Czechoslovakia (Director: Prof. P. Lukl). Dr. I. Krč was working with a grant at the Blood Res. Found. Center, Tortona/Italy.

[3] Dr. D. Micu is Chief of the Division on Cytology and Cytochemistry, Institut of Int. Med., Academy of Medicine, Bucarest/Romania (Director: Prof. I. Bruckner). Dr. D. Micu is working with a grant at the Blood Res. Found. Center, Tortona/Italy.

2. Investigations

The enzymatic inhibition of blastogenesis is certainly a fascinating topic, also because it might be connected with a possible immuno-suppressive property of L-asparaginase [10, 11]. Different hypothesis concerning the mechanism of the above-mentioned L-asparaginase inhibition have been suggested. We proposed that human peripheral blood lymphocytes need L-asparagine or other amino-acids essential for their blastic transformation [8]. On the contrary, DARTNALL and BAIKIE [12] have pointed out that the inhibition of blastogenesis caused by L-asparaginase could result from a direct toxic effect of that drug on lymphocytes. Our original interpretation is now strongly supported by the results of the experiments by WEINER et al. [13], and our interpretation that L-asparaginase is an immuno-suppressive agent is also substantiated by the results of SCHULTEN et al. [14].

In any case, it seemed worthwhile to us to investigate some points relating to the blastogenesis inhibition induced by L-asparaginase, such as:

2.1. The relationship between the L-asparaginase dosage and the extent of the lymphocyte blastogenesis inhibition in the PHA-culture.

2.2. The time after the onset of culture at which the addition of the enzyme can still induce the inhibition.

2.3. Whether L-asparaginase might inhibit PHA-blastogenesis by acting as an antagonist of the PHA itself.

2.4. Whether L-asparaginase inhibits only PHA-blastogenesis, or also that caused by other agents such as mitogen pokeweed, which stimulates lymphocytes similarly to PHA, as well as the blastogenesis which occurs in a more specific immunological system, such as that of the mixed lymphocyte cultures. The latter is in fact taken into account as a histo-compatibility test.

2.5. The behaviour of blastogenesis inhibition of lymphocytes periodically removed from subjects after i. v. administration of L-asparaginase.

2.6. Whether L-asparaginase brings about its effect directly on lymphocytes (viz., by damaging these cells primarily), or via a serum action (viz., by the presence of the inhibiting agent in the serum).

2.7. Whether the addition to the L-asparaginase PHA-culture medium of some important amino-acids decreases the inhibiting effect of the above-mentioned enzyme on the lymphocyte blastogenesis.

3. Results

According to the results of our investigation, we could answer the above-mentioned questions as follows:

3.1. One IU of L-asparaginase/ml of culture medium is effective in causing the maximum extent of blastogenesis inhibition. In fact, the above-mentioned enzyme dosage causes degrees of inhibition not significantly different from the extents of inhibition caused by doses of 5—10 IU of L-asparaginase/ml culture medium. Quantities up to 0.1 IU/ml are in general practically ineffective, whereas the dose of 0.5 IU/ml gives about 50% of the maximum extent of inhibition (Table 1). Furthermore, the S.D. with a dose of 0.5 IU is quite high, thus showing that different

L-asparaginase sensitivity does exist among the lymphocytes from the different donors.

3.2. The addition of L-asparaginase to the lymphocyte culture, either at the very beginning of the culture or at any time within one hour after its onset, causes the maximum extent of blastogenesis inhibition. This inhibition is still high when the culture is added to the enzyme 6 hours after the onset of incubation. Then, the increase in the extent of blastogenesis parallels the delay in the addition of the enzyme to the culture. In other words, the blastic transforming process was stopped approximately at the extent reached at the time the enzyme was added to the culture (Table 2). The fact that L-asparaginase is completely inhibitory for blastogenesis still one hour after the onset of the PHA-culture suggests that the enzyme inhibits the blastic transformation of lymphocytes not only via a cell surface mechanism, but also by acting via a metabolic mechanism.

Table 1. *Percentages of activated lymphocytes in the 3-day PHA-cultures added to different doses of E. coli L-asparaginase in respect to the control PHA-cultures taken as 100*

Asparaginase doses (IU/ml)	0.00 Control	0.01	0.05	0.10	0.50	1.00	2.50	5.00	10.00
Per cent of activated Lymphocytes	100	88.3 ± 9.1	87.8 ± 11.1	87.7 ± 13.3	34.0 ± 23.0	11.0 ± 3.1	7.8 ± 1.9	8.5 ± 1.9	5.9 ± 0.6

Table 2. *Percentages of activated lymphocytes in the 3-day PHA-cultures added to E. coli L-asparaginase at different hours from the onset of culture in respect to the control PHA-cultures taken as 100*

Time of asparaginase addition	0 hr (onset of culture)	1 hr	6 hrs	12 hrs	24 hrs	36 hrs	48 hrs	No Asp. add. (control)
Per cent of activated Lymphocytes	5.3 ± 1.9	4.4 ± 1.5	17.0 ± 5.1	43.4 ± 12.3	60.3 ± 10.6	70.9 ± 12.5	80.2 ± 10.0	100

3.3. The lymphocyte cultures to which to 1—10 IU of L-asparaginase/ml of culture medium were added always showed the same maximum effect of blastogenesis inhibition with different doses of PHA [15]. The following doses of PHA were tested; the standard PHA dose of 0.01 mg/ml of culture medium as well as 2, 4, 8, and 16 times the above-mentioned standard dose. The results here mentioned suggest that no antagonism takes place in the L-asparaginase inhibition of PHA-blastogenesis. (In this experiment, as well as in all the other experiments mentioned in this paper, PHA x 5 was employed and it was a highly purified non-commercial product.)

3.4. The experiment carried out with the addition of L-asparaginase to cultures with mitogen pokeweed showed that this enzyme definitely also inhibits the pokeweed blastogenesis (Fig. 1). Furthermore, experiments studying the effect of L-asparaginase on the lymphocyte blastogenesis occurring in the mixed cultures showed that the tested enzyme has the capacity to inhibit this type of blastogenesis. This latter study was carried out on 14 normal volunteers whose peripheral blood lymphocytes were randomly mixed in pairs and put into L-asparaginase cell culture (1 IU of L-asparaginase/ml culture medium). The observation made after 7 days of culture incubation showed an extent of $16.8 \pm 7.8\%$ immunologically activated lymphocytes in the control mixed cultures, whereas the extent of the activated lymphocytes was $0.6 \pm 0.14\%$ in the same cultures when 1 IU of *E. coli* L-asparaginase/ml of culture medium was added (Fig. 2).

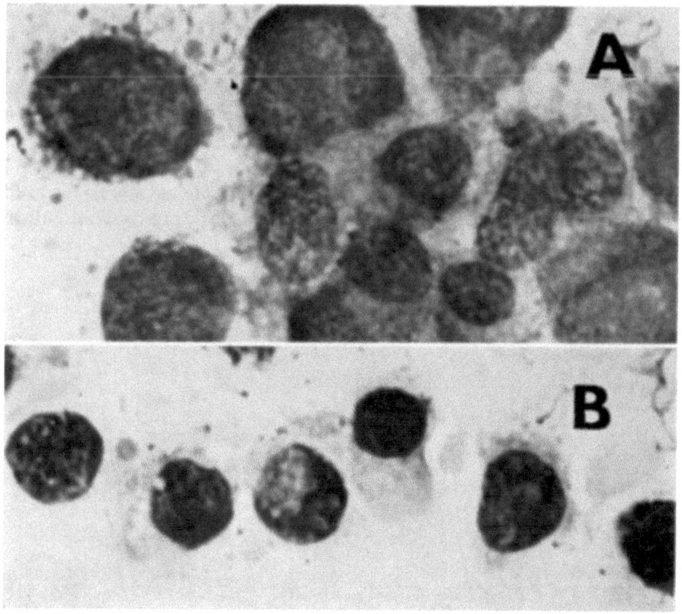

Fig. 1. Normal blastogenesis in the 3-day mitogen pokeweed cultures (A) and inhibition of blastogenesis in the same cultures by 1 IU of *E. coli* L-asparaginase/ml culture medium (B)

3.5. Daily culture controls of the PHA-responsiveness of the blood lymphocytes removed from volunteers injected i. v. with a single dose of L-asparaginase (800 IU/kg b. w.) showed that they remain PHA-*non* responsive for several days (Fig. 3).

3.6. Cross experiments carried out on normal volunteers [16] showed that: a) peripheral blood lymphocytes from i. v.-asparaginase injected subjects set up in a PHA-culture medium with blood serum from non-injected subjects undergo a normal extent of blastogenesis; and b) peripheral-blood lymphocytes from non-injected subjects set up into PHA-culture medium added to blood serum from i. v. asparaginase-injected subjects are inhibited in their blastic transformation (Fig. 4).

This study was carried out on 6 pairs of normal volunteers. They were injected with a single dose of 800 IU of L-asparaginase/kg b. w. and the lymphocytes, respectively the serum, were removed 1—2 days after the enzyme administration.

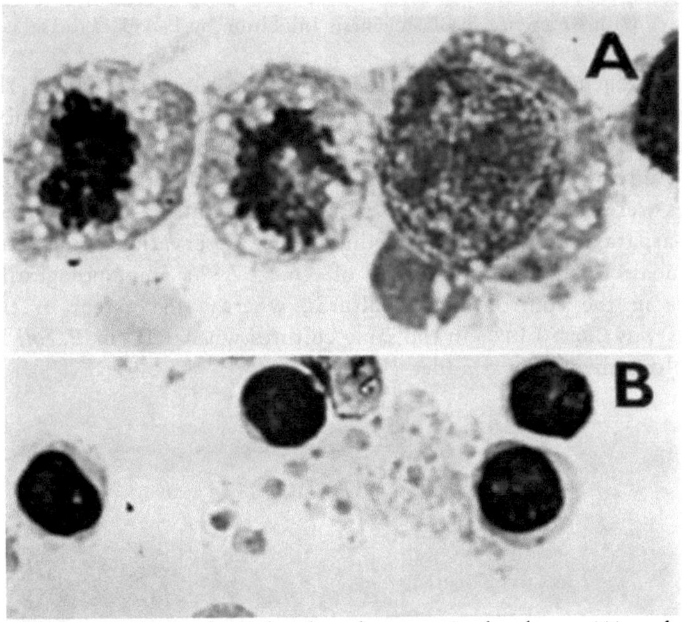

Fig. 2. Normal blastogenesis in the 7-day lymphocyte mixed cultures (A) and inhibition of blastogenesis in the same cultures by 1 IU of *E. coli* L-asparaginase/ml culture medium

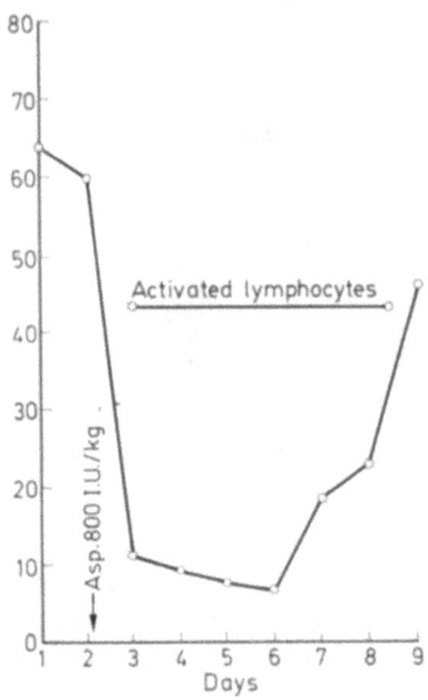

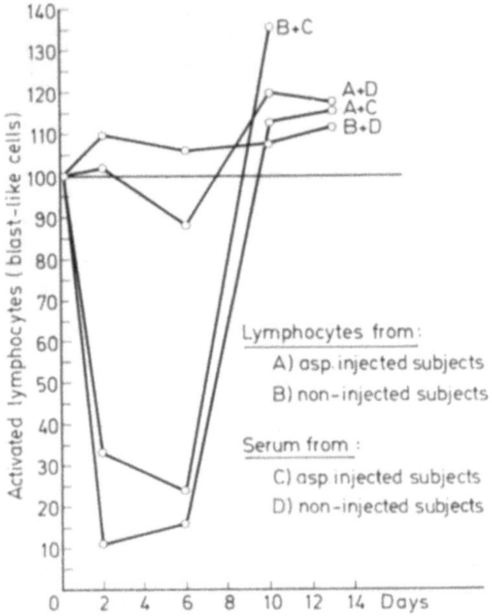

Fig. 3.

Fig. 4.

Fig. 3. Behaviour of the PHA-responsiveness of blood lymphocytes daily removed from a volunteer after i. v. injection of *E. coli* L-asparaginase

Fig. 4. Behaviour of the PHA-responsiveness of: 1) blood lymphocytes removed from volunteers after i. v. injection of *E. coli* L-asparaginase and cultivated in autologous [A+C] and heterologous serum [A+D] and 2) blood lymphocytes from non-injected subjects cultivated in serum obtained from volunteers injected i. v. with *E. coli* L-asparaginase [B+C]. Initial values taken as 100

In both types of cultures the serum was added in the quantity of 20% to the total culture medium.

These results suggest that lymphocytes from asparaginase-injected volunteers were not damaged in respect to their capacity of PHA-blastogenesis, but that blastogenesis was inhibited just by the asparaginase present in the serum of the injected subjects.

3.7. The addition of some important amino-acids to the L-asparaginase PHA-cultures produced an increase of the lymphocyte blastogenesis. Doses of 1—5 mg of glutamine/ml of culture medium, of 0.5—1 mg of asparagine, and of 0.2 mg of aspartic acid were tested in this experiment, carried out on the lymphocytes from 9 to 18 different donors for each aminoacid. The results of this study are shown in Table 3.

Table 3. *Percentages of activated lymphocytes in the 3-day L-asparaginase PHA-cultures supplemented with some aminoacids (control PHA-cultures taken as 100)*

	Without L-asparaginase	With L-asparaginase 1 IU/ml	5—10 IU/ml
PHA alone (control)	100	2.9 ± 2.7	
PHA + Glutamine (1—5 mg/ml)	86.0 ± 15.3	31.3 ± 16.7	28.3 ± 14.8
PHA + Asparagine (0.5—1 mg/ml)	86.5 ± 13.0	28.3 ± 18.5	24.0 ± 5.3
PHA + Aspartic ac. (0.2 mg/ml)	84.3 ± 11.0	24.8 ± 18.6	15.2 ± 5.7

It shows that each of the above-mentioned amino-acids may reduce the L-asparaginase inhibition of the lymphocyte blastogenesis. Nevertheless, it is quite clear that none of the tested aminoacids, at least at the doses we employed, can reverse completely the blastogenesis-inhibiting effect of L-asparaginase. This might depend on the fact that L-asparaginase was still present in the culture medium. In other words, the enzyme preparation contained in the culture system had to be continuously depleting asparagine, and not only the asparagine content of the original medium, but also—at least in part—the quantity of asparagine and/or asparagine-precursors which were added to the medium in that experiment.

4. Conclusions

From the results, taken as a whole, it appears that:

L-asparaginase causes marked inhibition of the blastogenic transforming process of human peripheral blood lymphocytes in cell culture.

The above-mentioned inhibition happens either when lymphocytes are stimulated with PHA or mitogen pokeweed, as well as in the mixed lymphocytes cultures.

The dose of 1 IU of L-asparaginase/ml culture medium is effective in causing the maximum extent of blastogenesis inhibition, and similar results are obtained with higher doses, such as 5—10 IU. On the other hand, the dose of 0.5 IU/ml gives about 50% of the maximum extent of inhibition, whereas the dose of 0.1 IU/ml is practically ineffective.

L-asparaginase is completely inhibitory for blastogenesis not only when added at the very beginning of the culture, but also when added any time within one hour after the onset of the culture. This suggests that the enzyme inhibits blastogenesis not, or not only, via a cell surface mechanism, but also by acting via a cellular metabolic mechanism.

Lymphocyte blastogenesis is inhibited also when L-asparaginase is administered i. v., and lymphocytes are removed and put into the PHA-cell culture system.

The i. v. L-asparaginase administration does not damage human blood lymphocytes in respect of their capacity of PHA-blastogenesis. In fact, these lymphocytes put into PHA-cell culture added to serum from subjects not injected with L-asparaginase, do undergo blastogenesis to normal extents.

The addition to the L-asparaginase PHA-cultures of doses of 1—5 mg glutamine/ml culture medium or of 0.5—1 mg of asparagine, or of 0.2 mg of aspartic acid partially restores lymphocyte blastogenesis. Nevertheless, complete reversal of the blastogenesis-inhibiting effect of L-asparaginase was never obtained.

Acknowledgment

We wish to thank Dr. J. M. HILL, Wadley Institutes of Molecular Medicine, Dallas/Texas, USA, for his kind supply of *E. coli* L-asparaginase, and Dr. A. H. GRIFFITH, Clinical Res. Dep., Wellcome Res. Lab., Langley, Beckenham, Kent/U.K., for his kind supply of the purified PHA compound.

These studies were carried out in part with a grant from "A. NATTERMANN", Cologne-Braunsfeld, Germany.

References

1. SCHRECK, R., DOLOWY, W. C., AMMERAAL, R. N.: L-asparaginase: Toxicity on normal and leukemic human lymphocytes. Science **155**, 329 (1967).
2. BROOME, J. D.: Studies on the mechanism of tumor inhibition by L-asparaginase. Effects of the enzyme on asparagine levels in the blood, normal tissues, and 6C3HED lymphomas of mice: Differences in asparagine formation and ultilization in asparaginase-sensitive and -resistant lymphoma cells. J. exp. Med. **127**, 1055 (1968).
3. ADAMSON, R. H., FABRO, S.: Embryotoxic effect of L-asparaginase. Nature (Lond.) **218**, 1164 (1968).
4. BECKER, F. F., BROOME, J. D.: L-asparaginase: Inhibition of early mitosis in regenerating rat liver. Science **156**, 1602 (1967).
5. GRUNDMANN, E., SEIDEL, H. J.: Die reparative Parenchymregeneration am Beispiel der Leber nach Teilhepatektomie. Hdbch. allgem. Pathol. Bd. VI/2. Springer-Verlag Berlin, Heidelberg, New York 1969, S. 129—243.
6. BOLL, I., RECKERS, V.: Die Beeinflussung der Proliferationskinetik normalen menschlichen Knochenmarks in vitro durch L-asparaginase. Paper delivered at the Internationale Arbeitstagung über Chemo- und Immunotherapie der Leukosen und malignen Lymphome. Wien, March 24—26, 1969.
7. OEKERMANN, H., HIRSCHMANN, W. D.: Experimentelle Untersuchungen zur Wirkung der Asparaginase. Paper delivered at the Internationale Arbeitstagung über Chemo- und Immunotherapie der Leukosen und malignen Lymphome. Wien, March 24—26, 1969.
8. ASTALDI, G., BURGIO, G. R., KRČ, I., GENOVA, R., ASTALDI, A. A., JR.: L-asparaginase and Blastogenesis. Lancet **1969 I**, 423.

9. McElvain, T. J., Hayward, S. K.: L-asparaginase and Blastogenesis. Lancet **1969 I,** 527.
10. Astaldi, G., Burgio, G. R., Krč, I., Astaldi, A., Jr., Krčova, V., Genova, R.: L-asparaginase as an inhibitor of the blastic transformation of human lymphocytes in cell culture. 7th Meeting of Tissue and Organ Culture Study Group of the Eur. Com. for Hum. Tumor Caract. Prague 1969, May 7th. Published in: Med. Klinik **65,** 451 (1970),
11. Astaldi, A., Jr., Burgio, G. R., Krč, I., Genova, R., Astaldi, G.: Inhibition of the PHA-response by L-asparaginase. Discussion at the workshop session: Effect of inhibitors and cell derived factors on blastogenesis. The 4th Leukocyte Culture Conference (Abstracts). Dartmouth Med. School, Hanover, N.H., USA, June 26—28, 1969. Published in: Haematologia (Hungarica) **3,** 395 (1969).
12. Dartnall, J. A., Baikie, A. G.: L-asparaginase and blastogenesis. Lancet **1969 I,** 1098.
13. Weiner, W. S., Waithe, W. J., Hirschhorn, K.: L-asparaginase and blastogenesis. Lancet **1969 II,** 748.
14. Schulten, H. K., Giraldo, G., Boise, E. A., Oettgen, H. F.: Immunosuppressive action of L-asparaginase. Lancet **1969 II,** 644.
15. Ferfoglia, L., Astaldi, A., Jr., Krč, I., Biscatti, G.: Could L-asparaginase be an antagonist of phytohaemagglutinin? Abstract Book of the Vth Congr. Asian-Pacific Soc. Haematol. Sept. 1—6, 1969. Istanbul/Turkey.
16. Astaldi, G., Burgio, G. R., Biscatti, G., Astaldi, A., Jr., Ferfoglia, L.: L-asparaginase and blastogenesis. Lancet **1969 II,** 643.

Some Clinical Observations on the Treatment with L-Asparaginase of the Acute Leukemias

A. M. Marmont and E. E. Damasio

Centre of Haematology and II Medical Division
Ospedali Civili Genova-Sampierdarena, Italy

With 9 Figures

Introduction and Review of the Literature

The history of this new type of enzymatic depletion of the amino acid asparagine, which has been shown to be indispensable for the growth most particularly of the early cellular stages of the lymphatic system and, to a lesser degree, of some other tissues, has passed through several distinct investigational phases. The first stage was, characteristically, purely biological, starting with Clementi's [17] preliminary report in 1922 of the richness in asparaginase of guinea pig serum, comprising Kidd's [30] pioneering observations in 1953 on the suppression of certain transplanted lymphomas of mice and rats by guinea pig serum and finally including Broome's [13] experimental demonstration that the enzyme L-asparaginase (L-ase) was the growth-inhibitory fraction of guinea pig serum, a finding later confirmed by the demonstration by Mashburn and Wriston [34] that L-ase derived from *Escherichia coli* had the same effect as that from guinea pig serum. This important discovery, together with the additional demonstration that L-ase derived from *E. coli* exists in two forms, known as EC-1 and EC-2 [16], of which only the second was active against 6C3HED lymphoma in mice [39, 40], opened up the possibility of large-scale production for clinical trials.

The commencement of the second phase may be traced to Hill's [25] and Old's [36] treatment of dog lymphosarcoma with L-ase. Leaving apart the endeavour to treated a case of acute leukemia (AL) with L-ase-rich agouti serum (de Barros et al. [18]), the first human patient with AL to receive L-ase is apparently the patient reported by Dolowy et al. [20] in 1966, in whom some laboratory and clinical improvement was noted. Soon after (1967) Hill and co-workers [27] reported the favourable results obtained in 3 cases of acute lymphoblastic leukemia (ALL). These investigators already made use of an *in vitro* test of asparagine dependency, adapted from the C^{14}—tagged L-valine procedure described by Sobin and Kidd [46], subsequently modified by Gallmeier et al. [21], and described the development of clinical sensitization to L-ase. In the same year there appeared an important report by Oettgen et al. [38], reporting on the results obtained in 9 patients, 2 of whom with lymphosarcoma (LSA), 4 with ALL and 3 with acute myeloblastic leukemia (AML). An inhibitory effect on the leukemic process was found in all 4 cases of ALL, in 1 of the 3 patients with AML and in none of the patients with LSA. In their material there was good agreement between the *in vitro* L-ase dependency tests and the clinical outcome following L-ase administration. Perusal of their charts shows the abruptness of lymphoblastic fall and serum uric acid augmentation in the responsive cases.

Subsequently, in a series of papers presented at the XII Congress of the International Society of Hematology (New York 1968), other important aspects and results could be established. It could be conclusively demonstrated that asparagine blood levels decreased very rapidly at the start of treatment in patients with L-ase, falling to zero when relatively high levels of enzyme were present [41]. In transplanted mouse leukemia it was found that L-ase, in contrast with conventional agents such as cyclophosphamide, was more effective in a single dose on days 5 or 7 than on day 0, producing a doubling of survival time at a time when bioassay demonstrated large numbers of leukemic cells in the brain tissue [14]. Injections of L-ase were markedly effective against intracerebrally inoculated leukemia [14], and a synergistic effect between L-ase and BCNU, VLB and C-ARA could be demonstrated [15].

Clinically, the much greater responsiveness of ALL could be confirmed on a larger material; however, it was claimed by Hill's group [26] that similar results could be also obtained in AML by augmenting most markedly (up to 50 times and to 18,000 IU/kg) administration schedules. The initial hopes of disposing of a long-awaited chemotherapeutic agent in diffusing malignant melanoma (MM), which has been founded on a solitary responsive case, had to be abandoned in view of the consistent negative results in all the other cases [15]. Also the blastic transformation of chronic myelogenous leukemia (CML-Bl. T.) proved to be refractory to L-ase, with very few exceptions. The topics of pharmacologic impurities, clinical side-effects and sensitization phenomena all received great interest, but will be gone into later.

A third phase in the clinical (and biological) investigations with L-ase has started with the always greater large-scale production of the enzyme by comparatively numerous pharmaceutical firms, so that the number of clinical trials has become very large indeed. This phase, which we are living at present, has been initiated in practice with the multicentric clinical trial of the Paul-Ehrlich-Gesellschaft, as recently (March 1969) reported by Begemann [7]. Summing up their experience, 61 cases of ALL were treated with 200 IU/kg of L-ase over a period of more than 14 days ("adequate treatment": since it has been shown that bone marrow remission will not take place before this time), and 19 (33%) went into complete remission. Patients with ALL had a remission rate of 45%, and children with ALL attained a 60% remission rate. A highly interesting finding, which had already been signalled by Schmidt and Gallmeier [43, 44], was that 2 out of 5 patients with acute promyelocytic leukemia (APL) went into remission, thus displaying an initial remission rate of 40%. Contrarywise, no remission at all could be obtained in 14 adequately treated cases of AML and 3 of CML-Bl. T. [7].

When the haematologic parameters of 13 cases of ALL (11 of ALL, 2 of APL) that went into remission after L-ase were compounded in a composite chart, the abruptness and sharpness of the fall of leukemic cells stood out impressively. This was paralleled by a fall of the neutrophil survivors, whose increase started gradually only after two weeks. The platelets showed a slow and moderate decrease over the first week, a moderate increase over the second and a sharp increase subsequently, which appeared to be the most consistent sign of incipient remission. It was confirmed that the disappearance of leukemic cells from the bone marrow took place only after the first two weeks of treatment; however, the most detailed bone marrow studies to date appear to be those of Astaldi et al. [4], who pointed out the appearance of numerous smudge cells in the bone marrow of ALL patients at the beginning of treatment, and the subsequent appearance first of great sheets of erythroblasts and later on of granulocytoblasts and megakaryocytes. They also described the appearance in the bone marrow of "monocyte-like" cells, which however do not appear in the photomicrographs.

The fastness of action of L-ase, its several toxic side-effects and the not infrequent appearance of side-effects all indicate that this enzyme should be considered as a potent induction agent, to be followed by conventional maintenance treatment. However, the interest focussing on the duration of unmaintained remissions as a yardstick for evaluating the degree of destruction of leukemic cells has been conducive to non-administration of maintenance treatment in some L-ase remitters. In a case of ALL treated by Schmidt and Gallmeier [43] the unmaintained remission has lasted more than 14 months.

Among the wide array of side-effects caused by L-ase the most frequent and severe have been shown to depend from a damage of liver function. Hypoalbuminaemia, hypocholesterinaemia, hyperbilirubinaemia, hypergammaglobulinaemia, augmentation of serum transaminases and alkaline phosphatase and fall of the prothrombin complex are all biochemical symptoms of hepatotoxicity, while pancreatic damage has been found in much rarer cases. The hemostatic mechanism appears to be also a primary target of L-ase toxicity, especially as a consequence of the fall of platelets and, even more markedly and consistently, of fibrinogen. Three mechanisms for these changes have been postulated by Stier et al. [47, 48], namely an intravascular coagulation process *("Verbrauchskoagulopathie")*, an activation of fibrinolysis and an impairment of the hepatic biosynthesis of blood clotting factors, especially of fibrinogen.

Finally, other important biologic acquisitions have contributed to ameliorate our present knowledge of the mechanism of action of L-ase. After it had been demonstrated that L-ase-resistant cells and cell-lines are endowed with a high asparagine-synthetase activity, and that the acquisition of resistance is paralleled by an enhancement of asparagine-synthetase, it was assumed that the L-ase sensitivity of the responsive cases of ALL and other neoplastic disease was due to an enzymatic deletion in the genome of these cells [28]. In other words, it was hoped that herein one had at last pinpointed a true metabolic, biochemically-based diversity between normal and leukemic cells, the sensitive leukemia cells being viewed as an auxotrophic mutant [28]. However, it was shown quite early that L-ase inhibited the early wave of mitoses occurring in rat liver approximately 30 hours after hepatectomy [6], and that it exerted embryotoxic effects in NZW mice [1]. In addition, Astaldi et al. [5] demonstrated most conclusively that the PHA-induced blastogenesis of normal human peripheral-blood lymphocytes can be inhibited by L-ase, a finding which is in full agreement with the experimental demonstration that the graft-versus-host reaction, as measured by the spleen-index, is depressed by L-ase [23]. Obviously, there appears to be a whole spectrum of L-ase sensitive tissues and cells, so that one is not dealing with an all-or-none mutation process.

Additional informations may be found in some recent review papers [1, 4, 8, 9, 22, 33, 43].

Materials and Methods

The L-ase used in these clinical studies was an EC2-derived preparation kindly supplied by Bayer Laboratories. The isolation and purification procedures of the enzyme, as well as its biochemical characterization, have been described in two other papers presented at this same Symposium. The specific activity of the preparation was 156 International Units (IU)/mg of protein. Besides the usual pharmacological testing procedures, a skin test was performed in each patient at the start of treatment and every 10 days subsequently by means of an intradermic injection of 100 IU of the enzyme, which was dissolved in 0.9% NaCl. The enzyme preparation was administered by drip intravenous infusion.

No tests for leukemic cells' L-ase requirements *in vitro* were performed because of the lack of the appropriate facilities.

In addition to clinical observations with measurements of liver, spleen, lymph gland and/or tumor masses when present, the following laboratory investigations were performed before, during and after L-ase treatment: haemoglobin determination, red and white corpuscles' enumeration, platelet and reticulocyte counts, bone marrow examination, lymph node needle aspiration, serum and urine uric acid determination, serum glutamic oxaloacetic (GO) and pyruvic (GP) transaminase, alkaline phosphatase, bilirubin, electropherograms, fibrinogen dosage and thrombo-elastograms.

35 patients were treated with L-ase in this study with a total of 38 treatments, since some cases received more than one course in subsequent relapses. Of these, 29 were affected with AL, 2 with LSA and 3 with MM. 19 had ALL; of these, 6 were over 15 years of age ("adults"), and 13 under ("children"); 10 of these last cases were treated by Prof. L. Massimo at the University's Paediatric Department directed by Prof. R. Bulgarelli; their results were kindly placed at our disposal and are accordingly tabulated in Table 1 and Fig. 1. All cases received "adequate" treatments, viz. 14 days or longer, according to the Ehrlich-Gesellschaft's criteria, except 2 cases of ALL: the first of these cases (Fig. 4) was considered a failure despite a treatment of only 4 days for the reasons that will be specified later; the second case received a small dose (200 IU/kg) of L-ase for only 2 days, and is *not* included in any tabulation, but is quoted here because it enabled to make some clinical observations on the enzyme's hepatotoxicity.

Results

1. Remissions and failures. The clinical results of this study are reported on Table 1. Since a consistent percentage of complete remissions was obtained only in the ALL cases, a closer scrutiny of this material seemed justified. It was found

Table 1. *L-asparaginase treatment in 30 cases of acute leukemia and other solid tumors*

Disease	N. cases	Treatments	Complete remissions	Incomplete remissions	Partial failures	Total failures
Acute lymphoblastic leukemia — Adults (> 15 y.)	5	8	2	4	2	—
Acute lymphoblastic leukemia — Children (< 15 y.)	13 [a]	15	10	3	—	2
Acute myeloblastic leukemia	5	5	—	—	1	4
Acute promyelocytic leukemia	4	4	—	—	—	4
Blastic transformation of CML	3	3	—	—	—	3
Lymphoblastic lymphosarcoma	2	2	1	1	—	—
Malignant melanoma (diffuse)	3	3	—	—	—	3

[a] 10 cases treated at the University's Paediatric Clinic.

accordingly that the percentage of complete remissions in the whole clinical material (adults *and* children) amounted to 66.6%, the percentage of children's remissions on the total was 52.7%, of adults' remissions on the total 11.1%, of children's remissions on the children's total 76.9% and of adults' remissions on the adults' total 40%.

In the occasion of this Symposium it was also believed of some interest to put together these results with those obtained in other Italian centres active in the clinical treatment of leukemia: these include, besides those directly concerned in the present study, the Istituto di Patologia Medica Universitaria of Modena (directed by Prof. E. Storti), the Clinica Pediatrica Universitaria of Pavia (directed by Prof. R. Burgio) and the Ospedale Civile of Tortona (directed by Prof. G. Astaldi). The clinical material was assembled in about one year. The L-ase dosage was comprised between 200 and 1000 IU/kg. Two centers (Pavia and Tortona) made use of L-ase prepared in the Wadley Institutes of Molecular Biology of Dallas, U.S.A. In this unofficial tabulation (Table 2) partial and total failures were epitomized under the sole entry "failures". Percentages were affixed when thought to be really significant.

2. *Remission patterns and illustrative case reports.* Without anticipating the comment section, we should here like to describe three different types of remission patterns we have observed in our responsive cases of ALL.

The first occurred exclusively in cases with high to very high peripheral lymphoblastosis, indifferently from age, and was characterized by a precipitous fall of circulating lymphoblasts associated with extreme hyperuricaemia and very high uric acid excretion. A brief summation of a representative case follows.

Table 2

	Cases	Complete remissions	Partial remissions	Failures
ALL	53	24 (45%)	13	16
Other AL	16	1 [a]	1	14 (87%)
CML Bl. Cr.	5			5 (100%)
LSA	5	2	1	2

[a] This was a case of cytochemically confirmed acute monocytic leukemia (Dr. D. QUAGLINO, Modena).

This 32 year old male taxi driver was first admitted to another hospital at the end of november, 1968, because of a swelling of the inguinal lymph nodes. A peak of 36,000 leukocytes×ml was found during this period; diffuse "lymphatic" infiltration of the bone marrow was also found. A diagnosis of chronic lymphatic leukemia was made, and 40 mgrs per day of prednisone over less than one month were given. The patient left the hospital with a normal leukocyte count and with regression of the lymph nodes enlargement, and felt well for a short period.

On January 25, 1969, he was admitted to the Sampierdarena General Hospital with diffuse lymph gland enlargement and moderate splenomegaly. His leukocytes were 200,000× ml, with > 90% small lymphoblasts and almost total lymphoblastic replacement of the bone marrow. A diagnosis of ALL was made, and treatment with L-ase (200 IU/kg) was started on Jan. 29, 1969, and continued as shown on the chart (Fig. 1).

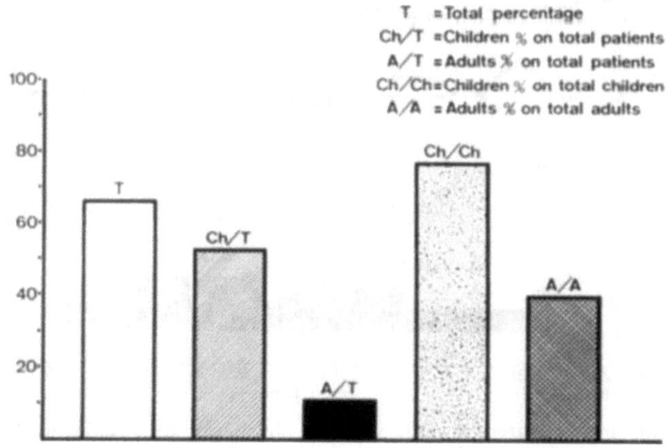

Fig. 1. Percentage of complete remissions obtained in 18 cases of ALL. The greater responsiveness in children is clearly apparent

The absolute circulating lymphoblast count dropped to 1350×ml (from an initial 180,000) in 3 days; the uric acid serum level attained mgs 21%, and 3 Gms in the urines. This case received L-ase for 28 days, went into complete remission and was dismissed with maintenance parental intermittent methotrexate (MTX: 30 mg/m^2) treatment.

The patient did well until July 4, 1969, when he was again admitted because his WBC count had reached 40,000×ml, with 58% lymphoblasts. There was also an extensive lymphoblastic infiltration of the bone marrow. He was again treated with L-ase, this time at the dose of 500 IU/kg. The WBC dropped to 4500×ml on day 6, but on the same day the usual L-ase drip infusion was followed after the first drops by an extremely severe shock, with sudden loss of vision and peripheral pulses and upper airway obstruction. Massive epinephrine and corticosteroid administration were immediately resorted to and proved effective. It may still be mentioned that the circulating WBC were 160,000×ml 2 days after day 6, when L-ase treatment was discontinued, and reached 300,000 4 days later, notwithstanding that 2 mgs of vincristine (VCR) and 40 of daunomycin (DMC) had been given on the 3rd day after the shock, and 1 mg of VCR plus 40 mgs of DMC on the 4th. The subsequent course of this patient was extremely stormy, and a high of 1,000,000 lymphoblasts× ml was observed at some time of the disease. He proved refractory to the conventional

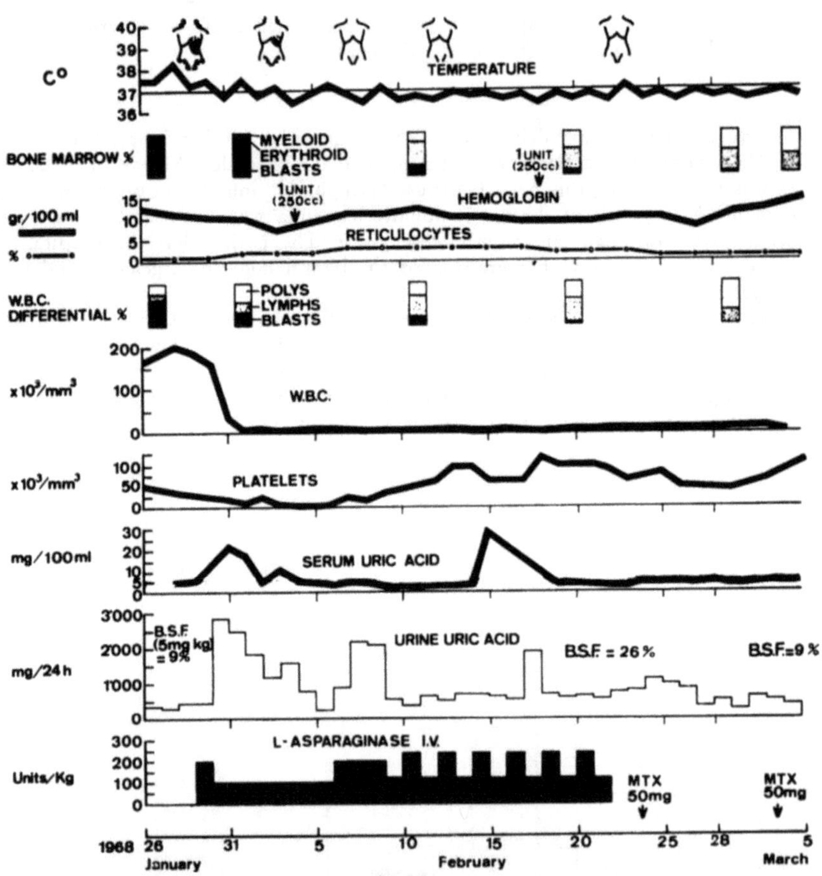

Fig. 2. ALL in an adult treated with L-ase. The sharp fall of circulating lymphoblasts and the high values both of serum and urine uric acid are evident. Because of the limited supply of the drug at that time and in order to avoid dispersing it an alternate "high-low/day" regimen had been instituted. S. S. 33 yr. ♂ acute lymphoblastic leukemia

VCR-DMC-prednisone treatment, to MTX, 6-MP and cyclophosphamide, responding eventually to a course of cytosine arabinoside (C-ARA) at a dosage of mg 3/kg for 7 days. He has been dismissed in complete remission on November 8, 1969, and is on a MTX-6MP maintenance treatment.

The second pattern occurred chiefly in leukopenic ALL in adults, and was characterized by extreme pancytopenia necessitating—at least in our hands—the intermittent discontinuation of treatment. Again, a brief report of an illustrative case follows.

This 28 year old married female was first diagnosed as affected with ALL in August, 1967. In November, 1967 she received the conventional VCR-DMC-prednisone treatment, and achieved an incomplete remission, since there was still a 10% to 20% lymphoblastic infiltration in the bone marrow. She experienced severe jaw pain and polyneuritic dysbasia following VCR. She was subsequently maintained with corticosteroids, MTX and 6-MP and did comparatively well at home for almost all of 1968. On July 24, 1968, a bone marrow examination was essentially normal (M 1). However, at the end of 1968 multiple lymph node enlargements could be felt, skeletal pains, fever and pancytopenia developed, and she was hospitalized and repeatedly treated with VCR-DMC-prednisone, achieving each time incomplete remissions. She was again hospitalized on December 30, 1968, and treated with VCR and prednisone. On January 31st, 1969 her haematocrit was 25%, WBC 3500×ml with 78% lymphoblasts and 37,000 platelets. She was given 200 IU/kg of L-ase on two consecutive days (Jan. 31 and Feb. 1st); the day after (Feb. 2nd) the haematocrit was 27%, WBC 800×ml with a sharp drop of lymphoblasts and platelets 50,000. L-ase treatment was discontinued on the same day, but WBC levels reached their nadir on Feb. 5 (4 days after discontinuation of treatment) with 200 WBC×ml and virtual disappearance of lymphoblasts, and platelets were 60,000×ml, having first gone down to a low 20,000 on Feb. 3rd. Leukopenia under 1000 WBC×ml lasted 9 days; on Feb. 13, with 1000 WBC and 100,000 platelets, treatment with L-ase was resumed for 3 days, and again followed by a leukopenia of 800 WBC with 85,000 platelets. L-ase treatment was however continued for other 21 days, with total disappearance of the enlarged lymph nodes and the obtainance of an incomplete remission, which was subsequently maintained with corticosteroids and MTX.

The patient was again admitted on July 2nd 1969 because of relapse, and treated for 2 days with 300 IU/kg of L-ase and 600 IU on the 3rd day. Her progress is shown on Fig. 2. Leukocytes went down to 550×ml on the 5th day after discontinuation of treatment, with total disappearance of blasts but also a concomittant fall in neutrophils from 2300×ml before treatment to 150×ml on the 2nd day after discontinuation. L-ase was started again 11 days after discontinuation, but had to be interrupted again after 3 days because of a severe anaphylactic shock. The patient went again into an incomplete remission, had subsequently other relapses and incomplete remissions, and finally died on November 5th, 1969 with a leukopenia of 250×ml lasting more than 20 days having supervened after 600 mgs of cyclophosphamide given over a period of 3 days.

The third pattern was the simplest and the most straightforward, occurring most predominantly in children with pancytopenic ALL. In these cases there was no early reduction of platelet levels, but a gradual thrombocytic increment took place from the very first start of L-ase treatment, generally heralding complete remission. A typical example of this pattern of response is shown on Fig. 4 These cases displayed the earliest medullary remission; in this case an erythroblastosis of more than 75% was discernible already one week after the inception of treatment.

Contrasting with these remissions patterns were those cases of ALL in which the disease followed its course quite independently from L-ase treatment. Especially in ALL, where an early response had always been the rule in responsive cases, it was felt that this behaviour expressed refractoriness to the enzyme, as exemplified in the following case.

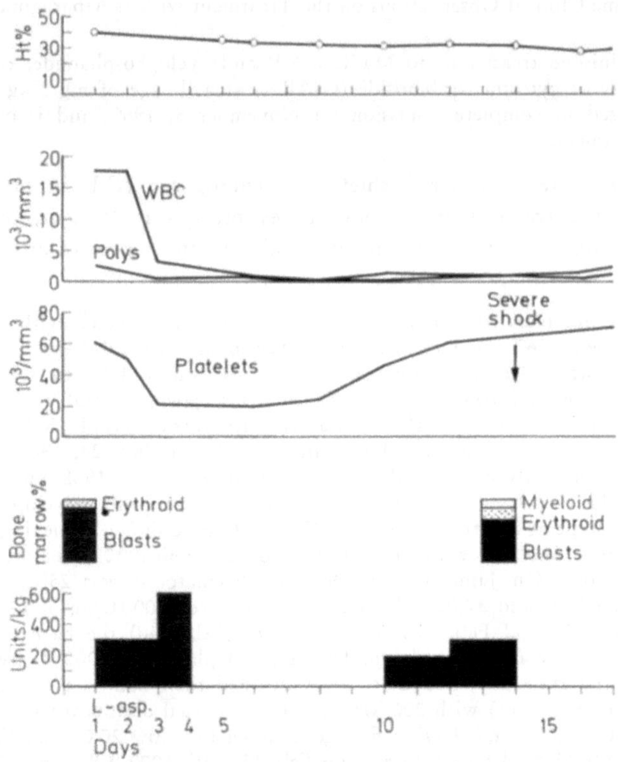

Fig. 3. Pancytopenic ALL showing extreme leukopenia after L-ase, necessitating temporary discontinuation of treatment. This was subsequently abandoned after an anaphylactic shock. D.A. yr. ♀ acute lymphoblastic leukemia

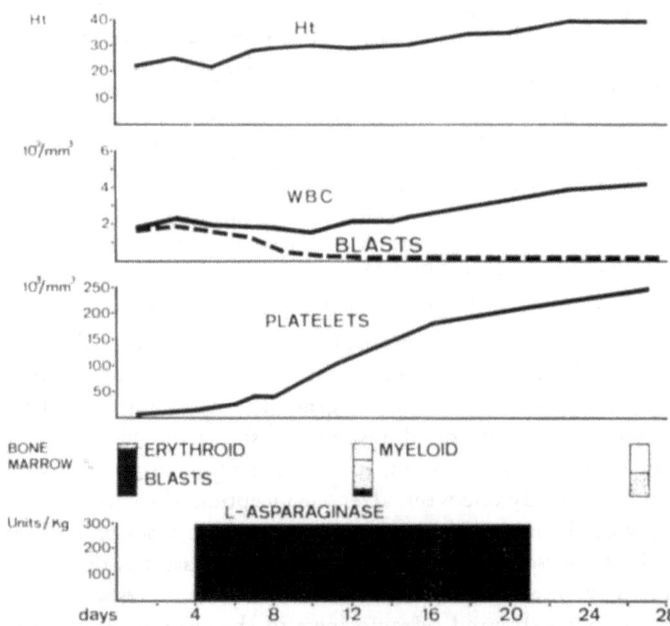

Fig. 4. Optimal response (pattern III) of ALL to L-ase. In this case there was no initial thrombocytopenia, and there occurred the earliest medullary remission that was observed in this series. B.C. 11 yr. ♂ acute lymphoblastic leukemia

This 14 year old girl had been admitted to the Sampierdarena General Hospital because of ALL on March 28, 1969. She started L-ase treatment (200 IU/kg) on March 31. Since the WBC more than doubled in 4 days, L-ase was discontinued on April 3rd, and a conventional VCR-DMC-prednisone treatment was given (Fig. 4). The patient went into complete remission, and was subsequently maintained with MTX, 6-MP and steroids until August 1969. At that time her parents put a stop to medical supervision in order to place her under the ministrations of a charlatan. On November 4, 1969 she was admitted in severe relapse and with leukemic infiltration of the central nervous system, and died, notwithstanding systemic and intrathecal therapy, on Nov. 10.

The only other remission pattern worthy of reporting concerns LSA, as in the following case.

This 68 year old married male had been diagnosed as affected with generalized lymphoblastic lymphosarcoma in 1962, and had been repeatedly treated with radiation, corticosteroids, alkylating agents (trisethylene-iminbenzoquinone, cyclophosphamide), VCR and blood transfusions over a period of 6 years. During all this period the circulating blood had

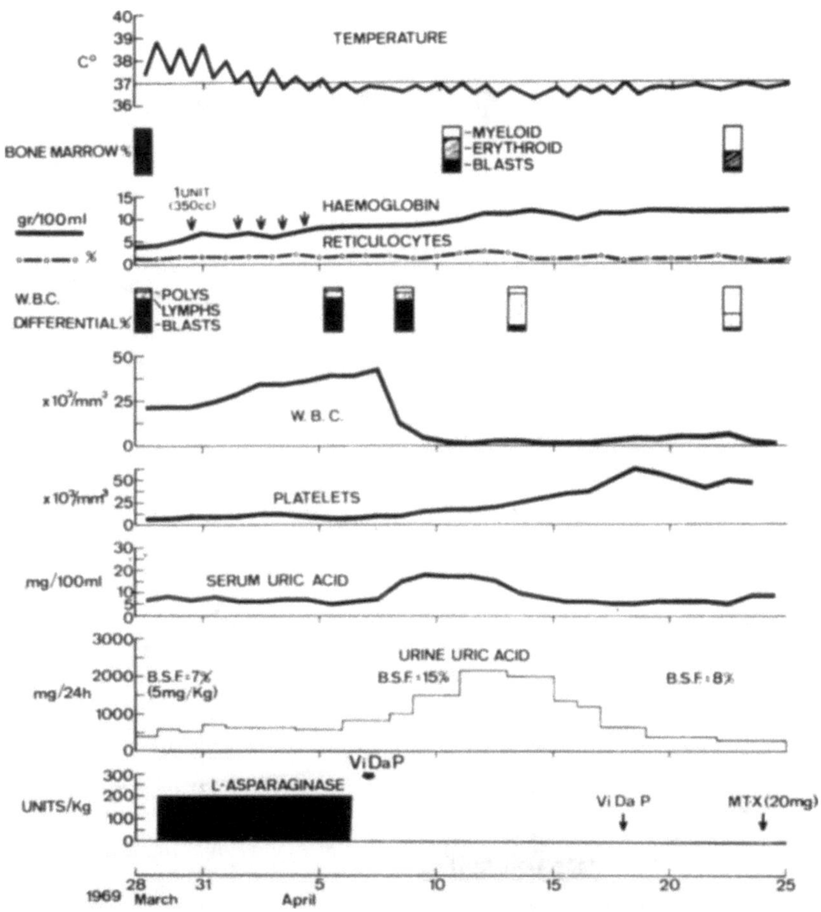

Fig. 5. ALL refractory to L-ase. Circulating lymphoblasts doubled while on treatment. Lymphoblastic drop and massive uric acid excretion took place only after vincristine-daunomycin-prednisone (ViDaP) treatment. B.R. 14 yr. ♀ acute lymphoblastic leukemia

been free from all but minimal numbers of lymphosarcoma cells, and the bone marrow had never shown more than 5% of the same.

The patient was again admitted on April 4, 1969 because of diffuse, marked enlargment of lymph glands, which varied between the aequivalents of walnuts to large plums. The spleen was however not palpable. Haematocrit was 32%, WBC 4200×ml with a normal differential and platelets 115,000×ml. The bone marrow showed about 5% lymphosarcoma cells.

L-ase treatment was started on April 17, 1969 at the dosage of 500 IU/kg, and continued for 15 days, with some increments to 1000 IU/kg (Fig. 5). It was attended by a marked shrinkage of the lymph nodes, which was already discernible on the 3rd day of treatment. There was a marked increase both of serum and urine uric acid. The haematocrit gradually

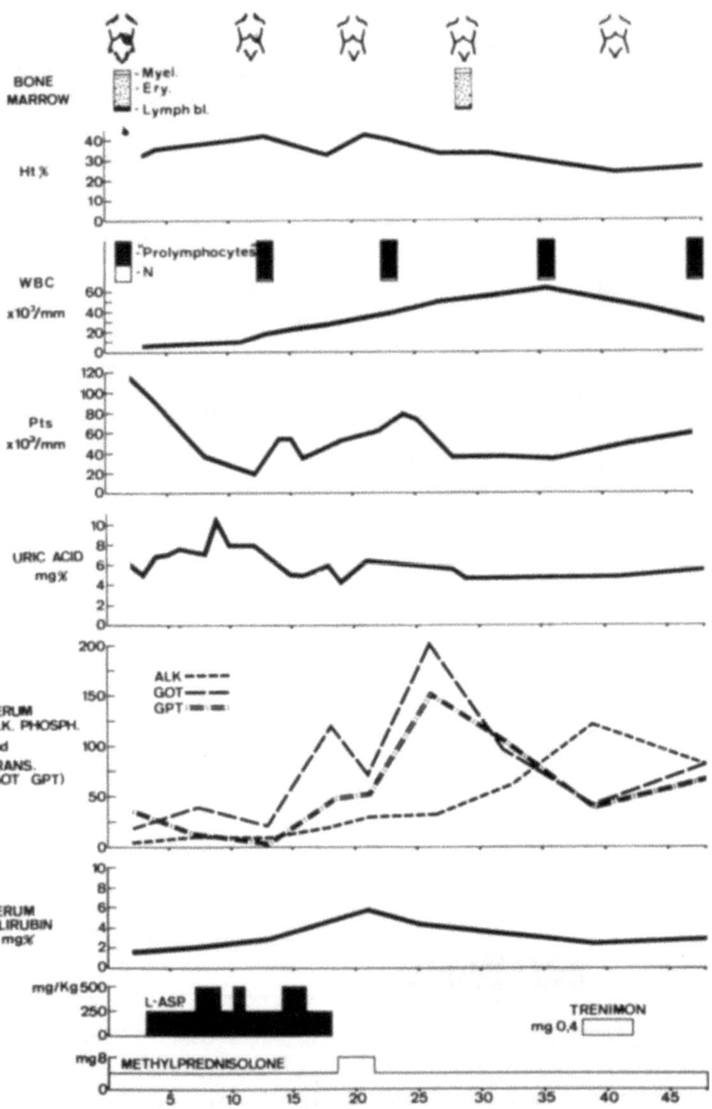

Fig. 6. Lymphoblastic lymphosarcoma treated with L-ase. Remission was accompanied by severe liver failure, that eventually caused patient's death

increased up to a maximum of 41% on the 12th day of treatment. The WBC also rose gradually from the initial 4500 to a high of 63,000×ml, a number which was reached 33 days from the start of treatment and 18 after its completion; semimature lymphocytes made up the bulk of this leukocytosis. The blood platelets gradually decreased to a nadir of 21,000 on the last day of treatment, than gradually went up again but never attained the initial values.

In this case a very marked deterioration of liver function took place quite early in treatment, and was the reason of its early discontinuation. Serum bilirubin and alkaline phosphatase were the first parameters to increase (Fig. 5), soon followed by the transaminases GO and GP. Fibrinogen fell to a minimum of 150 mg-%, but thrombodynamic studies suggested an even greater impairement (Fig. 6) Bromsulphalein retention went from 5% before treatment to 29% 41 days after discontinuation of treatment. The patient was dismissed on June 14, 1969, but went on to present marked hypoalbuminaemic oedemas of the whole body, which responded only partially to intravenous crystallized albumin, and died at home at the end of July, 1969, in a condition which was felt both by the attending physician and by one of us, who was called as consultant, as a severe chronic liver insufficiency.

3. Laboratory studies and side effects. The changes in the figurate components of circulating blood have been already described, and are apparent in the case reports and graphs.

The first change detectable in bone marrow aspirates was a transition from the hypercellular lymphoblastic sheets to a markedly hypoplastic, sometimes almost desertic picture. In these early post-L-ase aspirations no marrow particles could be generally isolated, and adequately cellular preparations could be obtained only by gentle centrifugation. At this stage a certain number of "smudge" cells (Gumprecht's shadow-like cells) could be seen, but this aspect was far from constant, and did not differentiate clearly from pre-L-ase samples. After a few days isolated or aggregated erythroblasts, generally in nest-or island-like arrangements, could be seen, most generally belonging to the late or polyorthrochromatic stages. However, when marrow examinations were made after one week of treatment in responsive cases, proerythroblasts and basophilic erythroblasts could also be observed. Megakaryocytes were the second cellular lineage that showed restoration, generally antedating granuloblasts. Finally, generally after about two weeks of treatment, the granulocytoblastic lineage became abundant, and the whole bone marrow's cellularity appeared to be restored. Hyperplasia of lymphatic follicles and collections of *mature* lymphocytes were also found in some marrow samples. None of these changes could be found in the marrow of the refractory cases [1].

The effect of L-ase on the circulating blood platelets was best studied in 3 cases of disseminated MM, one of which had extensive malignant cell invasion of the sternal bone marrow, but in whom aspirations from both iliac crests showed a normal composition. The explorable bone marrow in the other 2 cases was found normal. In all 3 cases, that proved completely refractory to L-ase but had severe subjective disturbances from the treatment, a sharp drop, up to 50%, of the circulating platelets could be determined [2] (Fig. 7).

[1] In the bone marrow of one of our cases of blastic crisis of CML abundant sheets of Gaucher-like cells were found. This finding, originally described by M. Albrecht [3] and subsequently confirmed by others, [29], [45] has not yet been reported in the Italian literature.

[2] Platelet counts were made according to our modification [32] of the original Feissly-Lüdin method. In the healthy adult a mean value of capillary platelets was found to be 235,000/ml, with a standard deviation (σ) of $\pm 0.11 \times 10.5$, and a coefficient of variation (C.V.) of $\pm 5.3\%$.

Fibrinogen levels were examined in all cases, and consistently displayed a moderate to marked fall during and after L-ase treatment, then reverting to normal, more sharply and promptly in children and young adults, more slowly in elder persons. The results of serial dosages in 6 cases of ALL that went into remission following L-ase treatment are shown in Fig. 8.

The thrombodynamic (thromboelastographic) examination of these cases showed a consistent major change, that is a marked reduction of the maximal amplitude (ma). When this change was more specifically investigated by means of parallel determinations on platelet-rich and platelet-poor (30′ high speed centrifugation) plasma in cases of nonleukemic patients (LSA and MM), it was found that the

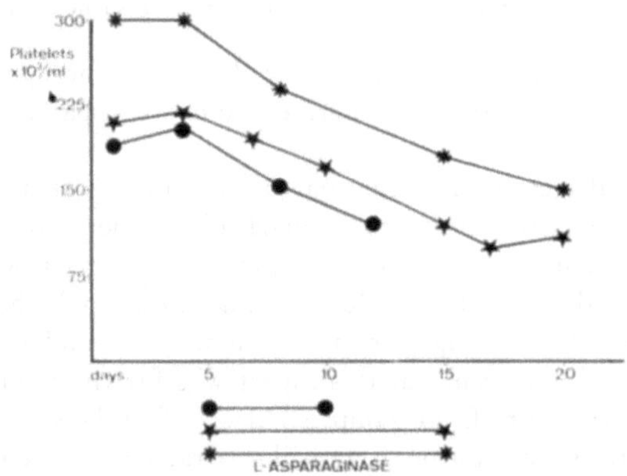

Fig. 7. Platelet levels in non-leukemic patients treated with L-ase. Platelets were enumerated by a direct phase-contrast method (see text)

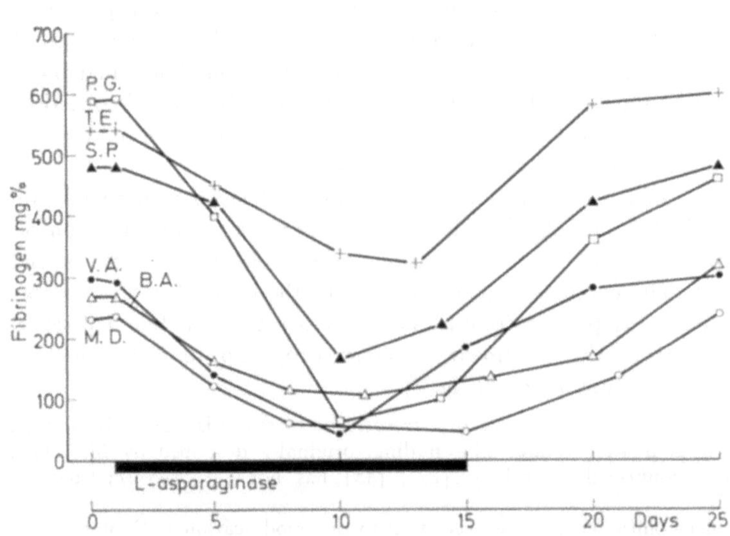

Fig. 8. Fibrinogen levels in 6 cases of ALL treated with L-ase. Fibrinogen fall occurred quite independently from the evolution into remission

alteration was chiefly expressed in the platelet-poor samples, thus reflecting the reduction in fibrinogen. A typical pattern is shown on Fig. 9, but it should be emphasized that these extremely hypocoagulable, amplitude-deficient thromboelastograms were a typical feature of the late phase of L-ase treatment of all patients.

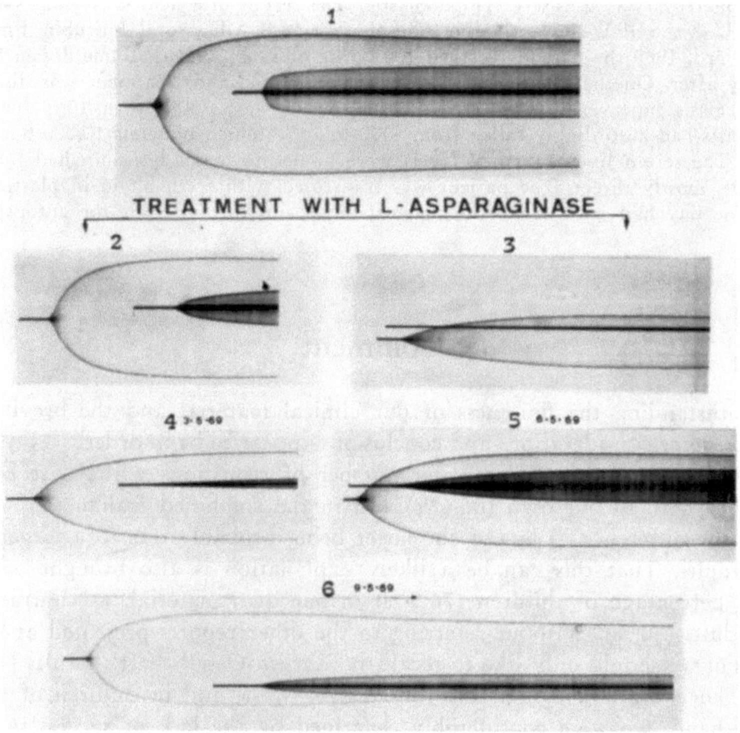

Fig. 9. Thrombodynamic changes in the case of LSA before and during L-ase treatment. Two tracings were recorded on each determination, one with platelet-rich (non-centrifuged) and the other with platelet-poor (centrifuged) plasma. While the maximal amplitude (ma) of the latter expresses only fibrinogen values, the difference between ma of PRP and PPP reflects platelet activity ("platelet amplitude"). As it can be seen, both values are affected, but mostly the PPP value, thus clearly indicating the fibrinogen defect. P. Giov. 67 y. ♂

The most definite side effects of this clinical material, leaving apart general or subjective disturbances such as nausea, malaise, vomiting, depression and the like, all of which were observed particularly in the elderly, affected liver function. Elevation of serum transaminases, alkaline phosphatase, conjugated and unconjugated bilirubin, drop of prothrombin and fibrinogen (as already remarked), augmentation of BSF retention were all observed, and sometimes constituted a limiting factor to the continuation of therapy. Besides the already reported case of LSA with pronounced liver toxicity another case will be briefly reported.

This 19 year old single male had been diagnosed as affected with ALL in the summer of 1969, had been admitted to another hospital and treated with corticosteroids only. He achieved an incomplete remission, and was subsequently admitted to the Sampierdarena Hospital on October 29, 1969 because of a severe relapse.

On admission the patient was moderately febrile, pale and with some disseminated petechiae. There was a bilateral, firm, extremely marked enlargement of the parotid glands, thus displaying a typical Mikulicz's syndrome. Both the liver and spleen were enormously enlarged, their lower margins almost attaining the iliac cristae.

The haematocrit was 30⁰/₀, WBC 10,000×ml with 43⁰/₀ lymphoblasts, platelets 11,000. The bone marrow was diffusely lymphoblastic. The serum uric acid was 20 mgs-⁰/₀. SGOT was 20 W.U.-⁰/₀, SGPT 18 U, alkaline phosphatase 56 K.A.U., total bilirubin 1 mg-⁰/₀. On November 3rd, 1969 the patient received 200 IU/kg of L-ase, and the same dosage was given on the day after. On the same day he appeared subicteric, and treatment was discontinued. A haematemesis supervened. On Nov. 5, 1969 WBC were 7500, with 10⁰/₀ lymphoblasts (lymphoblasts had accordingly fallen from 4300 to 750×mmc), platelets 10,000 but haematocrit 18⁰/₀. The serum liver enzymes' levels were unmodified, but bilirubin had increased to 5,90 mgs-⁰/₀, mostly direct. The patient was transfused with fresh blood in plastic bag, but on the same day had another profuse haematemesis and died. Permit for autopsy was not given.

Comment

Notwithstanding the finiteness of our clinical material and the brevity of our experience, some considerations and conclusions appear to be in order.

Firstly, the expected much greater number of remissions with L-ase in ALL is brought out both in our own (66.6⁰/₀) and in the combined Italian (45⁰/₀) clinical material, the difference in less of the latter being probably due to a larger proportion of adults. That this can be a likely explanation is also brought out by the remission percentage of children (76.9⁰/₀) in our own material, as contrasted with that of adults (40⁰/₀). Without referring to the other reports presented at this same Symposium, we should only like to recall the Ehrlich-Gesellschaft's results [7], which furnished an overall remission rate for ALL of 45⁰/₀, and in children of 60⁰/₀. On the other hand, we were considerably chagrined by the lack of success in APL, in which the German report [7] had given the surprising remission rate of 40⁰/₀. Perhaps it should be remarked that, in reality, there were 2 remissions out of 5 cases, which considerably reduces its statistical significance, especially when contrasted with our 4 failures (100⁰/₀). We should still like to point out the lack of success, at least at the dosages that were employed, in AML and in the blastic transformation of CML. Indeed, in these last cases, which include a category of severely debilitated and chronically ill patients, not rarely chronically intoxicated by busulphan, we have been so impressed by the bad tolerance of L-ase together with its complete lack of efficacy, that we have altogether avoided further trials with the enzymatic treatment.

Even in ALL, and notwithstanding the intrinsic interest of the results obtained with an entirely new principle of therapy, they still must be contrasted with the much higher remission rates obtainable by means of the standard vincristine-corticosteroid (with minor alterations) treatments. However, a redeeming point is the possibility of obtaining remissions in cases become refractory to conventional treatments. In addition, our experience fully supports Mathé's et al. [35] contention that the chances of obtaining a remission with L-ase are clearly apparent even after one only week of treatment, so much so that we have discontinued treatment after a few days in the face of a markedly increasing lymphoblast count.

Although it has been claimed that the selectivity of L-ase enables its safe administration also in severely pancytopenic cases [4, 35], more often than not this has *not* been our experience. Side by side with those rare cases in which an early thrombocytosis heralded the onset of complete remission, generally in children, there have been others with severe progredient neutropenia which demanded discontinuation of treatment. Illustrative case reports of both occurrences have been briefly presented. We shall revert to this and other similar aspects when we shall discuss GRUNDMANN's [23] "gradient of asparagine-dependency" concept.

Another clinical aspect we should like to stress is the sensitivity to L-ase of LSA and of the ALL-syndrome which may supervene in the late stages of LSA. These are extremely severe conditions, seldom responsive to conventional treatments, which may greatly benefit from L-ase. Unfortunately, an important drawback is caused by the fact that, again, these are chronically ill, often elderly patients, in whom, as we have found, profound hepatotoxicity is prone to develop.

The most important side-effects of L-ase have affected, in our material, the blood platelets, fibrinogen and liver function. The most demonstrative effect of L-ase on platelets was found in our non-thrombocytopenic patients with MM, which nevertheless displayed a clear-cut and marked decrease during treatment. A combination of factors is held to be responsible for L-ase induced thrombocytopenia; however, it should be noted that the administration of heparin is very seldom effective [19, 47, 48], that no fibrin- or fibrinogen split products are found in the blood [47, 48], that the half-life of infused platelets is not reduced [19], so that a damaging effect on the megakaryocytes would appear as the most probable cause.

The fall of fibrinogen levels is due most probably to a closely similar mechanism, that is damage of the hepatic cell. Thrombodynamic alterations, also described by DEUTSCH and WEISSMANN [19], are a reflection of both thrombocytic and fibrinogen changes (besides other coagulation factors), but principally of fibrinogenopenia. We have, however, also observed the appearance of frank jaundice, hyperbilirubinaemia, hypertransaminasaemia, elevation of serum alkaline phosphatase, constant and marked bromosulphalein retention, hypoalbuminaemia with sometimes dyscrasic pitting oedema, hypocholesterinaemia and hypoprothrombinaemia. There can be no doubt that L-ase profoundly affects the liver cell. We should like to emphasize that the most adverse effects have been seen in elderly patients, already debilitated for years by disease and remedies, while in children and young adults the impairement of liver function could be found only as laboratory disturbancies. However, if vincristine must be considered a potential poison of the peripheral and autonomic nervous system and daunorubicin of the heart, L-ase is undoubtedly a potent liver poison, and hepatotoxicity is a potential hazard to be reckoned with in all treatments. In fact, we believe L-ase should not be given altogether in patients with evidence of liver damage or a history of chronic hepatitis. In such conditions there may develop a situation somewhat comparable to the inhibition of early mitoses in regenerating rat liver [6], where it has been postulated that the reduced amount of asparagine after treatment with L-ase may be critically low for processes essential for cell growth, particularly for the synthesis of large amounts of new protein.

Although this last point introduces our final comments on the rationale and the mechanism of action of L-ase in the AL, we should first still like to make a brief comment on the incidence of sensitization to this bacterial, and therefore highly antigenic enzyme. We have met with two major sensitization accidents, both of them during a second course of asparaginase. Both occurred during the drip infusion and in both the clinical picture was of acute systemic anaphylaxis. The most severe case was near-fatal, involving acute circulatory failure necessitating massive epinephrine and corticosteroid administration, though, curiously enough, no disturbance whatever had been experienced on the preceding day infusion. The second case pointed out more clearly to the effect of homocytotropic antibodies of the IgE class, since the clinical pattern was manifested chiefly by urticaria and angioneurotic oedema.

The gravity and potential danger of such reactions, besides drastically curtailing the enzyme's continuation in the affected cases, clearly points out to the necessity of an unceasing "sensitization surveillance", be it under the form of more frequent skin testing, or, perhaps better, by means of *in vitro* tests to be developed in the near future.

The initial hope that treatment of malignant neoplasms with L-ase might represent "the first clear example of therapy based on a specific nutritional difference between certain malignant and normal cells" [27] has been considerably shaken by later experimental and clinical acquisitions. Besides acting on leukemic lymphoblasts [42], it was soon shown that L-ase was detrimental to the metabolism of widely differring tissues as regenerating rat liver [6], NZW mice embryos [1] and the graft-versus-host reaction in mice [23]. In addition, it was also demonstrated that the regeneration of human erythroblasts and granulocytoblasts is inhibited by L-ase in tissue cultures [10], and that there is cytochemical evidence of a global damage of haemopoiesis following L-ase treatment [24, 37]. It would appear that there is a "gradient of sensitivity" [22] to L-ase in different tissues, according to the efficiency of the asparagino-synthetase apparatus, and that the enzyme has not an absolute cancer cell selectivity, but exerts also a global ("aspecific") myelotoxicity. This important aspect has not only a fundamental theoretical significance, but must be borne in mind by the clinical haematologist.

Even the fact that L-ase is so extremely active in ALL is most probably the consequence of the fact that the metabolic machinery of the actively growing and reproducing lymphoid cell is devoid of, or extremely poor in, asparagino-synthetase. This is clearly brought out by ASTALDI and co-workers' [5] demonstration that L-ase can intensely inhibit blastic transformation of human peripheral blood lymphocytes in the PHA-culture system. In other words, the asparagine-depriving enzyme appears to be active not against the "malignant change" of the lymphatic cells, but on the metabolic requirements associated with their "blastic" transformation, be it leukemic or immunologic in nature. There is no need to stress the significance of these assumptions, which, while curtailing some excessively optimistic hopes that had been entertained originally, open at the same time the vast field of immunodepression.

Finally, L-ase appears to be shifting from its original position as the mainstay of treatment of otherwise refractory cases of ALL to an important component of anti-leukemic polychemotherapy. However, until we shall not have more accurate and consistent information on the effects of L-ase on "quiescent", "sleeper" [31] or Go lymphoblasts, its utilization as a complementary chemotherapeutic agent in the "invisible" or "low-logarithm" phase of ALL is still uncertain.

Summary

Over a period of about 1 year 35 patients were treated with L-ase in this study, of whom 29 were affected with AL, 2 with LSA and 3 with MM. An overall remission rate of 66.6% was obtained in ALL, with better results in children than in adults. No remissions were obtained in AML, not even in the promyelocytic variety, which had been reported to respond in a recent multicentric report.

Three different patterns of remissions were seen in the responding cases of ALL, the first occurring in highly leukemic cases with massive lympholysis, the second in leukopenic cases in which extreme pancytopenia followed necessitating discontinuation of treatment, and the third characterized by an early thrombocytosis, which was not found in the other patterns and generally heralded remission. The chief side-effects affected the liver especially of older patients, while fibrinogenopenia, also demonstrated by means of thromboelastography, was a constant finding of the late stages of treatment.

Although it had been originally postulated that L-ase acted through an enzymic defect (lack of asparagino-synthetase) characteristic of malignant cells, subsequent studies are in favour of its activity through a veritable "gradient of asparagine-dependency", which appears foremost in the immature cells of the lymphoid lineage, irrespective of their reactive, homeostatic (immunologic) or anhomeostatic (neoplastic) nature.

References

1. Adamson, R. H., Fabro, S.: Embryotoxic effect of L-asparaginase. Nature (Lond.) **218**, 1164 (1968).
2. — — Antitumor activity and other biologic properties of L-asparaginase (NSC-109229). A review. Cancer Chemother. Rep. **52**, 617 (1968).
3. Albrecht, M.: „Gaucher-Zellen“ bei chronisch myeloischer Leukämie. Blut **13**, 169 (1966).
4. Astaldi, G., Burgio, G. R., Severi, F., Genova, R., Curtoni, E., Bruschelli, M., Astaldi, A. A.: Osservazioni preliminari sul trattamento della leucemia linfatica acuta del bambino con L-asparaginasi. Haemat. lat. (Milano) **11**, 311 (1968).
5. — — Krc, J., Genova, R., Astaldi, A. A., Jr.: L-asparaginase and blastogenesis. Lancet **1969 I**, 423.
6. Becker, F. F., Broome, J. D.: L-asparaginase : inhibition of early mitosis in regenerating rat liver. Science **156**, 1602 (1967).
7. Begemann, H.: Behandlungsergebnisse mit L-asparaginase bei akuten Leukämien. In: Chemo- und Immunotherapie der Leukosen und malignen Lymphome. Ed.: A. Stacher. Wien: Bohmann 1969, p. 293.
8. Boiron, M., Jacquillat, Cl., Weil, M., Tanzer, J., Bernard, J.: L'asparaginase. Presse méd. **76**, 2099 (1968).
9. — — Bernard, J.: L'asparaginase. In: Actualités Hématologiques. Ed.: J. Bernard. Paris: Masson 1969, p. 115.
10. Boll, I., Reckers, U.: Die Beeinflussung der Proliferationskinetik normalen menschlichen Knochenmarks in vitro durch L-asparaginase. In: Chemo- und Immunotherapie der Leukosen und malignen Lymphome. Ed.: A. Stacher. Wien: Bohmann 1969, p. 41.
11. Boyse, E. A., Old, L. J., Campbell, H. A., Mashburn, L. T.: Suppression of murine leukemias by L-asparaginase. J. exp. Med. **125**, 17 (1967).
12. — — Stoeckert, E.: Inhibitory effect of guinea pig serum on a number of new leukemias in mice. Nature (Lond.) **198**, 800 (1963).
13. Broome, J. D.: Evidence that the L-asparaginase activity of guinea pig serum is responsible for its antilymphoma effects. Nature (Lond.) **191**, 1114 (1961).
14. Burchenal, J. H., Dollinger, M. R.: L-asparaginase in transplanted mouse leukemia. XII. Congr. Int. Soc. Hemat., New York 1968 (Abstr. C-6).
15. — Karnofsky, D. A., Murphy, M. L., Oettgen, H. F.: Effects of L-asparaginase on leukemias and other neoplasms. XII. Congr. Int. Soc. Hemat., New York 1968 (Abstr. C-7).

16. Campbell, H. A., Mashburn, L. T., Boyse, E. A., Old, L. J.: Two L-asparaginases from Escherichia coli B. Their separation, purification and antitumor activity. Biochem. **6**, 721 (1967).
17. Clementi, A.: La désamidation enzymatique de l'asparagine chez les différentes espèces animaux et la significance physiologique de la présence dans l'organisme. Arch. int. Physiol. **19**, 369 (1922).
18. De Barros, T., Cunha Filho, M., Ferreira de Santana, C., Valenca, M., Pereira da Silva, M., Guedes, J., de Carvalho, A. R. L.: Utilizaçao da L-asparaginase em paciente humano portador de neoplasia maligna. An. Fac. Med. Recife **25**, 21 (1965).
19. Deutsch, E., Weissmann, A.: Therapie der haemorrhagischen Komplikationen bei Leukosen. In: Chemo- und Immunotherapie der Leukosen und malignen Lymphome. Ed.: A. Stacher. Wien: Bohmann 1969, p. 261.
20. Dolowy, W. C., Henson, D., Cornet, J., Sellin, H.: Toxic and antineoplastic effects of L-asparaginase. Study of mice with lymphoma and normal monkeys and report on a child with leukemia. Cancer **19**, 1318 (1966).
21. Gallmeier, W. M., Schmidt, C. G., Stier, H. W.: In vitro-Testung von Zellen auf Asparaginmangelempfindlichkeit. In: Chemo- und Immunotherapie der Leukosen und malignen Lymphome. Ed.: A. Stacher. Wien: Bohmann 1969, p. 30.
22. Grundmann, E.: L-asparaginase und Leukämie. Klin. Wschr. **47**, 61 (1969).
23. — Grundlagen der L-asparaginase-Therapie. In: Chemo- und Immunotherapie der Leukosen und malignen Lymphome. Ed.: A. Stacher. Wien: Bohmann 1969, p. 23.
24. Heller, A., Gross, R.: Zytochemische Veränderung der Leukosen unter Asparaginasetherapie. In: Chemo- und Immunotherapie der Leukosen und malignen Lymphome. Ed.: A. Stacher. Wien: Bohmann 1969, p. 323.
25. Hill, J. M.: Avances en el tratamiento de las neoplasias de tejido linfoiedo. 17. Nat. Ass. Smg., Mexico City, Nov. 14, 1966.
26. — Loeb, E., Roberts, A., Mac Lennan, A., Khan, A., Hill, N. O.: L-asparagine therapy of leukemia. XII. Congr. Int. Soc. Hemat., New York 1968 (Abstr. C-14).
27. — Roberts, J., Loeb, E., Khan, A., Mac Lennan, A., Hill, R. W.: L-asparaginase therapy for leukemia and other malignant neoplasms. Remission in human leukemia. J. Amer. med. Ass. **202**, 882 (1967).
28. Horowitz, B., Mapras, B. K., Meister, A., Old, L. J., Boyse, E. A., Stockert, E.: Asparagine synthetase activity of mouse leukemia. Science **160**, 533 (1968).
29. Kattlove, H. E., Williams, J. C., Gaynor, E., Spivack, M., Bradley, R. M., Brady, R. O.: Gaucher cells in chronic myelocytic leukemia: an acquired abnormality. Blood **33**, 379 (1969).
30. Kidd, J. G.: Regression of transplanted lymphomas induced in vivo by means of normal guinea pig serum: I. Course of transplanted cancers of various kinds in mice and rats given guinea pig serum, horse serum or rabbit serum. J. exp. Med. **98**, 565 (1953).
31. Killmann, S. A.: Acute leukemia: development, remission-relapse pattern, relationship between normal and leukemic hemopoiesis, and the "sleeper-to-feeder" stem cell hypothesis. Ser. Hemat. **1**, 103 (1968).
32. Marmont, A. M., Giacca, S.: A technical improvement of direct platelet counting by phase-contrast microscopy: a special "thin-bottom" counting chamber. Acta haemat. **17**, 169 (1957).
33. Marquardt, H.: L-asparaginase — das erste spezifische Cytostaticum. Arzneimittel-Forsch. **18**, 1380 (1968).
34. Mashburn, L. T., Wriston, J. C., Jr.: Tumor inhibitory effect of L-asparaginase from *Escherichia coli.* Arch. Biochem. **105**, 451 (1964).
35. Mathé, G., Amiel, J.-L., Schwarzenberg, L., Schneider, M., Cattan, A., Schlumberger, J.-R., Hayat, M., de Vassal, F., Jasmin, C., Rosenfeld, C.: Essai de traitement de la leucémie aigue lymphoblastique par la L-asparaginase. Presse méd. **77**, 461 (1969).
36. Old, L. J., Boyse, E. A., Campbell, H. A., Brodey, R. S., Fidler, J., Teller, J. P.: Treatment of lymphosarcoma in the dog with L-asparaginase. Cancer **20**, 1066 (1967).
37. Oekermann, H., Hirschmann, W. D.: Experimentelle Untersuchungen zur Wirkung der Asparaginase. In: Chemo- und Immunotherapie der Leukosen und malignen Lymphome. Ed.: A. Stacher. Wien: Bohmann 1969, p. 316.

38. OETTGEN, H., OLD, J., BOYSE, E. A., CAMPBELL, H. A., PHILIPS, F. S., CLARKSON, B. D., TALLAL, L., LEEPER, R. D., SCHWARTZ, M. K., KIM, J. K.: Inhibition of leukemias in man by L-asparaginase. Cancer Res. **27**, I, 2619 (1967).
39. PRAGER, M. D., ROBERTS, J., BACHYNSKY, N.: Immunity to the 6C3HED ascites tumor following treatment of tumor-bearing mice with *E. coli* L-asparaginase. J. Immunol. **98**, 1045 (1967).
40. ROBERTS, J., PRAGER, M. D., BACHYNSKY, N.: The antitumor activity of *Escherichia coli* L-asparaginase. Cancer Res. **26**, 2213 (1966).
41. SALSER, J. S., MILLER, H. K., BALIS, M. E.: Amino acid levels following L-asparaginase therapy. XII. Congr. Int. Soc. Hemat., New York 1968 (Abstr. C-30).
42. SCHREK, R., DOLOWY, W. C., AMMERAAL, R. N.: L-asparaginase toxicity to normal and leukemic human lymphocytes. Science **155**, 329 (1967).
43. SCHMIDT, C. G., GALLMEIER, W. M.: Zur Enzymtherapie der Leukämien. Dtsch. med. Wschr. **48**, 2299 (1968).
44. — — Klinik der Asparaginasetherapie bei Leukämien. In: Chemo- und Immunotherapie der Leukosen und malignen Lymphome. Ed.: A. STACHER. Wien: Bohmann 1969, p. 305.
45. SMITH, W. C., OKANESHIRO, M. M., GOLDSTEIN, B. D., PARKER, J. W., LUKES, R. J.: Gaucher cells in chronic granulocytic leukemia. Lancet **1968 II**, 780.
46. SOBIN, L. H., KIDD, J. G.: A metabolic difference between two lines of lymphoma 6C3HED cells in relation to asparagine. Proc. Soc. exp. Biol. Med. **119**, 325 (1965).
47. STIER, H. W., GALLMEIER, W. M., SCHMIDT, C. G.: Über Störungen des Blutgerinnungssystems im Verlaufe der Enzym-Therapie maligner Tumoren und Hämoblastosen. Dtsch. med. Wschr. **94**, 253 (1969).
48. — SCHMIDT, C. G., GALLMEIER, W. M.: Das Blutgerinnungssystem während der Leukämiebehandlung mit L-asparaginase. In: Chemo- und Immunotherapie der Leukosen und malignen Lymphome. Ed.: A. STACHER. Wien: Bohmann 1969, p. 310.

Clinical Trials of Asparaginase in Chemotherapy-Resistant Acute Leukemias

M. GOUDEMAND and F. BAUTERS *

Service des Maladies du Sang, Hôpital A. Calmette, Centre Hospitalo-Universitaire, Lille, France

The place of asparaginase in the strategy of acute leukemia treatment has not yet been defined because experience with this agent is too recent. Thus we present our own results, despite the very small number of patients (14 cases). These results seem highly significant, in so far as asparaginase, being in short supply, was strictly reserved for patients who had previously proved to be resistant to different anti-mitotic drugs.

Treated Patients

The categories of patients were:

Acute Lymphoblastic Leukemia (A. L. L.): 10.

Acute Myeloblastic Leukemia (A. M. L.): 4.

The average age was 9 years for A. L. L. for nine of them (only one was an adult 50 years of age). The four A. M. L. patients were young adults (18 to 25 years).

Asparaginase [1] was never used as the first agent. It was always tried after conventional chemotherapy had proved unsuccessful, either during the first phase of the disease or during relapses.

In every case of A. L. L., asparaginase was only used in relapse (Table 1). Previously every patient had been treated according to schedule Paris 04 LA 65 (Unité de Chemiothérapie, Hôpital Saint-Louis, Professor JEAN BERNARD): combination of prednisone and vincristine for the induction course or schedule Paris 06 LA 66: combination of rubidomycin with the other two drugs. Later on, the remission maintenance therapy combined 6-mercaptopurine and methotrexate with periodical reinduction courses of prednisone, vincristine and rubidomycin. All patients in relapse scheduled for an asparaginase trial were completely resistant to a prolonged induction course with vincristine and rubidomycin. The patients with A. M. L. were treated with asparaginase twice during the first phase of the disease and twice during a relapse but only after conventional chemotherapy had been unsuccessful (rubi-

* With the assistance of B. LERCHE and M. T. CAULIER.

[1] Laboratories SPECIA.

domycin in the first trial, then cytosine-arabinoside alone or in combination with cyclophosphamide and vincristine).

In all cases, before asparaginase treatment there was a heavy leukemic infiltration of the bone marrow with more than 50% blast cells. The blood showed various changes. In five patients, leucopenia (less than 1500/mm^3) and thrombocytopenia (less than 100,000/mm^3) were observed.

Modalities of Treatment

a) *Asparaginase* was always used as *induction* therapy.

The dose was 1000 units/kg/day injected intravenously in isotonic dextrose solution.

The average duration of treatment was 27 days (from 15 to 43 days). Blood examination was performed twice a week, bone marrow examination once a week.

In case of a remission, asparaginase was continued for eight days after the return to normal of blood and bone marrow. When treatment was unsuccessful, the course was continued for at least one month.

For ten patients, asparaginase was the only treatment which influenced the course of the disease. Five times the enzyme was used alone (4 A. L. L., 1 A. M. L.) because of severe pancytopenia. The bone marrow was characterized by decreased numbers of normal myeloid cells and by the presence of blast cells. In five other patients (3 A. L. L., 2 A. M. L.) asparaginase was added to antimitotic drugs which had previously been ineffective in spite of a long period of treatment (thus the results were attributable to asparaginase only).

In the last four patients (3 A. L. L., 1 A. M. L.), on account of a massive bone marrow infiltration by blast cells, we added cytosine-arabinoside and cyclophosphamide (100 mg/m^2/d of each) to asparaginase. These antimitotic drugs were used for the first time in these patients and their own effects must be considered in the discussion of the results.

b) In the most favorable cases (complete remission) a remission maintenance therapy was added immediately, with 6-mercaptopurine (2,5 mg/kg/d p. o.) and methotrexate (10 mg/m^2/week i. m.). At regular intervals (1, 2, 4 months after complete remission) *reinduction courses* of eight days' duration were performed. These courses included combinations of prednisone-vincristine-rubidomycin + amethopterin intrathecally) for A. L. L. and of prednisone (40 mg/m^2/d), cytosine-arabinoside (100 mg/m^2/d), cyclophosphamide (100 mg/m^2/d) (+ amethopterin intrathecally) for A. M. L.

Results

1. Immediate Results (Table 1)

a) Complete remissions (C. R.) were obtained in 6 out of 10 cases of A. L. L. and in 2 out of 4 cases of A. M. L. The term C. R. is defined by a normal clinical condition, normal blood and cerebrospinal fluid and less than 5% of blast cells in a bone marrow of normal density. These results must be attributed to asparaginase only, except for one case of A. L. L. and one case of A. M. L. where treatment with antimitotic agents was started at the same time as treatment with asparaginase.

b) Incomplete remission (I. R.) was observed in 2 cases of A. L. L. treated with a combination of asparaginase and two antimitotic drugs (cytosine-arabinoside and cyclophosphamide). I. R. is defined by a normal clinical condition, normal blood and C. S. F., but 10—15% of blast cells in the bone marrow.

c) No remission. The treatment was unsuccessful in 2 cases of A. L. L. and in 2 cases of A. M. L. Bone marrow hypoplasia was too severe in these cases for combining antimetabolites with asparaginase. In three patients the infiltration of the bone marrow with leukemic cells remained unchanged, and death occurred shortly after asparaginase therapy was terminated. In one patient the peripheral blood became normal but the bone marrow showed the persistence of more than 50% blast cells.

d) Leukemia-meningitis: In an A. L. L. patient in whom asparaginase produced an incomplete remission, a leukemic meningitis occurred at the same time with a large number of blast cells in the C. S. F., but it responded well to amethopterin given intrathecally.

2. Late Results (in Cases of Remission)

Remission remained complete in 4 out of 8 patients (Table 1): 2 with A. L. L. (one was treated with cytosine-arabinoside and cyclophosphamide in addition to asparaginase) and 2 with A. M. L. (one received the same combination).

In 4 patients with A. L. L. in whom a complete remission was obtained with asparaginase relapse occured before the end of two months. The disease appeared completely resistant to antimitotic drugs and death soon occurred in three of them.

With respect to the patients who achieved an incomplete remission, one of them is now in complete remission but only for a few weeks. In the second patient relapse occurred about two weeks after asparaginase was discontinued, with leukemic infiltration of the bone marrow and the meninges. The patient died soon afterwards.

Table 1. *Results of therapy by L-asparaginase in chemo-resistant acute leukemias*

		Immediate results			Late results (in case of remission)		
		C.R.	I.R.	No remission	Persistent C.R. 2 months	Relapse 2 months	Case too recent
A.L.L.	1st occurrence						
	2nd occurrence	1	1 [a]	1		2	
	3rd occurrence	1		1	1		
	4th occurrence	2+1 [a]	1 [a]		1 [a]	2	1
	5th occurrence	1				1	
A.M.L.	1st occurrence	1		1	1		
	2nd occurrence			1			
	3rd occurrence	1 [a]			1 [a]		
Total		8	2	4	4	5	1

[a] Patients where Asparaginase was combined with Cytosine-Arabinoside and cyclophosphamide—see text.

Side Effects

Clinically, the drug was well tolerated except for one patient, where gastro-intestinal complications (anorexia, nausea) made it necessary to discontinue treatment after only two weeks.

However, biochemical determinations have revealed some disturbances.

a) Fibrinogen and Prothrombin Complex

In 7 out of 10 patients we saw, after about ten days, a slight degree of hypofibrinogenemia (about 2 g/liter) which quickly disappeared after the end of the course. On one occasion, fibrinogen fell to 0.8 g/l after two weeks of asparaginase therapy without clinical consequences. When treatment was discontinued the fibrinogen levels returned to normal. In two patients the fibrinogen remained normal throughout.

With respect to other coagulation factors, only factors of the prothrombin complex were explored. These factors were always normal, except in two patients where we observed 35 and 40%. One of them, however, was affected by a Pyocyanic bacillus septicemia with endotoxin shock.

b) Liver Function

Bilirubinemia

In 11 out of 13 patients the serum bilirubin, which was normal at the beginning, increased during the course of asparaginase (1, 5 to 4 mg/100 ml of total bilirubin with a larger part of direct bilirubin). This hyperbilirubinemia was transient. It disappeared quickly when asparaginase was stopped.

Serum Alkaline Phosphatasis

Hyperbilirubinemia was always associated with an increase of alkaline phosphatasis (from 20 to 50 Bodansky units or more) with return to normal (under 15 U) after the end of the asparaginase course.

Serum Transaminases

Transaminases (SGOT and SGPT) were normal in 6 out of 13 patients and slightly increased (80 U to 150 U) in 6. In the other patient, the rate reached 400 U (SGOT) and 900 U (SGPT) after two weeks and returned quickly to normal during the asparaginase course.

Flocculation Tests, Serum Protein Electrophoresis

No significant changes were observed.

c) Pancreatic Function

Amylase levels were always normal in blood and urine.

d) Lipid Metabolism

In three cases the serum lipids were normal (total lipids between 5.5 and 8 g/l, cholesterol between 1.7 and 2.3 g/l), in three cases there was a slight decrease (total

Table 2. *Lipid balance*

	Normal	Patients during treatment (21—30 days)			Patients after stopping asparaginase				Without asparaginase
		P. Jean	F. Jacques	D. Pierre	D. Pierre 15 days	LEG. 2 months	ARN. 2 months	AG. 3 months	PELL.
Total lipids (g/l)	4 à 7	24.80	12	10.40		6.85			10.55
Glycerides (g/l)	0.50 à 1.75	12.30	4.20	5.26	4.30	1.15	0.75	3.16	2.35
Phospholipids (g/l)	1.5 à 2.50	8.90	2.82	2.70	2.50	2.12	1.95	2.68	2.05
Total cholesterol (g/l)	< 2.50	6.10	2.10	1.93	2.10	2.52	2.10	3	2.35
E/T	75%		68%	61%	58.5%	68%	62%	56.5%	43%
Lipidogram (cellulose acetate)									
— chylo	0	+		0	0	0	0	0	0
— β	+++	++	+++	+++	+++	+++	+++	+++	+++
— pre β	± (à +)	++++	++	+++	+++	+	±	++	++
— α	++	0	0	±	+	++	++	+	++
β/pre β	$\gg 1$	0.45	0.88	0.6	0.40	3.4	$\gg 1$	1	1.4
Lipidogram (paper)									
Index of α lipo (optical density)	14	0	1.9	3.7		12.5			7.4

lipids between 4.5 and 5.5 g/l, cholesterol between 1.2 and 1.7 g/l) and in seven cases an increase was observed (lipids above 8 g/l, in three cases above 15 g/l with milky appearance of the serum, cholesterol between 2.3 g and 6 g/l).

We can only given preliminary results of a more elaborate study of the serum lipids. It showed that, in hyperlipidemia, there was essentially a large increase of triglycerides. The lipidograms revealed an increase of "pre-β-lipoprotein" and disappearance of α-lipoproteins. These changes were already less pronounced two weeks after the treatment was stopped. They disappeared completely after two months. They were never seen in acute leukemia not treated with asparaginase, but receiving corticosteroids or other chemotherapy (Table 2).

Discussion

The small number of our cases does not allow us, of course, to draw definite conclusions. However, we may consider the following points with respect to L-asparaginase:

The enzyme has an undisputed effect on acute leukemia: we obtained 8 complete remissions in 14 treated patients. Even if there is some doubt about 4 cases because a combination of asparaginase and antimitotic drugs was used, the fact remains that 6 complete remissions can be attributed exclusively to asparaginase. These results were obtained in patients who had proved resistant to several antimitotic drugs, most of them in their second, third or fourth relapse. Increasing resistance to drugs as the disease progresses is a well-known feature of acute leukemias.

The results also show that there is no cross-resistance between asparaginase and antimitotic drugs, which is probably due to fundamental differences in their mechanisms of action.

Asparaginase is said to be more effective against A. L. L. than against A. M. L. For this reason we have treated mainly A. L. L. cases (with 6 C. R. out of 10). Nevertheless we obtained two C. R. in 4 A. M. L. cases.

The late results were not as good. The remission seems to be transient: Only four persisted for more than two months in spite of maintenance therapy with other drugs.

Although inconstant and transient, these results are very interesting. Some of them were obtained in patients with severe bone marrow aplasia. Such an aplasia means, first, that earlier drugs were unsuccessful and secondly, that all antimitotic compounds must be stopped. So before asparaginase no treatment would have been possible. With asparaginase, thoses patients can be treated since this enzyme is not toxic to the normal hematopoietic cells.

The enzyme seems to be tolerated rather well. Systematic biochemical determinations have revealed only slight metabolic alterations, although the course lasted longer than one month. These disturbances were always completely reversible. They concerned particularly the liver function. No important cellular alteration was seen in our patients. The symptoms were chiefly of cholestasis. Even the serum lipid abnormalities can be considered as a hepatic disturbance for, in retention icterus, identical symptoms such as disappearance of α-lipoproteins and increase of pre-β-lipoproteins are observed. Thus asparaginase seems to provoke a toxic hepatitis of the cholostatic type, which is reversible after a course of treatment limited to four or five weeks.

Another biochemical disturbance that has been reported is the decrease of fibrinogen. Perhaps the hypofibrinogenemia is related to the hepatic deficiency, but it might also indicate a selective disturbance of fibrinogen synthesis.

Further experience will show if the liver toxicity is due to impurities or to the enzyme itself.

In spite of these favorable aspects, asparaginase therapy has been somewhat disappointing because the remissions were rather transient.

More experience is required. Some suggestions may be made:

use of longer courses or higher doses (although then the treatment may be more toxic);

combination with antimitotic drug.

Lastly, other enzymes should be tried.

References

ADAMSON, R. H., FABRA, S.: Antitumor activity and other biologic properties of L-asparaginase. A review. Cancer Chemother. Rep. **52**, 617—626 (1968).

BERNARD, J., BOIRON, M., JACQUILLAT, C., WEIL, M., NAJEAN, Y., THOMAS, M.: Traitement des leucémies aiguës lymphoblastiques de première atteinte par une association de Prednisone-Vincristine-Rubidomycine. Path. Biol. **15**, 919—920 (1967).

BOIRON, M., JACQUILLAT, C., WEIL, M., TANZER, J., BERNARD, J.: L-asparaginase. Presse méd. **76**, 2099—2101 (1968).

— Bilan de L-asparaginase. Journées d'Hématologie, Paris, Octobre 1969.

BROOME, J. D.: Factors which may influence the effectiveness of L-asparaginase as tumor inhibitors. Brit. J. Cancer **22**, 595—602 (1968).

HENDERSON, E. S.: Treatment of acute leukemia. Seminars in Hematology **6**, 271 (1969).

HILL, J. M., ROBERTS, J., LOEB, E., KHAN, A., MACLELLAN, A., HILL, R.: L-asparaginase therapy for leukemia and other malignant neoplasms: remission in human leukemia. J. Amer. med. Ass. **202**, 882—888 (1967).

JACQUILLAT, C., WEIL, M., BOIRON, M.: La méthode de réinduction dans le traitement des leucémies aiguës. Actual. Hémat. deuxième série. Paris: Masson 1968, pp. 12—19.

MATHÉ, G. et coll.: Essai de traitement de la leucémie aiguë lymphoblastique par la L-asparaginase. Presse méd. **77**, 461 (1969).

OETTGEN, H. F., OLD, L. J., BOYSE, E. A., CAMPBELL, H. A., PHILIPS, F. S., CLARKSON, B. D., TALLAL, L., LEEPER, R. D., SCHWARTZ, M. K., KIM, J. H.: Inhibition of leukemias in man by L-asparaginase. Cancer Res. **27**, 2619—2631 (1967).

Use of Asparaginase in Conjunction with Cytosine Arabinoside in Acute Leukemia in Children

R. M. Hardisty and T. J. McElwain

London, England

With 3 Figures

We should like to report the results of treating a small number of children with acute lymphoblastic leukemia in relapse, with a course of cytosine arabinoside followed immediately by a course of L-asparaginase. Although the number of patients in this study is too small to draw any definite conclusions, the results that we have obtained are sufficiently encouraging to suggest the need for further studies of this type of treatment.

Nine patients with acute lymphoblastic leukemia, aged between two and eleven years, were treated. All had previously received other antileukemic drugs and all were in their second or subsequent relapse, with the exception of one patient who was in her first relapse, but whose disease was refractory to vincristine, prednisone, 6-mercaptopurine, methotrexate and cyclophosphamide. Details are shown in Table 1. At

Table 1. *Treatment summary*

Patient	Age	Sex	No. of relapse	Time since diagnosis (weeks)	Ara-C 3 mg/kg i. v. daily No. of days treatment	L-asparaginase 1000 IU/kg daily. Days treatment	Result
1	2	F	1	17	10	21	Remission
2	5	M	3	71	14	14	Remission
3	11	M	2	78	7	21	Remission
4	5	M	4	100	8	21	Remission
5	6	M	3	101	10	28	Remission
6	6	F	3	119	10	18	Remission
7	5	F	4	98	9	21	Remission
8	5	M	4	50	13	14	Remission
9	6	F	3	73	5	9	Failed Blast count continued to rise on Ara-C and asparaginase

the time of relapse seven of the patients had between 12.5% and 94.5% of leukemic cells in the marrow. Of the other two, whose marrow was not examined at this stage, one had 60,000 and the other 13,000 leukemic cells per mm³ of peripheral blood (Table 2).

Fig. 1 shows the method of treatment. This was started with cytosine arabinoside 3 mg/kg i. v. daily, the courses ranging from 5 to 14 injections, given over 5 to 24 days. Following this treatment the bone marrow was examined and treatment with L-asparaginase 1000 IU/kg intravenously daily was begun. It can be seen from Table 2 that following treatment with cytosine arabinoside no patient was in remission, although in some the percentage of blast cells in the bone marrow had been reduced, and indeed in many all leukemic had disappeared from the peripheral blood. No patient had less than 10% of leukemic cells at the time of starting L-asparaginase treatment. L-asparaginase was given for 9 to 28 days, and treatment was continued until there was a sustained rise in the patients' neutrophil and platelet counts. The bone marrow was then re-examined and if it showed less than 5% blasts and the patient was clinically in remission the drug was stopped. It can be seen from Fig. 1

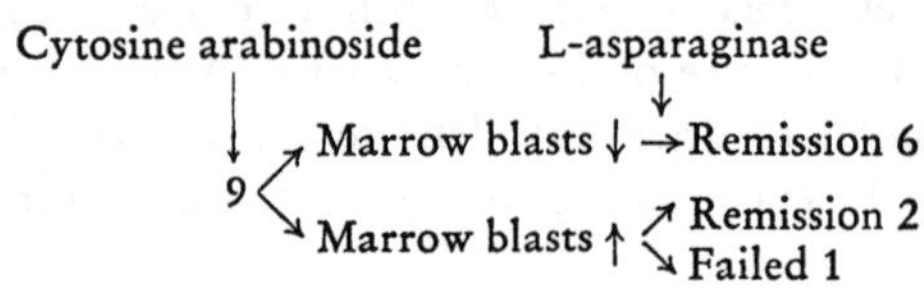

Fig. 1. Results of treatment

and Table 2 that these patients fall into 3 groups. In six patients the proportion of leukemic cells in the marrow was reduced by cytosine arabinoside, but complete remission did not occur while it was being given; in two patients the leukemic cell count actually rose in the marrow during treatment with cytosine arabinoside, and in one patient the blast count in the blood continued to rise during both cytosine arabinoside and L-asparaginase treatment, and the combined treatment failed to produce a remission. However, the other eight patients achieved remission following treatment with L-asparaginase. Fig. 2 shows the typical course of one such patient. It can be seen that following treatment with cytosine arabinoside the marrow leukemic cell percentage had been reduced from 84% to 37% although at no time during cytosine arabinoside treatment did the leukemic cells actually disappear from the peripheral blood. Furthermore there was an effect that we observed in all patients successfully treated: this was a considerable degree of hypoplasia of normal bone marrow elements, accompanied by a profound blood neutropenia and thrombocytopenia, at times as low as 100 neutrophils per cubic millimetre and 10,000 platelets per mm³. It was this side-effect of cytosine arabinoside which made us stop treatment and change to L-asparaginase, even though there were signs that further treatment with cytosine arabinoside might have produced a remission. It was felt that to continue with cytosine arabinoside would have been unreasonable because of the risk of infection, particularly when we had, in L-asparaginase, a drug which would permit us to treat a patient who was severly neutropenic and in whom the normal bone marrow reserves were severely depleted. It can be seen from Fig. 2 that following

Table 2. *Bone marrow findings*

Case	Before Ara-C Cellularity	Blasts %	After Ara-C Cellularity	Blasts %	After L-asparaginase Cellularity	Blasts %	Subsequent [a] Cellularity	Blasts %
1	Increased	84	Decreased	37	Decreased	2.5	Normal	3.5 (6)
2	Normal	84	Decreased	68.5	Decreased	0.5		
3	Leukemic cells 13,000/cu. mm. in blood		Decreased	30	Normal	0.5	Normal	4.5 (5)
4	Increased	47	Decreased	11	Decreased	6		
5	Increased	94.5	Decreased	20.5	Normal	0.3	Increased	2 (9)
6	Normal	50	Decreased	19	Decreased	0.5		
7	Increased	12.5	Increased	99	Normal	2		
8	Normal	20.5	Increased	86.5	Decreased	0.5	Normal	1.5 (2)
9	Leukemic cells 60,000/cu. mm. in blood		Increased	79	Leukemic cell count in blood rose on treatment			

[a] Weeks after end of L-asparaginase shown in parentheses

treatment with L-asparaginase, the neutrophil and platelet counts returned to normal and remission occurred. This confirms the now well-known finding that L-asparaginase is virtually non-toxic to normal bone marrow elements.

The remissions obtained with this combination of drugs were maintained in a variety of ways so that the patients are not comparable on this basis. The choice of maintenance agent was often difficult since the majority of the patients were at a late stage of their disease. The length of remissions ranged from 6 to 21 weeks and all of the eight patients have now relapsed.

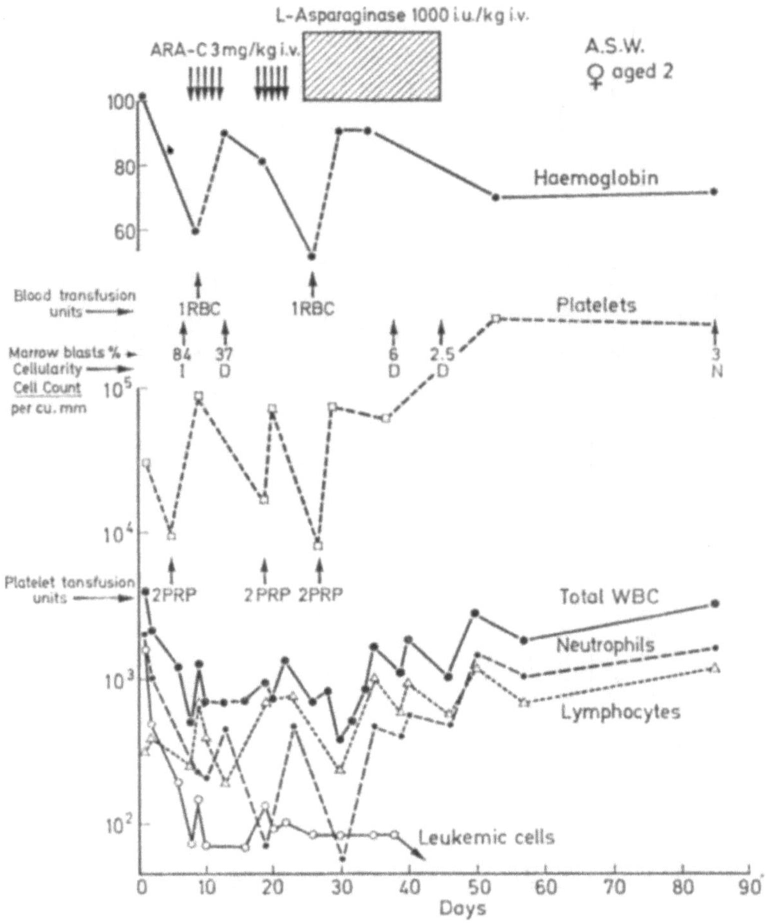

Fig. 2

We feel that this is an encouraging result and it is perhaps worth speculating on the mechanics of using cytosine arabinoside followed by L-asparaginase in this sequential fashion, particularly in view of Dr. Burchenal's findings, that prior treatment with cytosine arabinoside followed by L-asparaginase prolongs survival in EARAD 1 mice with L5178Y/CA55 leukemia. One possible way in which this effect might be produced is by the hypoplasia of normal marrow elements produced as a side effect of cytosine arabinoside treatment. The removal of normal cells from the marrow may reduce cross-feeding of leukemic cells with L-asparagine which is not accessible to the action of circulating L-asparaginase. Another possibility is that cytosine arabinoside may synchronise the mitotic cycle of leukemic cells following inhibition of reproduction, thus making them more sensitive to other anti-tumor agents. This has been shown to occur in HeLa cells by KIM and others and a similar effect has been observed in leukemic cells by LAMPKIN.

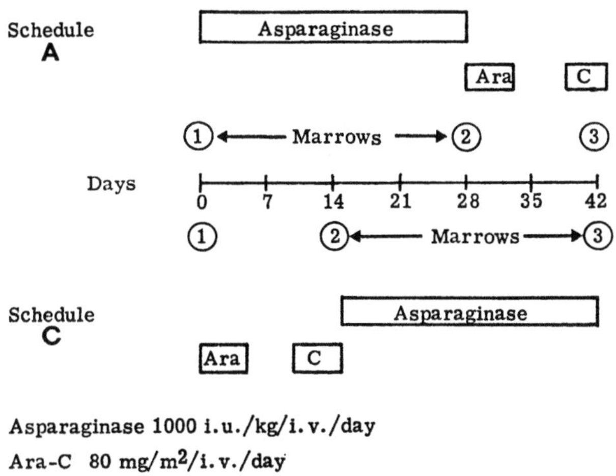

Fig. 3. Trial of L-asparaginase and cytosine arabinoside

It was felt that a controlled trial of this form of treatment was necessary and this is now in progress under the auspices of the Medical Research Council. Fig. 3 shows the design of the trial. Children with acute leukemia in relapse are randomised into two groups. One group receives cytosine arabinoside followed by L-asparaginase, and the other group receives L-asparaginase followed by cytosine arabinoside as shown. Seventeen patients have been studied so far. Ten have received L-asparaginase first. None of these achieved complete remission following one month's L-asparaginase at a dose of 1000 IU/kg i. v. daily, although one of these remitted when given cytosine arabinoside. Seven patients received cytosine arabinoside followed by L-asparaginase and five of these were in remission at the end of the course of L-asparaginase. We are a little worried about the lack of remissions in the asparaginase-first group, but this may be due to the late stage of the disease in the patients and the small numbers treated. It is probable that a more realistic remission rate will be seen in this group as more patients enter the trial. However, there can be little doubt that pre-treatment with cytosine arabinoside enhances the action of L-asparaginase in human leukemia and that it represents a useful form of treatment.

References

BURCHENAL, J. H.: Success and failure in present chemotherapy and the implications of asparaginase. Cancer Res. (in press).

ELLISON, R. R., HOLLAND, J. F., WEIL, M., JACQUILLAT, C., BOIRON, M., BERNARD, J., SAWITSKY, A., ROSNER, F., GUSSOFF, B., SILVER, R. T., KARANAS, A., CUTTNER, J., SPURR, C. L., HAYES, D. M., BLOM, J., LEONE, L. A., HAURANI, F. A., KYLE, R., HUTCHINSON, J. L., FORCIER, R. J., MOON, J. H.: Arabinosyl Cytosine: A useful agent in the treatment of acute leukemia in adults. Blood **4**, 507 (1968).

HORSFALL, F. L.: Personal communication, 1969.

HOWARD, J. P., ALBO, V., NEWTON, W. A., JR.: Cytosine arabinoside. Results of a cooperative study in acute childhood leukemia. Cancer **21**, 341 (1968).

KIM, J. H., EIDENDORFF, M. L.: Action of l- -d-arabinofuranosylcytosine in the nucleic acid metabolism and viability of HeLa cells. Cancer Res. **25**, 698 (1965).

LAMPKIN, B. C., NAGAO, T., MAUER, A. M.: Drug effect in acute leukemia. J. clin. Invest. **48**, 1124 (1969).

MCELWAIN, T. J., HARDISTY, R. M.: Remission induction with cytosine arabinoside and L-asparaginase in acute lymphoblastic leucemia. Brit. Med. J. **4**, 596—598 (1969).

TALLAL, L., OETTGEN, H.: Treatment of acute leukemia in children with L-asparaginase. Proc. Amer. Ass. Cancer Res. **9**, 70 (1968).

Clinical Studies with L-Asparaginase in Dermatomyositis

U. FINK and H. BEGEMANN

Städt. Krankenhaus München-Schwabing, I. Med. Abteilung, Germany

An immunosuppressive effect of L-asparaginase seems to be likely. Therefore it is interesting to investigate the effect of L-asparaginase in the treatment of human autoimmune disorders. We have treated a patient with dermatomyositis with L-asparaginase (Crasnitin) at a daily dose of 1000 units/kg body weight over a period of 35 days. Previously he did not respond to steroids at a dose of about 50 mg daily.

Ten days after beginning the asparaginase therapy skin alterations started to regress. After further application of the drug improvement of the skin lesions became more and more apparent.

It was interesting to study the changes in the blood cell counts and in the serum biochemistry produced by L-asparaginase, because in this case patient's haematological and metabolic serum findings had been found to be normal prior to the treatment.

1. Blood Cells

During the first 3 weeks the red cell counts remained unchanged. Between day 21 and day 28 the erythrocytes decreased by 1 million per mm^3 and remained stable afterwards. The reticulocyte counts increased threefold. The number of platelets was not affected.

During the first 7 days of treatment granulocytes decreased by more than 50%. They reached their initial values again on day 16 of treatment and remained at this level. The lymphocytes increased threefold up to the 13th day of treatment. Later they decreased but did not reach again their initial values. Bone marrow specimens did not show any remarkable alterations except for a slight increase of reticulum cells.

2. Serum Biochemistry

During the first 4 weeks activities of liver enzymes did not alter. On day 31 they increased slightly for the first time. Total serum protein, albumin as well as alpha and beta-globulin concentration diminished continously while the gamma globulin concentration rose.

Fibrinogen and cholesterol decreased until day 14 and returned gradually without reaching their initial values.

3. Lymphocyte Cultures

In lymphocyte cultures with PHA a total suppression of the blast transformation was observed, when the lymphocytes were incubated in autologous serum.

In summary: The alterations of blood cells and serum biochemistry in a patient with a probable autoimmune disorder treated with L-asparaginase did not differ very much from those alterations seen in leukemic patients. The most prominent changes were a transient decrease of the peripheral granulocyte count and of fibrinogen and cholesterol levels, a longer lasting decrease of the serum protein concentration and, on day 31, the appearance of the first signs of a more severely disturbed liver function.

In conclusion, L-asparaginase in a dosage of 1000 units per kg body weight produced a remarkable clinical improvement in a patient with dermatomyositis.

Blood Coagulation Changes under L-Asparaginase Therapy

E. DEUTSCH, M. FISCHER, H. FRISCHAUF, N. HONETZ, K. LECHNER, F. PESENDORFER, H. STYCH, and A. WEISSMANN

From the Department of Medicine, University of Vienna, Austria

With 8 Figures

Bleeding complications have been observed during the therapy of lymphoblastic leukemias with L-asparaginase. Frequently the platelet count is already low before treatment in these patients and may be reduced further during treatment, but is not sufficient to explain the observed bleeding tendency.

STIER and cow. observed that treatment with L-asparaginase induces a coagulation defect which, however, was not of the same pattern in all patients. They suggested that the decrease of fibrinogen which was the prominent feature of the coagulation defect, might be caused by consumption coagulopathy, primary fibrinolysis or inhibition of the production of clotting factors. DEUTSCH, KREPLER and STACHER, studying cases of acute leukemia found a decrease of fibrinogen and plasminogen following L-asparaginase therapy and discussed consumption coagulopathy or increased fibrinolysis as possibilities. GRALNICK and HENRY treating cases with acute leukemia also considered intravascular coagulation as cause of the coagulation defect. LECHLER observed a reduction of factor IX and suggested inhibition of the production of clotting factors, WHITECARE and coworkers observed a prominent decrease of fibrinogen but normal factors V and VIII.

Our experiments which will be reported here were designed with the scope to decide by which mechanism L-asparaginase induces the coagulation disturbance.

Material and Methods

Asparaginase was generously supplied by Bayer-Leverkusen (FB b 6366).

Collection of blood: Venous blood was obtained after clean venipuncture and mixed 1 : 10 with 3.8% sodium citrate solution in siliconized centrifuge tubes, centrifuged at 4,000 rpm for 30 min at room temperature in a MSE centrifuge. The plasma was divided in several samples most of them were quick frozen at once and stored at —20° C for the serial determination of factors II (DEUTSCH and SCHADEN), X (BACHMANN), VIII and IX (BARROW et al.), antithrombin III (HENSEN and

LOELIGER), Plasminogen, Plasmin and Antiplasmin (NORMAN). Thromboplastin time (QUICK), partial thromboplastin time with kaolin (PROCTOR and RAPAPORT), fibrinogen (CLAUSS), factor V (DEUTSCH and SCHADEN) and thrombin time (with 5 U/ml thrombin) were determined at once.

Standard and heated fibrin plates were prepared according to ASTRUP. Retraction was determined in citrated platelet rich plasma according to BENTHAUS. EDTA-venous whole blood (10 mg EDTA powder for 2 ml blood in a siliconized tube) was used for platelet counting (BRECHER and CRONKITE). Serum was obtained for the determination of fibrin degradation products (MERSKEY), total protein and albumin, BUN, creatinine, uric acid, cholesterol, GOT, leucin amino peptidase. Immune globulines and trace proteines were determined with Partigen plates (Behring-Werke). Capillary blood was used for the determination of blood sugar and platelet count (BRECHER and CRONKITE). Bleeding time was determined according to DUKE.

The survival of fibrinogen was determined with ^{125}I fibrinogen. Human fibrinogen (KABI) was labelled according to MACFARLANE. Labeled fibrinogen with approximately 2 mill. counts was injected and citrated whole blood samples were drawn at appropriate intervals, centrifuged and the plasma counted in a well type scintillation counter.

Design of the Study

Labelled fibrinogen was injected 72 to 96 hours before the first dose of L-asparaginase and samples for counting of the radioactivity were obtained at about eight hours intervals. Samples for the determination of the various parameters were drawn at least twice in the pretreatment period, every day before the infusion was given in the treatment period and daily for at least four days in the posttreatment period. L-asparaginase (FB b 6366) at a dose of 200 U/kg or 2000 U/kg diluted with saline was infused intravenously in the morning of the treatment days.

Four patients were in each group (for age, diagnosis, dose of asparaginase and duration of the treatment see Table 1).

Table 1

	In.	Sex	Age	Diagnosis	Daily dose of L-asparaginase	Duration of treatment	Total amount
1	Ly	f	69	Reticulosis	200 U/kg	4 days	48,000
2	Ba	m	77	Lung cancer	200 U/kg	6 days	76,000
3	Ul	m	67	Lung cancer	200 U/kg	6 days	84,000
4	Th	f	74	Myeloma	200 U/kg	14 days	168,000
5	Ta	f	68	Acute lymphoblastic leukemia	2000 U/kg	5 days	900,000
6	Le	f	63	Hysterocarcinoma with metastases	2000 U/kg	6 days	960,000
7	Kr	m	24	Lung cancer	2000 U/kg	4 days	610,000
8	Ne	f	58	Myeloma	2000 U/kg	3 days	280,000

Results

1. Coagulation Factors

The factors I, II, V, IX, X and antithrombin III decreased in all cases a few days after the initiation of the therapy. Factor IX was the first to be reduced, then followed factors II and X, V, antithrombin III and finally fibrinogen (Fig. 1). The degree of reduction of activity was similar for factors II, V and X with about 50%, then followed antithrombin III, fibrinogen and factor IX which showed the greatest loss of activity. Factor VIII behaved completely different. It was unchanged, showed a small reduction or was even increased after several days. An abnormal fibrinogen could not be detected by immune electrophoresis.

2. Fibrinolytic System

The plasminogen decreased rapidly and intensively. After the end of the therapy it started to increase again rapidly in several cases. The immediate antiplasmin was distinctly reduced in all cases, the reduction started slowly and continued after the

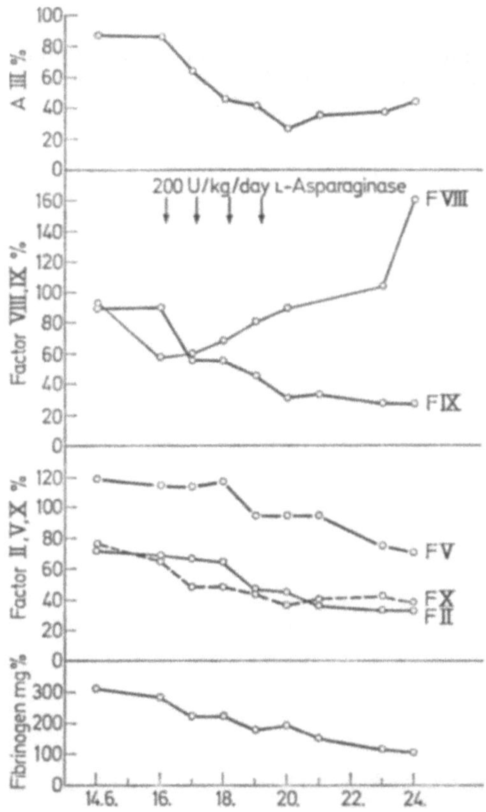

Fig. 1. Action of L-asparaginase on the blood clotting system. Ordinate: Activity of Antithrombin III, factors VIII, IX; II, V, X in % of normal, fibrinogen in mg-%. Abscissa: Time in days. Dose: 4×200 U/kg/day

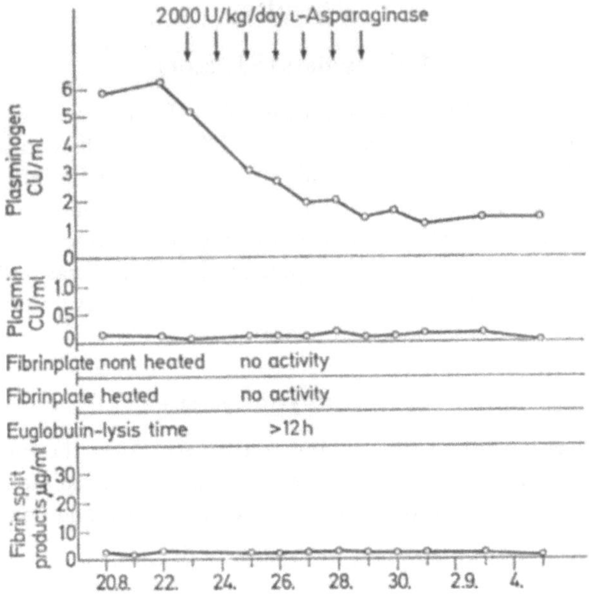

Fig. 2. Action of L-asparaginase on the fibrinolytic system. Ordinate: Plasminogen and plasmin in casein units/ml, Fibrin split products in µg/ml. Abscissa: Time in days. Dose: 7×2000 U/kg/day

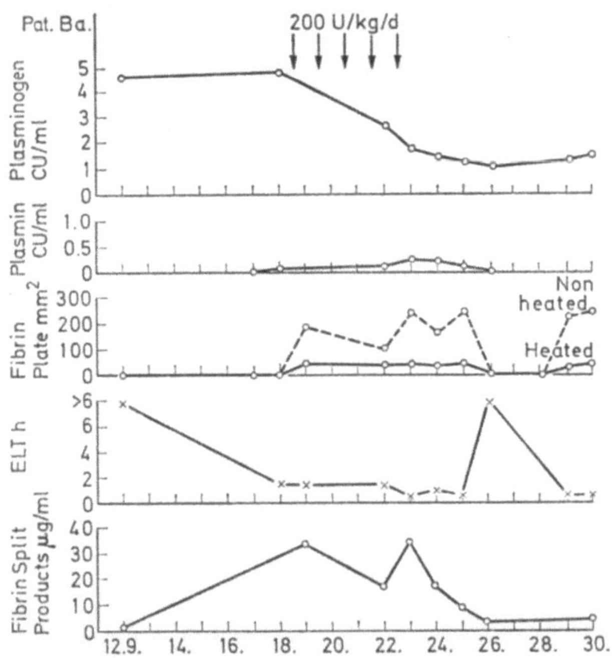

Fig. 3. Action of L-asparaginase on the fibrinolytic system in the only case with activation of fibrinolysis. Ordinate: Plasminogen and plasmin in casein units/ml, lysed area of standard and heated fibrin plates in mm², euglobulin lysis time in hrs, fibrin split products in µg/ml. Abszissa: Time in days. Dose: 5×200 U/kg/day. Diagnosis: Bronchus cancer

end of the treatment. The progressive antiplasmin was also reduced but to a lower extent (Fig. 2). No FDP could be found. Only one case of the lower dosage group showed a significant fibrinolytic activity in the euglobulin lysis time and on standard fibrin plates. This was also the only case where a plasmin activity of more than 0.2 U/ml was found. FDP could be detected in its serum (Fig. 3).

3. Survival Time of Labelled Fibrinogen

The survival time of labeled fibrinogen was between 48 hours and 94 hours in our patients during the pretreatment period. With one exception there was no increase of the disappearance rate during the treatment with L-asparaginase (Fig. 4, Table 2). In this one case the half-life was reduced from 94 to 67 hrs. This patient died a few days after the treatment was stopped. No radioactivity was found in the organs at necropsy.

The disappearance rate of fibrinogen determined with the method of Clauss was slower than the disappearance rate of the radioactivity in all cases.

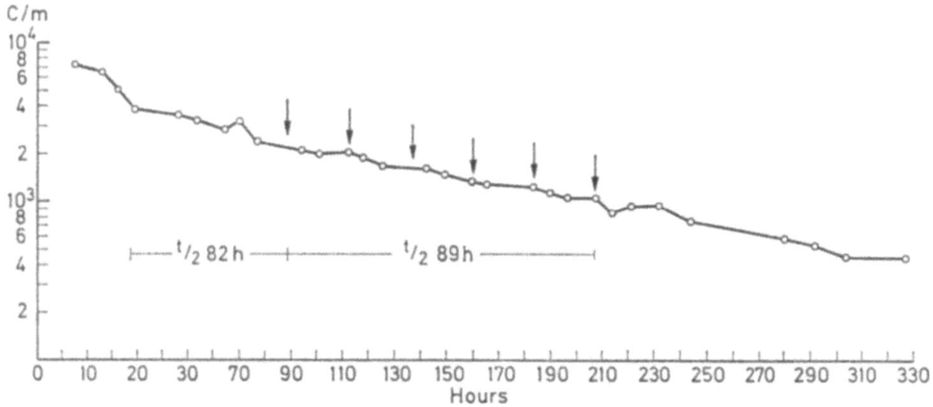

Fig. 4. Fibrinogen decay rate. Ordinate: counts/min. Abszissa: Time in hrs. Dose: 6×2000 U/kg/day. Patient: Le

Table 2. *t/2 of ^{125}I-labeled fibrinogen before and during therapy with L-asparaginase*

	Dosage	Before treatment	During treatment
Ly	200 U/kg/day	48 h	51 h
Th	200 U/kg/day	74 h	104 h
Pa	200 U/kg/day		67 h
Ul	200 U/kg/day	94 h	67 h
Ta	2000 U/kg/day	60 h	60 h
Ne	2000 U/kg/day	55 h	106 h
Le	2000 U/kg/day	81 h	89 h
Kr	2000 U/kg/day	47 h	69 h

4. Platelets

The platelets were counted by two independent observers from two different samples. The counts did not change significantly in any case (Fig. 5). In agreement with this observation the bleeding time and clot retraction did not change either.

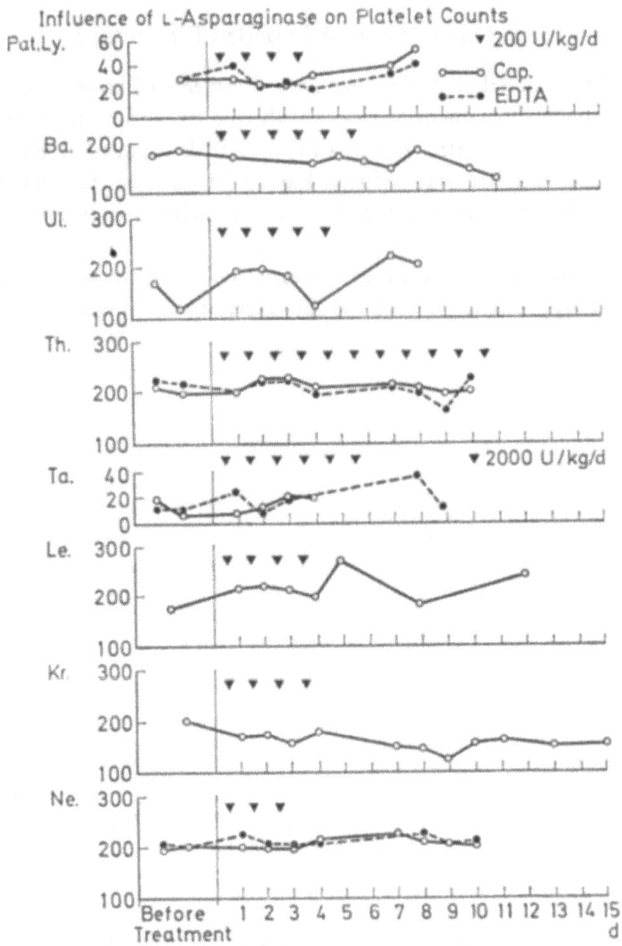

Fig. 5. Behaviour of platelets. Ordinate: Count ×1000. Abszissa: Time in days

5. Influence of the Dosage

The following parameters were calculated to compare the two treatment groups: The mean time interval necessary for a 25% reduction of an individual factor, the mean time, until the lowest level was reached and the mean of the maximal inactivation of an individual factor. It was found that the rate of reduction was a little slower in the lower dosage group for factors X, II and plasminogen (Fig. 6), but the

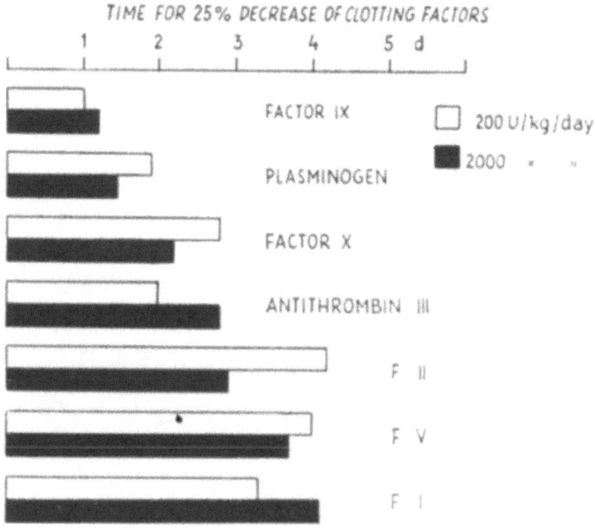

Fig. 6. Time necessary for a reduction of 25% of the initial value of the individual factors studied

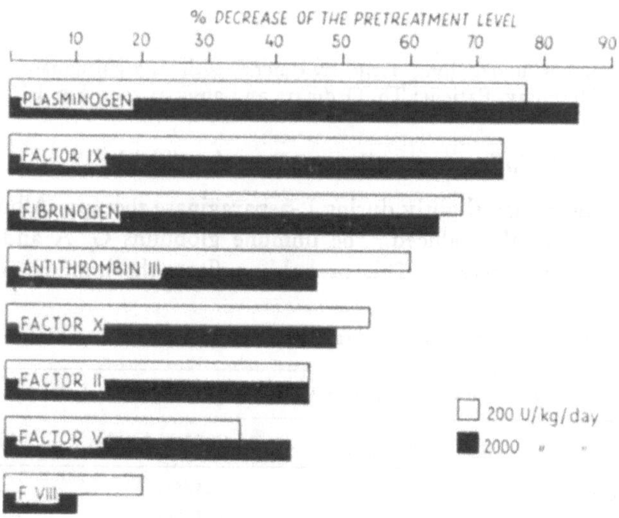

Fig. 7. Mean value of the maximal decrease of clotting factors in % of the initial value

extent of reduction did not differ significantly (Fig. 7). The decrease of the activity of the clotting factors continued after the end of therapy in the cases treated for a short time. In one case which was treated for 14 days the activity of the clotting factors started to increase during therapy (Fig. 8).

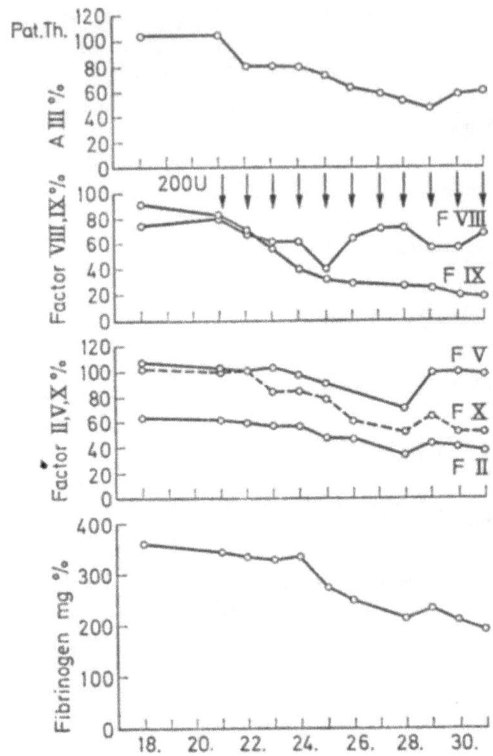

Fig. 8. Clotting factors under long term treatment with L-asparaginase. Dose: 11×200 U/kg/day. Patient: Th. Ordinate and abscissa as in Fig. 1

6. Influence on Serum Proteins (Table 3)

Total protein decreased slightly during L-asparaginase therapy. Albumin remained unchanged or was slightly reduced. The immune globulins G, A and M showed a definite increase during therapy. This probably reflects the immune response to the

Table 3. *Effect of L-asparaginase therapy on serum proteins*

	Decrease or increase in % of the pretreatment level		
	200 U/kg/day	2000 U/kg/day	All cases
Total protein	— 8%	—14%	—11%
Albumin	— 1%	—11%	— 6%
IgG	+58%	+88%	+75%
IgA	+18%	+95%	+86%
IgM	+28%	+23%	+29%
Ceruloplasmin	—49%	—65%	—58%
α_1-Antitrypsin	—46%	—45%	—45%
α^2-Macroglobulin	—31%	—40%	—36%
Transferrin	—48%	—77%	—65%

foreign protein. Other proteins as ceruloplasmin, a_1-antitrypsin, transferrin and a_2-macroglobulin showed a definite decrease similar to the clotting factors. These changes were more pronounced in the high dosage group.

7. Side Effects

All patients complained of headache, malaise, vomiting, and loss of appetite which was so intensive that it forced us to reduce the duration of the treatment as much as possible. Two patients developed overt bleeding. One case bled from the tumor and from hemorrhagic gastritis, the other developed multiple hematomas. The blood sugar showed a slight increase in three cases, but remained in the normal range. The cholesterol was distinctly reduced in four cases. An increase of urea nitrogen without accompanying increase of creatinine was observed in all cases. It was more pronounced in the higher dosage group. The bilirubin was slightly increased in two cases. The GOT increased in one patient to 265 U, this patient showed the highest bilirubin value and a distinct decrease in cholesterol. There was, however, already an increase of GOT and bilirubin in the pretreatment period. Therefore, it has to be doubted whether this increase was caused by the therapy. This case did not differ from other cases in the behaviour of clotting factors. The uric acid was increased in five cases.

Discussion

The coagulation defect induced by L-asparaginase was characterized by a reduction of clotting factors I, II, V, IX, X, antithrombin III, and by a reduction of plasminogen and antiplasmins in all but one case. Only factor VIII and the platelets behaved differently.

From the clinical point of view the hypofibrinogenemia is the most important change because it may reach dangerous levels. The other defects may contribute to but not cause a hemorrhagic diathesis.

The mechanism by which the clotting defect is caused is difficult to explain. Hypofibrinogenemia with reduction of antithrombin III and some reduction of factors II, V and X is found in cases with intravascular coagulation but the normal factor VIII and normal platelet counts are strong arguments against this explanation. On the other hand the combination of reduction of plasminogen, antiplasmin, fibrinogen and factor V, some reduction of factors II and X with a normal platelet count is characteristic for intravascular activation of fibrinolysis. However, factor VIII is normal and we succeded only in one case to demonstrate moderate fibrinolysis. We can not give an explanation, why this patient behaved differently. He had a cancer of the bronchus, at that time without clinically detactable metastasis. The most important argument against intravascular consumption of fibrinogen is the behaviour of the labeled fibrinogen whose decay rate is not accelerated during and after the L-asparaginase treatment. Bettigole et al. also demonstrated that the disappearance rate of labeled fibrinogen was not changed by asparaginase treatment.

In numerous experiments it has been demonstrated that protein synthesis is inhibited by L-asparaginase. Therefore, it should be considered that the decrease of clotting factors could be caused by an inhibition of their synthesis. In this sense argues that it was not possible to find any signs of increased consumption of clotting factors, especially of fibrinogen. Second, that the sequence of disappearance of clotting factors correlated roughly to their biological half life time. Third that the production of other proteins is also reduced. Amino acid analysis by others has demonstrated that prothrombin and factor X contain appreciable amounts of asparagin (Jackson and Hanakan, Laki and cow.). It can, therefore, be expected that a deficiency of asparagin could interfere with the synthesis of these clotting factors.

Our results are not necessarily at variance with those of Stier and cow. We studied patients with malignant diseases of different types including two cases with leukemias, both with low leucocyte counts. We feel that we have observed in these cases the pure effect of L-asparaginase. Stier and cow. studied cases of acute lymphoblastic leukemia with high cell counts. In these cases where many cell desintegrate following therapy with L-asparaginase it is certainly possible that other mechanisms, such as intravascular coagulation or fibrinolysis may complicate the situation and superimpose the coagulation defect induced by L-asparaginase. It seems, however, that these changes are secondary and are observed only in cases which are prone to intravascular coagulation or fibrinolysis even without therapy.

The effects of the two dosage schedules studied did not significantly differ, which agrees with the findings of Whitecare et al. The decrease of clotting factors was a little bit faster and the increase of urea nitrogen was much more distinct in the higher dosage group. Obviously 200 U/kg L-asparaginase suffice to suppress the protein synthesis. If the medication is extended over a longer period, the clotting factors may increase again. It is suggested that the cells become resistant to the action of L-asparaginase.

Summary

The action of 200 and 2000 U/kg/day of L-asparaginase on the blood clotting and fibrinolytic system in humans was studied. The factors I, II, V, IX, X, antithrombin III, plasminogen, and the antiplasmins are reduced, but not platelets, factor VIII, bleeding time, and retraction. This is most probably caused by an inhibition of the synthesis of these factors. The decay rate of labeled fibrinogen is not influenced. In cases, for other reasons prone to intravascular coagulation or fibrinolysis, these mechanisms may be induced and superimposed on the defect induced by L-asparaginase.

References

Astrup, T., Müllertz, S.: The fibrin plate method for estimating fibrinolytic activity. Arch. Biochem. Biophys. **4 a**, 346 (1952).

Bachmann, F., Duckert, F., Koller, F.: The Stuart Prower factor assay and its clinical significance. Thrombos. Diathes. haemorrh. (Stuttg.) 2, 24 (1958).

Barrow, E. M., Roberts, H. R., Pons, K., Graham, J. B.: Studies of the antihemophilic factor (AHF, Factor VIII) produced in von Willebrandt's disease. Proc. Soc. exp. Biol. (N. Y.) **115**, 760 (1964).

Begemann, H.: Als Berichterstatter der Arbeitsgemeinschaft L-Asparaginase in der Sektion Onkologie der Paul-Ehrlich-Gesellschaft für Chemotherapie: Behandlungsergebnisse mit L-Asparaginase bei akuten Leukämien. In: Chemo- und Immunotherapie der Leukosen und malignen Lymphome. Ed.: A. Stacher. Wien: Bohmann 1969, p. 293.

Benthaus, J.: Über die Retraktion des Blutgerinnsels. Thrombos. Diathes. haemorrh. (Stuttg.) **3**, 311 (1959).

BETTIGOLE, R. E., HIMELSTEIN, E. S., OETTGEN, H. F., CLIFFORD, G. O.: Hypofibrinogenemia due to L-asparaginase: Studies using ^{131}I-Fibrinogen. Clin. Res. **17**, 399 (1969).

BRECHER, G., CRONKITE, E. P.: Morphology and enumeration of blood platelets. J. appl. Physiol. **3**, 365 (1950).

CLAUSS, A.: Gerinnungsphysiologische Schnellmethode zur Bestimmung des Fibrinogens. Acta haematol. **18**, 373 (1956).

DEUTSCH, E., SCHADEN, W.: Zur Reinigung und Charakterisierung des VII. Blutgerinnungsfaktors. Biochem. Z. **324**, 266 (1953).

— WEISSMANN, A.: Therapie der hämorrhagischen Komplikationen bei Leukosen. In: Chemo- und Immunotherapie der Leukosen und malignen Lymphome. Ed.: A. STACHER. Wien: Bohmann 1969, p. 261.

DUKE, W. W.: The relation of blood platelets to hemorrhagic diseases. Description of a method for determining the bleeding time and report of three cases of hemorrhagic disease relieved by transfusion. J. Amer. med. Ass. **55**, 1185 (1910).

GRALNICK, H. R., HENRY, P. H.: L-asparaginase induced coagulopathy. Proc. Amer. Ass. Canc. Res. **10**, 32 (1969).

GRUNDMANN, E.: Grundlagen der L-Asparaginase-Therapie. In: Chemo- und Immunotherapie der Leukosen und malignen Lymphome. Ed.: A. STACHER. Wien: Bohmann 1969, p. 23.

HENSEN, A. E., LOELIGER, A.: Antithrombin, III. Thrombos. Diathes. haemorrh. (Stuttg.) **9**, 53 (1963).

JACKSON, C. R., HANAHAN, D. J.: Studies on bovine factor X. II. Characterization of purified factor X. Observations on some alterations in zone electrophoretic and chromatographic behaviour occuring during purification. Biochem. **7**, 4506 (1968).

LAKI, K., KOMINZ, D. R., SYMONDS, P., LORAND, L., SEEGERS, W. H.: The amino acid composition of bovine prothrombin. Arch. Biochem. Biophys. **60**, 276 (1954).

LECHLER, E., HIRSCHMANN, W. D., GROSS, R.: Führt die Asparaginasebehandlung zu einer Verbrauchskoagulopathie? 75. Tg. Dtsch. Ges. Inn. Med. Wiesbaden 1969, S. 484.

MACFARLANE, A. S.: In vivo behaviour of ^{131}J-Fibrinogen. J. clin. Invest. **42**, 346 (1963).

MERSKEY, C., LALOZARI, P., JOHNSON, A. J.: A rapid, simple, sensitive method for measuring fibrinolytic split products in human serum. Proc. Soc. exp. Biol. (N. Y.) **131**, 571 (1969).

NORMAN, P. S.: Studies of the plasmin system. I. Measurement of human and animal plasminogen. Measurement of an activator in human serum. J. exp. Med. **106**, 423 (1967).

PROCTOR, R. R., RAPAPORT, S. I.: The partial thromboplastin time with kaolin. Amer. J. clin. Path. **36**, 212 (1961).

QUICK, A. J.: Hemorrhagic diseases. Springfield: Thomas 1942.

STIER, H. W., GALLMEIER, W. M., SCHMIDT, C. G.: Über Störungen des Blutgerinnungssystems im Verlauf der Enzym-Therapie maligner Tumoren und Hämoblastosen. Dtsch. med. Wschr. **94**, 253 (1969).

— SCHMIDT, C. G., GALLMEIER, W. M.: Das Blutgerinnungssystem während der Leukämiebehandlung mit L-Asparaginase. In: Chemo- und Immunotherapie der Leukosen und malignen Lymphome. Ed.: A. STACHER. Wien: Bohmann 1969, p. 310.

WHITECAR, J. P., JR., HARRIS, J. E., BODEY, G. P., FREIREICH, E. J.: Host effects of L-asparaginase treatment. Clin. Res **17**, 408 (1969).

The Hemostatic Defect Induced by Treatment with Asparaginase in Leukemia

D. L. Heene and H. Löffler

Department of Medicine, University of Giessen, Germany

In order to evaluate the character of the hemostatic defect usually observed during therapy with asparaginase, coagulation studies were performed in 18 patients treated with asparaginase for different types of leukemia. With regard to the follow-up only 13 patients could be selected. The diagnosis in these cases was:

Type of leukemia	Number of patients
Promyelocytic l	1
Myeloblastic l	4
Blastic crises in chron. myelocytic l	3
Monocytic l	2
Lymphoblastic l	3

Methods

The coagulation studies included platelet count, thrombelastography, thromboplastin time, partial thromboplastin time, thrombin time, euglobulin lysis time and quantitative determination of individual plasma components such as fibrinogen, factors II, V, VIII and XIII as well as fibrinmonomer-complexes and fibrinogen degradation products. The analysis were performed daily or at least two-day intervals.

Results

As compared to the pretreatment values (100%) in all cases a significant decrease ($p < 0.05$) of fibrinogen (70%), factor V (69%), factor XIII (51%) and prolongation of the thromboplastin time (66%) were observed regularly between the 2nd and 5th day of therapy with asparaginase. Since loss of fibrinogen concentration, low factor V and XIII activity are considered as analytical criteria of consumption-coagulopathy, further differentiation was necessary with regard to the development of diffuse intravascular clotting, possibly induced by asparaginase. Circulating fibrinmonomer-complexes as indicators of diffuse intravascular coagulation were demonstrated repeatedly in 1 patient with myeloblastic and 1 patient with monocytic leukemia before and during treatment, the latter showed also secondary fibrinolysis detected by means of quantitative immunochemical analysis of fibrinogen degradation products, shortened euglobulin lysis time and prolongation of the thrombin time. Consumption-coagulopathy during treatment was observed in 1 patient with promyelocytic and 1 patient with lymphoblastic leukemia. Both cases responded to heparin administration. Otherwise, 1 patient with myeloblastic leukemia developed secondary fibrinolysis during therapy. Thus the manifestation of consumption-coagulopathy and secondary fibrinolysis coincided only in 3 cases with asparaginase treatment. The alterations of plasma factors were reversible after therapy was discontinued.

Conclusion

Consumption-coagulopathy and secondary fibrinolysis are eventually observed in cases with acute leukemia either spontaneous or related to cytostatic therapy [1, 2]. Hypofibrinogenemia, decrease of factors V and XIII are constantly observed during treatment with asparaginase and can be correlated to concommittant hypalbuminemia, probably due to defect proteinsynthesis in the liver [3, 4]. With regard to the relatively low coincidence of consumption-coagulopathy and secondary fibrinolysis in cases treated with asparaginase, which may occur in the same rate during cytostatic therapy in general, the typical decrease of plasma clotting factors should rather be explained as consequence of inhibition of protein synthesis than by increased turn-over due to diffusc intravascular clotting. However the latter always should be excluded and may be difficult to prove by analytical procedures in the presence of asparaginase induced hypofibrinogenemia [5].

References

1. Sultan, Y., Larrieu, M. J., Tschernia, G., Klener, P.: Fibrinopénie au cours des leucémies à promyelocytes. Traitement par l'héparine. Nouv. Rev. franç. Hémat. **8**, 119 (1968).
2. Lasch, H. G., Heene, D. L.: Diagnosis of intravascular coagulation and fibrinolysis. In: Platelets, their role in hemostasis and thrombosis. Ed.: K. M. Brinkhous. Stuttgart: Schattauer 1967, p. 351.
3. Stier, H. W., Gallmeier, W. M., Schmidt, C. G.: Über Störungen des Blutgerinnungssystems im Verlaufe der Enzymtherapie maligner Tumoren und Hämoblastosen. Dtsch. med. Wschr. **94**, 253 (1969).
4. Oettgen, H. F., Schulten, H. K.: Hemmung maligner Neoplasien des Menschen durch L-asparaginase. Klin. Wschr. **47**, 65 (1969).
5. Lechler, E., Hirschmann, W. D., Gross, R.: Führt die Asparaginasebehandlung zu einer Verbrauchscoagulopathie? 75. Kongr. Verh. dtsch. Ges. inn. Med. Wiesbaden 1969 (in press).

Dysmetabolic and Neurological Complications in Leukemic Patients Treated with L-Asparaginase

E. Storti and D. Quaglino

Institute of Medical Pathology, University of Modena, Italy

With 1 Figure

The usefulness and value of any new antileukemic drug is assessed not only on the basis of its efficacy in causing the disappearance of the abnormal blast cell population, but also of its toxicity and on the nature and extent of complications which may appear, when it is used at therapeutic levels.

The purpose of our paper is to present some unusual and intriguing side-effects, concerning lipid metabolism and the central nervous system, which we have observed in the course of our clinical trial with L-asparaginase.

The trial was carried out in 34 cases of acute leukemia, and the results are briefly summarized in Table 1.

Of the 23 cases of acute lymphoblastic leukemia (11 males and 12 females), 14 were children under 12 years of age. The dose used in this type of leukemia varied from 50 IU/kg/day to 200 IU/kg/day, while high doses of 400 and 500 IU/kg/day were used in cases refractory to the lower doses and in patients in relapse.

With regard to the use of high levels of L-asparaginase in acute lymphoblastic leukemia, it is our impression that if a case is sensitive to the enzyme, it will respond

Table 1. *Results*

	First treatment	Duration of remission
Acute lymphoblastic leukemia *23 cases* (Dosage from 50—500 IU/kg/day)	Complete remission = 8 cases (34%) Partial remission = 5 cases (21%) No response = 10 cases (45%)	From 4 to 20 weeks From 3 to 5 weeks
Acute myeloblastic leukemia 7 cases (Dosage: 200 IU/kg/day)	No response in all seven cases	
Acute monocytic leukemia 1 case (Dosage: 200 IU/kg/day)	Complete remission	12 weeks
Leukosarcoma 3 cases (Dosage: 200 IU/kg/day)	Complete remission = 1 case No response = 2 cases	8 weeks

rapidly both haematologically and clinically (one may in fact observe a reduction in the size of lymphnodes, liver and spleen, already 48 hours after starting treatment), with doses as low as 50 IU/kg/day, whereas no apparent improvement is observed in poorly responsive cases, even when using daily doses of 500 IU/kg.

In acute lymphoblastic leukemia we have obtained a complete remission (i. e. a total disappearance of blast cells from the bone-marrow and reappearance of normally maturing haemopoietic tissue) in 34% of our cases and a partial remission in 21%. It is worth mentioning that about half of our patients in this group had received prior treatment with anti-leukemic drugs, which did not seem to influence in any way the degree and speed of the response to L-asparaginase.

The average length of our remissions was 5—6 weeks, although in one case we had a remission lasting 20 weeks. In order to increase the duration of remissions, we have recently adopted the following therapeutic scheme: one week of treatment at relatively high doses (500 IU/kg/day) every three weeks. Such a procedure has already yielded satisfactory results in two cases, who have been in good remission for three months.

We can dismiss rapidly our seven cases of acute myeloblastic leukemia, in all of which the results were completely disappointing.

The unexpectedly good remission obtained in our single case of acute monocytic leukemia (the cytological diagnosis was based on the results of cytochemical investigations) seems to indicate that this type of acute leukemia can also be sensitive to L-asparaginase, in contrast with the original impression, which suggested that mainly the lymphoid and occasionally the myeloid type of leukemia responded favourably to the drug (Cardinali, 1969; Adamson and Fabro, 1969).

Finally our case material includes three patients with leukosarcoma (two were children under 12 years of age). A good haematological and clinical remission, lasting 8 weeks, was observed in one child, who had previously been treated with various antimitotic agents without success.

Having thus briefly summarized our therapeutic results, we will now consider the side-effects encountered.

To begin with, nearly all our patients complained of anorexia, nausea and vomiting. In four instances, our patients presented signs and symptoms of hypersensitivity, consisting in cutaneous eruptions, puffiness of the face, shock, oedema of the glottis. Similar features have been described before by other authors (Hill et al., 1967; Oettgen et al., 1967).

From the laboratory point of view, the most constant finding was the increased urinary excretion of uric acid, which sometimes (especially in cases entering a good remission) was found to be 5 to 10 times above the normal level.

In Table 2 are shown the other laboratory findings: i. e. a decrease in fibrinogen in all cases, a reduction in prothrombin time in 69% of our patients, a variable increase in transaminases and serum alkaline phosphatase activity, a decrease in the cholesterol level in 76% of our cases.

These findings are in agreement with those reported by other authors (Haskell et al., 1969).

In two of our patients, lipid metabolism appeared to become markedly deranged under the effect of L-asparaginase treatment.

The first case was an 11 year old child with acute lymphoblastic leukemia in relapse, who had been treated for four weeks with L-asparaginase at a daily dose of 200 IU/kg, together with small doses of prednisone (10 mg daily). The patient went into a good clinical and haematological remission, but towards the second week of treatment the serum of the patient started to have a slightly milky appearance, which became gradually more marked as shown in Fig. 1.

Table 2

Laboratory findings in 34 cases of acute leukemia	
Fibrinogen:	Decreased in 100% of cases. Levels lower than 100 mg-% in 46% of cases.
Prothrombin time:	Decreased in 69%
S.G.P.T.:	Increased in 17%
S.G.O.T.:	Increased in 24%
Alkaline phosphatase:	Increased in 41% Decreased in 11%
Cholesterol:	Decreased in 76%

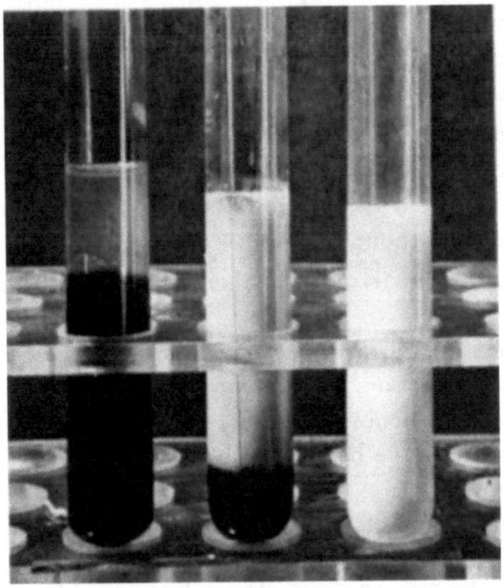

Fig. 1. Three test tubes showing from left to right normal human serum, the patient's serum and cow's milk

Measurement of the various lipid fractions, showed a general and marked increase (Table 3).

The patient was discharged from hospital on a maintenance dose of 5 mg prednisone daily and after one month her serum had assumed its normal appearance, which was confirmed by the findings shown again in Table 3.

Her remission lasted four months and when readmitted to hospital her leukemia proved refractory to L-asparaginase treatment even with doses of 500 IU/kg/day. During this period her lipid metabolism was repeatedly investigated, but showed a decrease in all fractions, a pattern similar to that seen in the majority of cases.

Table 3

	20-11-68 Before treatment	20-12-68 After 374,000 IU of asparaginase	7-2-69 One month after treatment
Total lipids (mg-%)	—	9950	1210
Triglycerides (mg-%)	—	3050	494
Total cholesterol (mg-%)	155	990	220
Phospholipids (mg-%)	—	1020	249
Lipoproteins β/α ratio	—	18.6	2.36
β+Chylomicrons/α ratio	—	36.1	3.93

The second patient was a case of leukosarcoma who had not responded to L-asparaginase and whose serum acquired a milky appearance 10 days after starting therapy. When the various lipid fractions were measured, the cholesterol level was found decreased, but total lipids, phospholipids, beta-lipoproteins, chylomicrons as well as triglycerides were found considerably increased.

With regard to the neurological complications observed, these were present in two of our cases.

The first case was a middle-aged woman, with acute lymphoblastic leukemia, who was treated with 200 IU/kg/day of L-asparaginase. A week after therapy was started, the patient began to show a progressive increase in muscular tone, affecting the whole range of movement and characterized by the so-called cog-wheel rigidity, typical of lesions of the extrapyramidal system. The disturbance in tone was first apparent in the cervical muscles spreading later to the other parts of the body. In addition the patient was also affected by tremor, more prominent at rest and consisting of coarse, regular, rhythmic movements at the rate of 5—6 per second, involving opposing muscle groups equally.

In other words, the patient presented a typical picture of parkinsonism, which disappeared with the interruption of treatment. However, when L-asparaginase was restarted one month later at twice weekly doses of 300 IU/kg/day an increase in muscular tone became again apparent.

It is conceivable that the neurological signs observed were related to the drug, since they disappeared completely when treatment was discontinued and also because a similar disturbance in muscular tone, as described above, was seen in three other patients, at a time when treatment had been prolonged beyond 25—30 days.

Neurological complications during the course of L-asparaginase treatment have recently been reported in adults by HASKELL and his colleagues (1969).

With regard to the mechanism by which L-asparaginase exerts a toxic effect on the central nervous system, the authors have suggested three possibilities: 1. L-asparaginase could interfere with central nervous system protein synthesis by depleting brain L-asparagine; 2. the increased levels of L-aspartic and L-glutamic acids, as a result of therapy, could affect brain metabolism; 3. the latter could also be altered by increased ammonia levels, as a consequence of liver dysfunction.

The authors favour this last hypothesis since ammonia may reach high levels during treatment with L-asparaginase (HILL et al., 1967).

In our second case, the neurological complications were apparently unrelated to L-asparaginase treatment, since they appeared three to four weeks after therapy had been discontinued, but, in our opinion, they deserve to be mentioned in connection with the problem of intracerebral administration of L-asparaginase and the question of the mode of action of the drug on leukemic lesions in the central nervous system.

Briefly, the patient, a woman of 34 with acute lymphoblastic leukemia in partial remission, was readmitted to hospital, having finished a course of treatment with L-asparaginase at a daily dose of 200 IU/kg about four weeks earlier.

On physical examination she presented signs of acute transverse lesion of the spinal cord, with retention and later overflow of urine, flaccid paralysis of the limbs, total sensory loss, loss of tendon reflexes and absence of plantar response. The patient was restarted on L-asparaginase at a dose of 500 IU/kg/day, but after 10 days no improvement in her neurological signs ensued. Being unaware at that time that L-asparaginase could be introduced intracerebrally, we did not attempt to inject the enzyme intrathecally and decided to change over to methotrexate intrathecally and vincristine intravenously. Little success was obtained and after two months the patient was discharged in a deteriorated condition.

From the experiments of BURCHENAL et al. (1968) on intracerebrally injected mouse leukemias EARAD 1 and L5178CA55 L-asparaginase was found active also by the intraperitoneal route, although at doses higher than those required for the same effect in the intraperitoneally or subcutaneously inoculated leukemias.

According to BURCHENAL and his colleagues, the antileukemic effect of L-asparaginase on cerebral lesions could be due either to penetration of L-asparaginase into the brain tissue or to the deprivation of brain tissue of asparagine by equilibration with the low levels of systemic asparagine. The latter hypothesis appears most likely since determinations of L-asparaginase levels in various organs, including the brain, 1 and 2 hours after injecting 1000 IU/kg showed no difference between treated animals and controls.

Finally TAN and OETTGEN (1969) have reported favourable results in cases of acute leukemia with neurological lesions by the intracerebral (intraventricular) introduction of L-asparaginase.

These results are of the greatest interest, since, with the exception of cortisone and methotrexate, all antileukemic drugs are completely ineffective against leukemic localizations in the central nervous system.

It therefore becomes a matter of great importance to decide whether the intracerebral introduction of L-asparaginase is a practical and worthwhile procedure or whether it is preferable to utalize the enzyme intravenously in association with methotrexate, given intrathecally.

If either method should prove of some value, a considerable advance towards the eradication of leukemia by chemotherapy would have been accomplished.

References

1. ADAMSON, R. H., FABRO, S.: Acta Vitamin. et Enzymol. **23,** III (1969).
2. BURCHENAL, J. H., LASH, E., SCHWARTZ, M., DOLLINGER, M.: Proc. Amer. Ass. Cancer Res. **9,** 37 (1968).
3. CARDINALI, G.: Il Policlinico **76,** 276 (1969).
4. HASKELL, C. M., CANELLOS, G. P., LEVENTHAL, B. G., CARBONE, P. P., SERPICK, A. A., HANSEN, H. H.: Cancer Res. **29,** 974 (1969).
5. — LEVENTHAL, J., BLOCK, J., CANELLOS, G. P.: Proc. Amer. Soc. Cancer Oncology, 5th Annual Scientific Meeting 1969, March 22, Comunication No. 15.
6. HILL, J. R., ROBERTS, J., LOEB, E., KHAN, A., MACLELLAN, A., HILL, R. W.: J. Amer. med. Ass. **202,** 882 (1967).
7. OETTGEN, H. F., OLD, L. J., BOYSE, E. A., CAMPBELL, H. A., PHILIPS, F. S., CLARKSON, B. D., TALLAL, L., LEEPER, R. D., SCHWARTZ, M. K., KIM, J. H.: Cancer Res. **27,** 2619 (1967).
8. TAN, C., OETTGEN, H. F.: Proc. Amer. Ass. Cancer Res. **10,** 92 (1969).

A Summary of the Clinical Status of Asparaginase

J. H. BURCHENAL

Division of Applied Therapy, Sloan-Kettering Institute for Cancer Research, New York, U.S.A.

Asparaginase is an agent for the treatment of leukemia which differs from other agents in that it takes advantage of a unique requirement of certain leukemic cells for asparagine, which most normal cells apparently do not have. It has been reported here to produce rapid remissions in acute lymphoblastic leukemia in from 40 to 100% of patients in small series and the average is probably in the order of 60%. There does not appear to be any real cross-resistance with any of the other active agents, but it may be that somewhat higher remission rates are achieved in the previously untreated cases. This seems not to be a question of cross-resistance but rather a reflection of the patient's better physical condition when seen soon after diagnosis has been made. In small series—and I stress small series because I am afraid of small numbers—approximately the same percentages of remissions are achieved with daily doses from 10 IU/kg to 5000 IU/kg. There may be some evidence, however, that longer unmaintained remissions are achieved by doses of 1000 IU/kg or higher. In acute lymphoblastic leukemia (ALL), children seem to respond perhaps somewhat better than adults. Asparaginase is also active against the meningeal manifestation of the disease, whether the drug is given intravenously or intrathecally.

In acute myeloblastic leukemia (AML) we have heard of results which vary from 0% to 50% remissions, again in small series. My guess would be that probably something in the order of 15% complete and good partial remissions are generally achieved in this form of the disease. It certainly appears from the work done in Dallas that in order to achieve remissions high doses are rather more essential in AML than they are in ALL.

The work of the Paul Ehrlich Group on acute promyelocytic leukemia (APL) is interesting: They reported a much higher percentage of remissions in APL than in AML, with up to 40% complete remissions in the patients who survived treatment for two weeks or more. We have not had this experience in our group, but we have not seen very many promyelocytic leukemias, and our diagnostic criteria may be different. This is certainly an area that should be examined further.

I believe that it was Dr. AMIEL who reported one complete remission in the blast crisis of chronic myelocytic leukemia. We have not seen any beneficial results as yet, but it is an area where most conventional agents are relatively ineffectual and where activity is certainly needed. There have been occasional reports of responses in lymphosarcoma, particularly leukemic lymphosarcoma. There was one patient with melanoma treated in 1967 whose disease responded to three different courses, and the investigators at the NCI also had one other partial remission in this disease. Other than that, the results in at least 50 patients with melanoma have been disappointing. Dr. HAMILTON FAIRLEY has suggested that something may be happening in melanoma treated with asparaginase which, although not readily apparent, may potentiate the effects of other drugs.

Certainly as far as the toxicity is concerned, this drug is not as non-toxic as it was originally hoped it would be. Apparently toxicity occurs at almost all the dosage levels, but my feeling, at least on the basis of the Memorial Sloan-Kettering work, is that most of the studies at low doses were done with rather impure preparations. Thus some of the toxicity seen at 10 or 100 IU/kg may well have been due to impurities rather than to asparaginase *per se*, and we have not accumulated enough toxicity data on these low doses since we have been using the pure material. It is our experience that 5000 IU/kg daily, certainly of the Merck preparation and probably of the Bayer preparation also, is too toxic for general use. 1000 IU/kg daily seem to be better tolerated, and if there is anything to the tissue gradient theory there might be an advantage in using 1000 IU/kg daily. Certainly there is toxicity with this drug, although I think those of us who have worked with the so-called cytostatic agents—and this includes nearly everyone in this room—realize that asparaginase toxicity is much less than that of most of the conventional agents.

The toxicity has been reported in great detail, and I will not elaborate on it now. I do think, however, that one of the questions which I will allude to later on might be mentioned now, that is, that it would be interesting to know whether the toxicity is indeed as great at a given dose with the Bayer preparation as with the Merck, inasmuch as the maintained blood levels differ considerably.

Then, in summary, asparaginase is active alone primarily in ALL and to a lesser extent in AML but generally the remissions are relatively short. Some remissions have lasted over a year, but these are very rare. Therefore ist would seem that asparaginase might beneficially be given in combination. It is possible that before going into strict combination, as far as potentiation of the therapeutic effect is concerned, we might consider the suggestion of a combination therapy which is designed to prevent both the liver toxicity and the CNS toxicity. It has been suggested that possibly giving asparagine or glutamine at the same time as asparaginase might cut down somewhat on the toxicity. In mice the therapeutic effect of very small doses of asparaginase can be blocked by very high doses of asparagine. If we increase the dose of asparaginase to 1000 IU/kg or greater, however, and then give big doses of asparagine the animals die rapidly of toxicity. This may be because the deamidation of the asparagine gives increased amounts of ammonia and aspartic acid, but whatever the cause, there is no doubt about the increased toxicity of the combinations, Thus, although it is possible that either one of these amino acids, asparagine or glutamine, might be beneficial in man, this should be undertaken with great caution because of the increased toxicity noted in mice.

There are two types of drugs which might be given in combination with asparaginase, (a) the so-called rational drugs such as the glutamine antagonists Azaserine, diazo-oxo-norleucine, azotomycin and 2-amino-4-oxo-5-chloropentanoic acid which interfere with the synthesis of asparagine or the metabolism of glutamine, and (b) the more empirical drugs, which in combination studies in mouse leukemia seem to have additive or potentiating effects. Perhaps the remark that Dr. MCELWAIN made, that these drugs may destroy some of the feeder cells which may be supplying asparagine to the leukemic cells even in the presence of asparaginase, would lift them out of the empirical status. At any rate, we must decide what drugs should be given in combination. In the mouse, there are a large variety of agents which seem to potentiate asparaginase such as cytosine arabinoside, 5-hydroxy-2-formylpyridine thiosemicarbazone, 6-mercaptopurine, thioguanine, methotrexate, Daunomycin, Adriamycin, Actinomycin, vincristine, vinblastine, and 4′-demethyl-epipodophyllotoxin-β-D-thenylidene glucoside. It is amazing how the addition of any one of so many agents can change a minor increase in life span to a complete cure. I cannot say which agent of this group would be preferable, and probably all should have some clinical trial. The work that has been presented so far on cytosine arabinoside by Dr. MCELWAIN and by several other groups including our own suggests that this drug may be useful in combination therapy.

If combinations are to be given another question is whether they should be given simultaneously or sequentially, and if sequentially, should asparaginase be given first to induce a remission followed by another drug for consolidation, or should the non-asparaginase drug be given first and followed by asparaginase. Our work in mice suggests that a drug like vincristine is perhaps better given, in our leukemia, before asparaginase, whereas Dr. MASHBURN, using a different and slower growing leukemia, feels very definitely that it is better to give asparaginase first and vincristine afterwards. Dr. BIERLING's data, I believe, also suggest that it would be better to give asparaginase first and the other drug afterwards. From our clinical studies on simultaneous combinations of asparaginase, vincristine, Daunomycin and prednisone where the toxicity of vincristine and Daunomycin was considerably increased and from the data that have been presented on the impairment of liver function by asparaginase, there might indeed be a rationale for giving the other drugs first, followed by asparaginase, in order that the toxicity of drugs which might be metabolized in the liver would not be increased by the asparaginase-produced impairment of liver function. The preceding is, however, merely a theoretical rationale, but we are now studying sequential combination therapy where the maximum tolerated course of the other drugs is given immediately before the course of asparaginase.

Let us now consider for a moment the evaluation of clinical combination therapy. In the evaluation of leukemia chemotherapy, we think a great deal of the median survival time as an indication of the results that are being achieved. Let us agree, however, that for the combination therapy to be most effective the patient's disease must be sensitive to each of the components of the combination. Thus, if we have three agents, each of which is able to induce remission in only 50% of the patients and if all three of these worked together, all leukemic cells might be destroyed, then we could only expect to have 50% of 50% of 50%, or 12.5%, of the patients whose disease would be sensitive to all three drugs simultaneously and in whom cure would result. Thus let us remember in combination studies not to concentrate entirely on the 50% survival time but rather to observe also the end of the curve. If it turns out that there are 10% of patients at the end of a year or two of unmaintained remission that are still without evidence of disease, this might be a significant results and not just an error of chance. I think that the value of unmaintained remission is important in determining the percentage of cells killed by a given treatment regimen. Oftentimes in acute leukemia we hesitate to stop treatment in patients but certainly the evaluation of a given combination which might be curative can be done much faster, if we give a course of therapy and then stop treatment and wait for relapse. Now to do this, one has to be an optimist because one has to assume that perhaps in some of these patients the combination therapy is going to be so successful that they are not going to relapse. Granted, this is being rather optimistic but still one can, I think, learn a great deal by the length of the unmaintained remissions. If one watches the unmaintained patient closely and detects the first sign of relapse one still may treat him with many other chemotherapeutic agents, including asparaginase.

I think that Dr. HAMILTON FAIRLY made a very good point, which is that asparaginase may be useful in sensitizing certain tumors, particularly acute myeloblastic leukemia, where we see some minor effect with asparaginase. This effect is not maintained but if asparaginase is used first and then a second and a third drug are given in combination, perhaps much better results will be achieved than with either agent alone. As Dr. HAMILTON FAIRLY has suggested, this might also be true with melanoma or other solid tumors where there is no visible effect with asparaginase alone but where there may be some disturbance of metabolic activity which might make the tumor specifically sensitive to another chemotherapeutic agent or to radiation.

Dr. CARBONE stressed the need for long duration of treatment. This is one of the problems with asparaginase, since it must be given intravenously or intramuscularly, and thus we tend to prefer short courses. It is certainly true that with some of the slow-growing tumors, which after all are the bulk of our cancer problem, long-term therapy is required. Thus I think we should take very seriously his suggestion that we consider intermittent therapy with immunosuppressive drugs to allow the repetition of asparaginase therapy at specific intervals without getting into difficulties due to sensitization. One of the striking aspects of some of our cases is that in the patients who have been treated with combination therapy or with asparaginase alone and then have remained in long-term unmaintained remissions, the relapse has oftentimes been manifested by meningeal involvement without a marrow relapse. Some patients have continued for a least six months with intermittent CNS relapses without any marrow relapse and without any treatment for the marrow—just intrathecal methotrexate for the meningeal disease. I do not know why should be or whether it is really more common with asparaginase than with other therapy, but we have certainly seen a great deal of CNS involvement after asparaginase therapy despite the fact that asparaginase, when used in treatment, is active against meningeal disease.

I mentioned the possible differences in toxicity that should be looked for between the Bayer and Merck compounds and I would add to that the Lilly preparation as well, but I think particularly we should look also for differences in therapeutic effect—Dr. SCHWARTZ's very preliminary data suggested that perhaps the Lilly preparation had an even shorter half-life than the Bayer preparation. Perhaps this is good. We do not really know whether it is the peak level or the maintained level of asparaginase which is necessary for the therapeutic effect. Perhaps the maintained level produces the toxic effect rather than the therapeutic effect. We do not have any data either way but I would suggest a careful comparison of the different types of asparaginase to see whether there are differences in therapeutic or in toxic effects.

Along that line I think that we will find in the next year that the new types of chemically altered asparaginase which are being worked on by Drs. IRION and ARENS at Bayer may be particularly interesting. So far there do not seem to have been any significant differences in therapeutic or toxic effects in mice, but just as different effects were found with the semi-synthetic penicillins, so perhaps either a different spectrum of activity or a better penetration into tissues may be achieved with these semi-synthetic asparaginases.

In closing I would like to suggest that we repeat this conference in one year to re-evaluate the effects of asparaginase when we have had more experimental and clinical experience and have had time to answer the following clinical questions posed at this conference:

1. The relation of dosage to the toxicity of pure preparations of asparaginase?
2. The relation of toxicity to maintained blood level?
3. The best drugs to give in simultaneous or sequential combination with asparaginase?
4. The best sequence for combination therapy?
5. The activating effect of asparaginase on other chemotherapeutic agents?
6. The value of immunosuppression to avoid immunological reaction to repeated courses of asparaginase?

Finally, I would like to take this opportunity to thank Dr. GRUNDMANN and the whole Bayer entourage for a very stimulating conference and one which has been most enjoyable for all of us.

Monographs already Published

1 SCHINDLER, R., Lausanne: Die tierische Zelle in Zellkultur. DM 16,—; US $ 4.40

2 Neuroblastomas — Biochemical Studies. Edited by C. BOHUON, Villejuif (Symposium). DM 16,—; US $ 4.40

3 HUEPER, W. C., Bethesda: Occupational and Environmental Cancers of the Respiratory System. DM 34,—; US $ 9.40

4 GOLDMAN, L., Cincinnati: Laser Cancer Research. DM 16,—; US $ 5.00

5 METCALF, D., Melbourne: The Thymus. Its Role in Immune Responses, Leukaemia Development and Carcinogenesis. DM 24,—; US $ 6.60

6 Malignant Transformation by Viruses. Edited by W. H. KIRSTEN, Chicago (Symposium). DM 32,—; US $ 8.80

7 MOERTEL, CH. G., Rochester: Multiple Primary Malignant Neoplasms. Their Incidence and Significance. DM 18,—; US $ 5.00

8 New Trends in the Treatment of Cancer. Edited by L. MANUILA, S. MOLES, and P. RENTCHNICK, Geneva. DM 32,—; US $ 8.80

9 LINDENMANN, J., Zürich, and P. A. KLEIN, Gainesville/Florida: Immunological Aspects of Viral Oncolysis. DM 18,—; US $ 5.00

10 NELSON, R. S., Houston: Radioactive Phosphorus in the Diagnosis of Gastrointestinal Cancer. DM 15,—; US $ 4.20

11 FREEMAN, R. G., and J. M. KNOX, Houston: Treatment of Skin Cancer. DM 15,—; US $ 4.50

12 LYNCH, H. T., Houston: Hereditary Factors in Carcinoma. DM 24,—; US $ 6.60

13 Tumours in Children. Edited by H. B. MARSDEN, and J. K. STEWARD, Manchester. DM 72,—; US $ 18.00

14 ODARTCHENKO, N., Lausanne: Production cellulaire érythropoïétique. DM 28,—; US $ 7.70

15 SOKOLOFF, B., Lakeland/Florida: Carcinoid and Serotonin. DM 24,—; US $ 6.60

16 JACOBS, M. L., Duarte/California: Malignant Lymphomas and their Management. DM 18,—; US $ 5.10

17 Normal and Malignant Cell Growth. Edited by R. J. M. FRY, Argonne, M. L. GRIEM, Argonne, and W. H. KIRSTEN, Chicago (Symposium). DM 56,80; US $ 14.20

18 ANGLESIO, E., Torino: The Treatment of Hodgkin's Disease. DM 24,—; US $ 6.60

19 BANNASCH, P., Würzburg: The Cytoplasm of Hepatocytes during Carcinogenesis. DM 32,—; US $ 8.80

20 Rubidomycin. A new Agent against Leukemia. Edited by J. BERNARD, R. PAUL, M. BOIRON, C. JACQUILLAT, and R. MARAL, Paris. DM 48,—; US $ 13.20

21 Scientific Basis of Cancer Chemotherapy. Edited by G. MATHÉ, Villejuif (Symposium). DM 28,—; US $ 7.00

22 KOLDOVSKÝ, P., Philadelphia: Tumor Specific Transplantation Antigen. DM 24,—; US $ 6.60

23 FUCHS, W. A., Bern, J. W. DAVIDSON, Toronto, and H. W. FISCHER, Ann Arbor: Lymphography in Cancer. DM 76,—; US $ 21.00

24 HAYWARD, J. L., London: Hormonal Research in Human Breast Cancer. DM 34,—; US $ 9.40

25 ROY-BURMAN, P., Los Angeles: Analogues of Nucleic Acid Components. Mechanisms of Action. DM 28,—; US $ 7.70

26 Tumors of the Liver. Edited by G. T. PACK and A. H. ISLAMI, New York. DM 56,—; US $ 15.40

27 SZYMENDERA, J., Warsaw: Bone Mineral Metabolism in Cancer. DM 32,—; US $ 8.80

28 MEEK, E. S., Bristol: Antitumour and Antiviral Substances of Natural Origin. DM 16,—; US $ 4.40

29 Aseptic Environments and Cancer Treatment. Edited by G. MATHÉ, Villejuif (Symposium). DM 22,—; US $ 6.10

30 Advances in the Treatment of Acute (Blastic) Leukemias. Edited by G. MATHÉ, Villejuif (Symposium). DM 38,—; US $ 10.50

31 DENOIX, P., Villejuif: Treatment of Malignant Breast Tumors: Indications and Results. DM 48,—; US $ 13.20

32 NELSON, R. S., Houston: Endoscopy in Gastric Cancer. DM 48,—; US $ 13.20

33 Experimental and Clinical Effects of L-Asparaginase. Edited by E. GRUNDMANN, Wuppertal-Elberfeld, and H. F. OETTGEN, New York (Symposium). DM 58,—; US $ 16.—

Special Supplement: Biology of Amphibian Tumors. Edited by M. MIZELL, New Orleans. DM 86,—; US $ 24.00

In Production

34 ENDO, H., Fukuoka, T. ONO, Tokyo, T. SUGIMURA, Tokyo: Chemistry and Biological Actions of 4-Nitroquinoline 1-oxide

35 PENN, I., Denver: Malignant Tumors in Organ Transplant Recipients

In Preparation

ACKERMANN, N. B., Boston: Use of Radioisotopic Agents in the Diagnosis of Cancer

BOIRON, M., Paris: The Viruses of the Leukemia-sarcoma Complex

CAVALIERE, R., A. ROSSI-FANELLI, B. MONDOVI, and G. MORICCA, Roma: Selective Heat Sensitivity of Cancer Cells

CHIAPPA, S., Milano: Endolymphatic Radiotherapy in Malignant Lymphomas

Cutane paraneoplastische Syndrome. Edited by J. J. HERZBERG, Bremen (Symposium)

GRUNDMANN, E., Wuppertal-Elberfeld: Morphologie und Cytochemie der Carcinogenese

IRLIN, I. S., Moskva: Mechanisms of Viral Carcinogenesis

LANGLEY, F. A., and A. C. CROMPTON, Manchester: Epithelial Abnormalities of the Cervix Uteri

MATHÉ, G., Villejuif: L'Immunothérapie des Cancers

NEWMAN, M. K., Detroit: Neuropathies and Myopathies Associated with Occult Malignancies

OGAWA, K., Osaka: Ultrastructural Enzyme Cytochemistry of Azo-dye Carcinogenesis

PARKER, J., and R. J. LUKES, Los Angeles: Lymphocyte Transformation in Neoplastic Disease

WEIL, R., Lausanne: Biological and Structural Properties of Polyoma Virus and its DNA

WILLIAMS, D. C., Caterham, Surrey: The Basis for Therapy of Hormon Sensitive Tumours

WILLIAMS, D. C., Caterham, Surrey: The Biochemistry of Metastasis

MIX
Papier aus verantwortungsvollen Quellen
Paper from responsible sources
FSC® C105338

If you have any concerns about our products,
you can contact us on
ProductSafety@springernature.com

In case Publisher is established outside the EU,
the EU authorized representative is:
Springer Nature Customer Service Center GmbH
Europaplatz 3, 69115 Heidelberg, Germany

Printed by Libri Plureos GmbH
in Hamburg, Germany